**INTERNAL MEDICINE
FOR ADVANCED
PHARMACIST PRACTITIONERS**

VOLUME II

INTERNAL MEDICINE FOR ADVANCED PHARMACIST PRACTITIONERS - VOLUME II

Copyright © 2024 by Huynh Wynn Tran

Cover: Artist Dinh Khai - Book designer: Tien Minh Nguyen

United Buddhist Publisher (UBF)

First printed in California, USA, September 2024

ISBN-13: 979-8-8693-0561-9

© All rights reserved. No part of this book may be reproduced by any means without prior written permission.

HUYNH WYNN TRAN, MD, FACP, FACR

INTERNAL MEDICINE
FOR ADVANCED
PHARMACIST PRACTITIONERS

VOLUME II

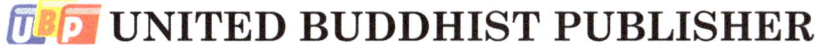 UNITED BUDDHIST PUBLISHER

This book is dedicated to all my patients, who have been my greatest teachers and sources of inspiration.

Additionally, I wish to dedicate this book to my parents, Ms. Nhung Huynh and Mr. Dang Tran, whose unconditional love has been a constant source of strength throughout my journey as a physician.

Preface

The role of the clinical pharmacist has evolved significantly in recent years, with California leading the way by establishing the first Advanced Practice Pharmacist (APh) separate license in 2017 through Bill SB493. This initiative has paved the path for pharmacists to assume expanded responsibilities and become integral members of primary care teams.

In 2020, Wynn Medical Center embarked on a groundbreaking collaboration with the University of Southern California and 986 Pharmacy to establish a pioneering APh residency program aimed at training PharmD residents to become fully-fledged healthcare providers within a physician clinic setting.

This comprehensive guide is designed to equip Advanced Practice Pharmacists and APh residents with a foundation of 350 common conditions encountered in primary care. Spanning across 24 chapters, this book addresses the APh profession, major disorders in internal medicine, common disorders in pregnancy and pediatrics, post-surgical and wound care, laboratory, imaging, biostatistics, and preventive measures.

I extend my heartfelt gratitude to a dedicated team of international expert reviewers, editors, and students who have contributed their time, expertise, and insights to the creation of this textbook.

Huynh Wynn Tran, MD, FACP
Assistant Professor of Medicine, Rheumatology/Dermatology, and Pharmacy
Founder/CEO of Wynn Medical Center Clinics, Los Angeles, USA

Reviewers:

Alvin Wong, MBBS, MD, MRCP
Consultant Dermatologist
NHS Stafford, United Kingdom

Dean Nguyen, MD, RN
Ottawa, Canada

Helen Tran, DO
Assistant Professor, Core Faculty, Department of Family Medicine
Charles R. Drew University of Medicine and Science
Los Angeles, California

Hoang Henry Nguyen, RPH, APh, MD, PhD, FACHE
Assistant Dean of Preclinical Education
Nova Southeastern University Dr. Patel College of Osteopathic Medicine, Tampa, Florida

Huynh Wynn Tran, MD, FACP
Assistant Professor of Medicine, Rheumatology/Dermatology, and Pharmacy
Founder/CEO of Wynn Medical Center Clinics, Los Angeles, USA

Ken Thai, PharmD, APh
Vice-President of National Community Pharmacist Association
CEO 986 Pharmacy Corporation
Los Angeles, California

Loan Vo, MD, RRT, ACCS
Clinical Instructor, Foothill College Respiratory Therapist Program
San Jose, California

Long To, PharmD, APh, BCPS
Program Director, Pharmacotherapy, Henry Ford Hospital
Detroit, Michigan

Micah Hata, PharmD, APh
Program Director, Pharmacy residency and fellowship
Western University College of Pharmacy
Pomona, California

Minh Do, MD
Attending Physician at Parkland Health
Dallas, Texas

Philip Phuc Tran, DO, FACC, FACOI
Associate Professor of Medicine and Cardiology, Midwestern University Phoenix, Arizona

Quan-Vinh Nguyen, MD, PhD
Professor and Attending Nephrologist
Fribourg, Switzerland

Quy Pham Nguyen, MD, PhD
Attending Oncologist, Chief Physician
Kyoto Miniren Central Hospital, Kyoto, Japan

Richard Dang, PharmD, APh
Program Director, PGY-1 Community Pharmacy Residency
University of Southern California Mann School of Pharmacy
Los Angeles, California

Sunil Prabhu, BPharm, PhD
Dean and Professor
Western University College of Pharmacy
Pomona, California

Tanya Thuy Nguyen, MD, FAAP
Attending Pediatrician at Wynn Medical Center
Los Angeles, California

Thanh Hoang, DO, FACP, FACE, CAP (US Navy)
Professor of Medicine and Endocrinology
Program Director, Endocrinology Fellowship, Uniformed Services
University Bethesda, Maryland

Tuan Nguyen, DO
Postdoc Clinical Fellow in Nephrology
UCLA Olive View Medical Center
Los Angeles, California

Student Editors:

Molynna Duong Nguyen, BS (Team Lead)
University of Toledo College of Medicine, Toledo, Ohio

Nidhi Lakshmanan, BS
Wynn Medical Center, Los Angeles, California

Tam Do (Tammy), BS
Wynn Medical Center, Los Angeles, California

Tri Huynh, BS
Western University College of Pharmacy, Pomona, California

CONTENTS

VOLUME II

Chapter 11: Nephrologic and Urological Disorders..................... 21
    11.1. Chronic Kidney Disease 22
    11.2. Acute Kidney Injury 25
    11.3. Kidney Stones 27
    11.4. Benign Prostatic Hyperplasia 29
    11.5. Prostatitis 31
    11.6. Urinary Incontinence 33
    11.7. Glomerulonephritis 35
    11.8. Polycystic Kidney Disease 37
    11.9. Interstitial Cystitis 39
    11.10. Hydronephrosis 41
    11.11. Hematuria 43
    11.12. Renal Artery Stenosis 45
    11.13. Renal Cyst 46
    11.14. Nephrotic Syndrome 48
    11.15. Nephritic syndrome 50
    11.16. Urinary Incontinence 52
    11.17. Erectile Dysfunction 55
    11.18. Overactive Bladder 58
    References 60

Chapter 12: Dermatologic Disorders 63
    12.1. Acne Vulgaris 64
    12.2. Atopic Dermatitis 66
    12.3. Contact Dermatitis 68
    12.4. Psoriasis 70
    12.5. Seborrheic Dermatitis 72
    12.6. Rosacea 74

- 12.7. Dermatophytosis 76
- 12.8. Scabies 78
- 12.9. Impetigo 80
- 12.10. Warts 82
- 12.11. Molluscum Contagiosum 84
- 12.12. Tinea Versicolor 86
- 12.13. Urticaria 89
- 12.14. Seborrheic Keratosis 91
- 12.15. Actinic Keratosis 93
- 12.16. Folliculitis 95
- 12.17. Cellulitis 97
- 12.18. Skin Abscess 98
- 12.19. Pruritus 100
- 12.20. Inversa Acne 102
- 12.21. Lichen Planus 104
- 12.22. Cutaneous Lupus 106
- 12.23. Oral Lesions 108
- 12.24. Vitiligo 109
- 12.25. Alopecia 111
- 12.26. Burn 113
- 12.27. Corticosteroid Prescribed Consideration 115
  - 12.27.1 Prescription Guidelines for the APh: 115
  - 12.27.2. Topical Steroid Classifications 116
  - 12.27.3. Systemic corticosteroid 117
- 12.28. Description of Skin Lesions 118
  - References 121

Chapter 13: Pediatric Disorders 123
- 13.1. Upper Respiratory Infections 124
- 13.2. Otitis Media 125
- 13.3. Asthma 127
- 13.4. Allergic Rhinitis 129
- 13.5. Dermatitis 131
- 13.6. Urinary Tract Infections 133

13.7. Febrile Seizures 135
13.8. Bronchitis 137
13.9. Croup 139
13.10. Constipation 141
13.11. Diarrhea 143
13.12. Conjunctivitis 145
13.13. Strep Throat 147
13.14. Acute Gastroenteritis 150
13.15. Sinusitis 152
13.16. Hand, Foot, and Mouth Disease 154
13.17. Pediatric Obesity 156
13.18. Rotavirus infection 158
    References 159

Chapter 14: Ophthalmologic Disorders 163
14.1. Refractive Errors 164
14.2. Cataracts 166
14.3. Glaucoma 168
14.4. Age-Related Macular Degeneration 170
14.5. Diabetic Retinopathy 172
14.6. Dry Eye Syndrome 174
14.7. Conjunctivitis 176
14.8. Blepharitis 179
14.9. Keratitis 181
14.10. Chalazion 183
14.11. Ptosis 185
14.12. Retinal Detachment 187
14.13. Uveitis 189
14.14. Floaters 191
14.15. Presbyopia 193
14.16. Corneal Abrasion 195
14.17. Subconjunctival Hemorrhage 197
14.18. Amblyopia 199
14.19. Pterygium 201

References 204

Chapter 15. Oncologic/Hematologic Disorders 207
    15.1. Breast Cancer... 208
    15.2. Lung Cancer... 210
    15.3. Colorectal Cancer... 212
    15.4. Prostate Cancer 214
    15.5. Melanoma... 217
    15.6. Basal Cell Carcinoma 219
    15.7. Squamous Cell Carcinoma... 221
    15.8. Bladder Cancer 223
    15.9. Pancreatic Cancer 226
    15.10. Ovarian Cancer 228
    15.11. Cervical Cancer.. 230
    15.12. Thyroid Cancer 232
    15.13. Leukemia 235
    15.14. Lymphoma 237
    15.15. Kidney Cancer 240
    15.16. Liver Cancer 242
    15.17. Esophageal Cancer 245
    15.18. Stomach Cancer 248
    15.19. Endometrial Cancer 250
    15.20. Brain Cancer 252
    15.21.Testicular Cancer 256
    15.22. Anemia 258
    15.23. Pancytopenia 261
    15.24. Thrombocytopenia 264
        References 266

Chapter 16. Obstetric and Gynecologic Disorders 269
    16.1. Intrauterine Pregnancy 270
    16.2. Ectopic Pregnancy 272
    16.3. Back Pain in Pregnancy 274
    16.4. Morning Sickness 276
    16.5. Gestational Diabetes Mellitus... 277

16.6. Preeclampsia 279

16.7. Iron-Deficiency Anemia 282

16.8. Pruritus Gravidarum 284

16.9. Striae Gravidarum 285

16.10. Melasma of Pregnancy 287

16.11. Miscarriage.. 290

16.12. Cholestasis of Pregnancy.. 292

16.13. Postpartum Depression 293

16.14. Multiple Gestation 296

16.15. Gestational Thyroid Disorders 298

16.16. Endometriosis 300

16.17. Uterine Fibroids 302

16.18. Pelvic Pain... 303

16.19. Vaginal Discharge 305

16.20. Infertility... 307

16.21. Irregular Menstruation 309

16.22. Ovarian Cysts 311

16.23. Abnormal Uterine Bleeding 313

16.24. Dysmenorrhea 316

16.25. Polycystic Ovary Syndrome 318

16.26. Sexual Discomfort 320

16.27. Menopause.. 322

16.28. Vaginitis 325

16.29. Amenorrhea 327

References 329

Part III: 331
Ancillary Services: Labs, Biostatistics, Wound Care, Surgical Care, and Imaging 331

Chapter 17: Blood Labs and EKG Interpretations 333

17.1. Complete Blood Count 333

17.2. Comprehensive Metabolic Panel 335

17.3. Urinalysis 337

17.4. Lipid Panel 339

17.5. Thyroid Panel 340
17.6. ANA Level 342
17.7. ESR/CRP Level 343
17.8. Lupus Panel 344
17.9. Rheumatoid Arthritis Panel 346
17.10. Cancer Markers 347
17.11. Vitamin D Level 349
17.12. Vitamin B12 Level 350
17.13. Hemoglobin A1c and Blood Sugar Level 352
17.14. Uric Acid Level 353
17.15. Protein and Urine Electrophoresis 354
17.16. Iron Panel 356
17.17. Sex Hormones Panel 357
17.18. Other Hormones 360
17.19. Hepatitis Panel 361
17.20. Sexually Transmitted Disease Panel 362
17.21. Prostate Panel 364
17.22. Basic EKG 365
References 366

Chapter 18: Basic Biostatistics for the APh 369
18.1. Introduction to Biostatistics 369
18.2. Descriptive Statistics 370
18.3. Inferential Statistics 373
18.4. Study Design and Research Methodology 375
18.5. A Good Clinical Study 378
References 379

Chapter 19: Wound Care Essentials 381
19.1. Wound Overview 382
19.2. Wound Assessment 384
19.3. Wound Dressing 386
19.4. Wound Complications 388
References 390

Chapter 20: Surgical Care Essentials 391

20.1. Pre-Operative Assessment 391
20.2. Anticoagulation for Dental Procedure 394
20.3. Post-Operative Complications 395
20.4. Post-Operative Concerned Symptoms 397
20.5. Post-Operative Monitoring 398
20.6. Post-Operative Pain Management 400
20.7. Post-Operative Nutrition and Rehabilitation 402
20.8. Post-Operative Medication Management 404
    References 406

Chapter 21: Post-Hospitalization Care 407
21.1. Transition of Care 407
21.2. Post-Discharge Monitoring 409
21.3. Patient Education on Self-care and Symptom Recognition ... 411
21.4. Coordination with Other Healthcare Providers 413
    References 415

Chapter 22: Imaging Modalities 417
22.1. X-ray (Radiography) 417
22.2. Computed Tomography 419
22.3. Magnetic Resonance Imaging 421
22.4. Ultrasound 423
22.5. Positron Emission Tomography 426
22.6. Fluoroscopy 428
22.7. Interventional Radiology 429
22.8. Nuclear Medicine 431
    References 432

Chapter 23: Preventive Measurements in Primary Care 433
23.1. Colon Cancer Screening 433
23.2. Cervical Cancer Screening 435
23.3. Breast Cancer Screening 436
23.4. Lung Cancer Screening 438
23.5 Prostate Cancer Screening 439
23.6. Osteoporosis Screening 440
23.7. Skin Cancer Screening 442

23.8. Depression Screening 444

References 445

Chapter 24: Medical Ethics for the Advanced Pharmacist Practitioners 447

24.1. Ethical Principles 447

24.2. Professional Integrity and Conflicts of Interest 449

24.3. Ethical Dilemmas in Pharmacy Practice 450

References 452

Chapter 11: Nephrologic and Urological Disorders

Reviewed by
Huynh Wynn Tran, MD, FACP

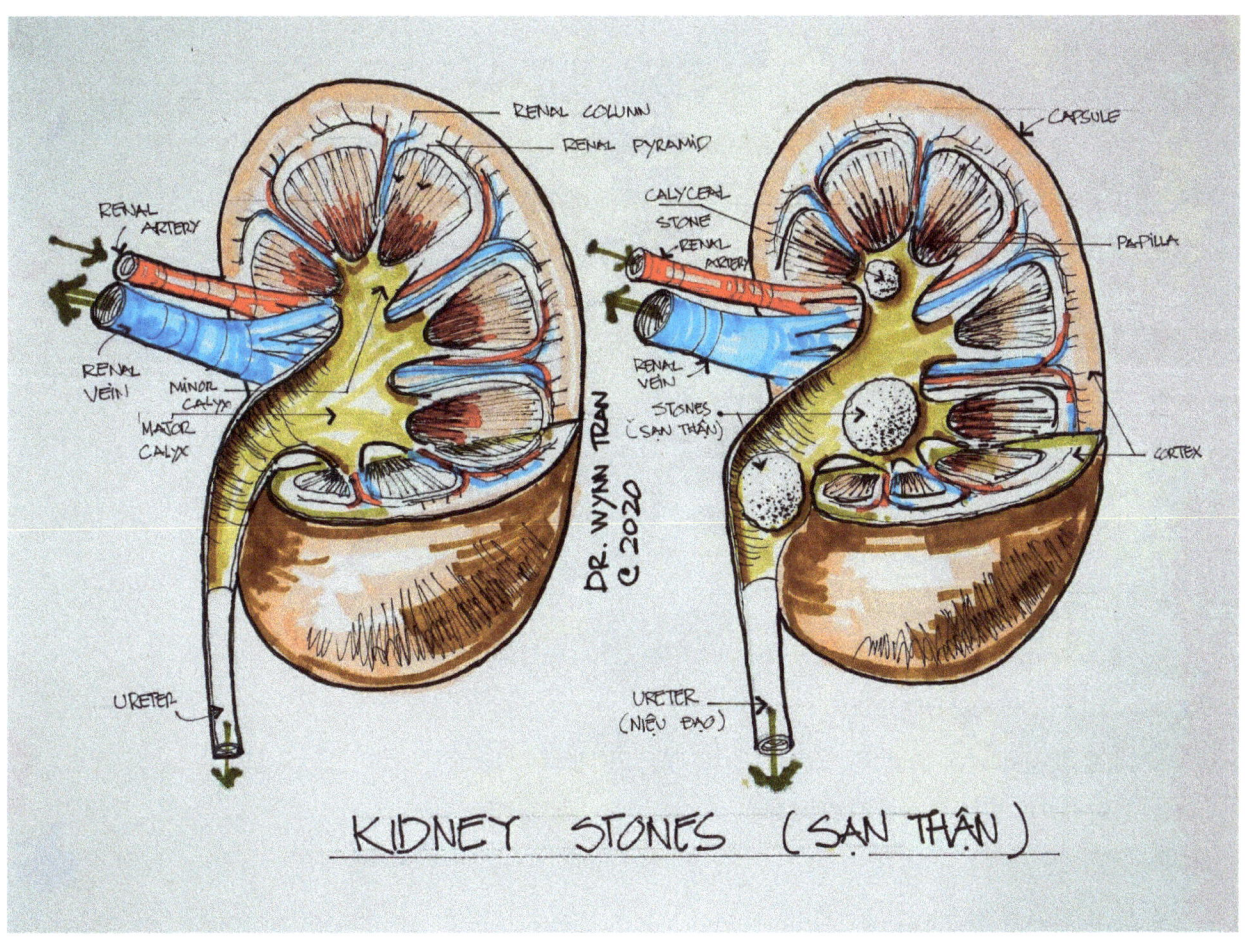

The APh should be familiar with the presentation, diagnosis, and management of these common nephrologic and urologic disorders to provide appropriate care and referral to the nephrologist/urologist when necessary.

11.1. Chronic Kidney Disease

> ➢ *Chronic kidney disease (CKD) is a progressive condition where the kidneys gradually lose function over time, leading to complications such as fluid retention, electrolyte imbalances, and cardiovascular disease.*
> ➢ *Common causes include diabetes, hypertension, and glomerulonephritis, with symptoms ranging from fatigue and swelling to nausea and decreased urine output.*
> ➢ *Management involves lifestyle changes, medications, and sometimes dialysis or kidney transplant for advanced stages.*

Symptoms:

Early stages of CKD may be asymptomatic or present with nonspecific symptoms such as fatigue, weakness, and difficulty concentrating.

As kidney function declines, symptoms may include:
- Fluid retention leading to edema in the legs, ankles, or around the eyes
- Increased or decreased urine output
- Hematuria
- Proteinuria
- Hypertension
- Persistent itching
- Nausea, vomiting, and loss of appetite
- Muscle cramps, particularly in the legs
- Difficulty sleeping
- Changes in urine color and frequency

Causes and Risk Factors:
- Diabetes mellitus and hypertension are the leading causes of CKD.
- Other risk factors include:
    - Older age
    - Family history of kidney disease
    - Cardiovascular disease
    - Obesity
    - Smoking

- Certain ethnicities (e.g., African American, Native American, Hispanic)
- Autoimmune diseases (e.g., lupus, vasculitis)
- Prolonged use of certain medications (e.g., NSAIDs, certain antibiotics)

Epidemiology:
- CKD is a global public health problem affecting millions of patients worldwide.
- The prevalence of CKD varies by country, with higher rates reported in low- to middle-income countries and among certain populations, such as older adults and those with diabetes or hypertension.

Diagnosis:
- <u>Evaluation of Kidney Function:</u> using estimated glomerular filtration rate (eGFR) calculated from serum creatinine levels.
- <u>Assessment of Urinary Albumin-To-Creatinine Ratio (ACR):</u> to detect proteinuria.
- <u>Kidney Imaging Studies:</u> (e.g., ultrasound) to evaluate kidney size and structure.

CKD Stage	
Stage 1: Kidney Damage with Normal or High GFR	- GFR: ≥90 mL/min/1.73 m² - Characteristics: Kidney damage is present, but the kidneys are functioning normally or above average.
Stage 2: Mild Loss of Kidney Function	- GFR: 60-89 mL/min/1.73 m² - Characteristics: There is mild reduction in kidney function, and evidence of kidney damage is still present.
Stage 3: Moderate Loss of Kidney Function	- Stage 3a: GFR 45-59 mL/min/1.73 m² - Stage 3b: GFR 30-44 mL/min/1.73 m² - Characteristics: Moderate reduction in GFR. Symptoms related to kidney dysfunction may start to appear in stage 3b.

Stage 4: Severe Loss of Kidney Function	• GFR: 15-29 mL/min/1.73 m² • Characteristics: Severe reduction in kidney function. This stage is often associated with symptoms of kidney failure and complications that require more intensive management.
Stage 5: Kidney Failure (End-Stage Renal Disease - ESRD)	• GFR: <15 mL/min/1.73 m² or on dialysis • Characteristics: Very low GFR indicating the kidneys have lost nearly all their ability to function effectively. At this stage, dialysis or a kidney transplant is necessary to sustain life.

Treatment:

Management of CKD aims to slow the progression of kidney damage, control symptoms, and prevent complications. Treatment strategies may include:

- Blood Pressure Control with Medications: such as ACE inhibitors and angiotensin II receptor blockers
- Glycemic Control: for patients with diabetes
- Dietary Modifications: to limit protein, sodium, and phosphorus intake
- Lifestyle Modifications: emphasizing smoking cessation, weight loss, and regular exercise
- Management of Complications: such as anemia, mineral and bone disorders, and cardiovascular disease
- Monitoring and Adjustment of Medications: to avoid nephrotoxicity
- Renal Replacement Therapy: including dialysis or kidney transplantation for end-stage kidney disease

11.2. Acute Kidney Injury

> ➢ *Acute kidney injury (AKI) is a sudden decline in kidney function over a short period, typically characterized by a rapid increase in serum creatinine and decreased urine output.*
>
> ➢ *It can result from various factors such as dehydration, infection, medications, or kidney trauma, leading to complications like electrolyte imbalances and fluid overload.*
>
> ➢ *Management involves addressing the underlying cause, supportive care, and sometimes renal replacement therapy in severe cases.*

Symptoms:
- Abrupt decreased urine output
- Edema in the legs, ankles, or around the eyes
- Fatigue and weakness
- Shortness of breath
- Confusion or altered mental status
- Nausea and vomiting
- Chest pain or pressure
- Fluid retention leading to weight gain

Causes and Risk Factors:
- Advanced age
- Pre-existing chronic kidney disease (CKD)
- Diabetes mellitus
- Hypertension
- Heart failure
- Liver disease
- Sepsis or severe infection
- Exposure to nephrotoxic medications (e.g., certain antibiotics, contrast agents, NSAIDs)
- Dehydration
- Major surgery or trauma
- Autoimmune diseases (e.g., lupus, vasculitis)

Epidemiology:
- AKI is a common and serious clinical condition that can occur in various settings, including hospitals, intensive care units (ICUs), and community settings.
- The incidence of AKI is increasing worldwide, particularly in hospitalized patients.
- Mortality rates associated with AKI can be high, especially in critically ill patients and those with underlying comorbidities.

Diagnosis:
- Changes in Kidney Function: Diagnosis of AKI is based on changes in kidney function, typically defined by:
    - Increase in serum creatinine levels within a short period (hours to days)
    - Decrease in urine output (oliguria)
- Additional Tests: to identify the underlying cause and severity of AKI. These can include urinalysis, kidney ultrasound, and blood tests to assess electrolyte levels and other markers of kidney function.

Treatment:

Management of AKI focuses on addressing the underlying cause, preventing complications, and supporting kidney function. Treatment strategies may include:

- Fluid Resuscitation: to restore intravascular volume and improve renal perfusion
- Discontinuation or adjustment of nephrotoxic medications
- Management of Electrolyte Imbalances: such as hyperkalemia or metabolic acidosis
- Renal Replacement Therapies: including hemodialysis or other therapies for severe or refractory cases
- Supportive Care: to address associated complications such as infection, sepsis, or electrolyte abnormalities

11.3. Kidney Stones

> ➤ *Kidney stones (nephrolithiasis) are hard mineral deposits that form in the kidneys and can cause severe pain as they pass through the urinary tract.*
> ➤ *Risk factors include dehydration, diet high in certain minerals, and family history, with symptoms ranging from flank pain and blood in urine to nausea and vomiting.*
> ➤ *Treatment involves pain management, hydration, and sometimes procedures to remove or break up larger stones.*

Symptoms:
- Severe pain: Sudden and intense pain in the back, side, abdomen, or groin, known as renal colic. Pain may fluctuate in intensity and may radiate to the lower abdomen and groin.
- Urinary symptoms: frequent urination, urgency, dysuria, and/or difficulty urinating. Hematuria may be visible or detected microscopically.
- Nausea and vomiting: Some patients may experience nausea and vomiting, particularly if the pain is severe.
- Fever and chills: Infection or inflammation associated with kidney stones may cause fever and chills.

Causes and Risk Factors:
- Dehydration: Inadequate fluid intake can lead to concentrated urine, increasing the risk of stone formation.
- Dietary factors: High intake of oxalate-rich foods (e.g., spinach, nuts), sodium, and animal protein may contribute to stone formation.
- Family history: increases the likelihood of developing them
- Medical conditions: Hyperparathyroidism, gout, urinary tract infections, and inflammatory bowel disease may predispose patients to kidney stones.
- Obesity: Obesity and metabolic syndrome are associated with an increased risk of kidney stones.
- Medications: Diuretics, calcium-based antacids, and certain antiretroviral drugs may increase the risk of stone formation.

Epidemiology:
- Kidney stones are a common condition, affecting approximately 10-15% of patients worldwide.

- The prevalence of kidney stones varies by geographic region, dietary habits, and genetic factors.
- Men are more commonly affected than women, with a peak incidence in the 30-50 age range.
- Recurrence rates are high, with up to 50% of patients experiencing another stone within 5-10 years of their initial episode.

Diagnosis:
- Imaging Studies:

    Non-contrast CT scan is the gold standard for diagnosing kidney stones due to its high sensitivity and specificity. Other imaging modalities include abdominal X-ray, ultrasound, and intravenous pyelogram (IVP).

- Urinalysis: Hematuria and crystalluria may be present. Urine pH and specific gravity may also be assessed.
- Blood Tests:

    Serum electrolytes, creatinine, calcium, uric acid, and parathyroid hormone levels may be measured to evaluate underlying metabolic abnormalities.

Treatment:
- Pain Management:

    Nonsteroidal anti-inflammatory drugs (NSAIDs), opioids, and/or alpha-blockers may be used to relieve pain and facilitate stone passage.

- Fluid Intake: Adequate hydration is essential to prevent stone formation and facilitate stone passage.
- Medical Expulsion Therapy: Alpha-blockers such as tamsulosin may be prescribed to help relax the ureter muscles and facilitate stone passage.
- Stone Removal:

    Larger stones or stones causing obstruction may require intervention, such as extracorporeal shock wave lithotripsy (ESWL), ureteroscopy with laser lithotripsy, or percutaneous nephrolithotomy (PCNL).

- Prevention Strategies:

    Dietary modifications, increased fluid intake, and medications to reduce stone formation (e.g., thiazide diuretics, citrate supplementation) may be recommended to prevent stone recurrence.

11.4. Benign Prostatic Hyperplasia

> ➢ Benign prostatic hyperplasia (BPH) is a non-cancerous enlargement of the prostate gland commonly affecting older men, leading to urinary symptoms such as frequent urination, urgency, and incomplete bladder emptying.
> ➢ It results from hormonal changes and can cause complications like urinary retention and urinary tract infections.
> ➢ Treatment options include medications, minimally invasive procedures, or surgery to relieve symptoms and improve urinary flow.

Symptoms:
- Urinary frequency: increased frequency of urination, especially at night (nocturia)
- Urgency: strong and sudden urge to urinate
- Weak urinary stream: decreased force and caliber of urine flow
- Incomplete emptying: feeling of incomplete bladder emptying after urination
- Straining: difficulty initiating or maintaining urination
- Dribbling: dribbling or leakage of urine after urination
- Hematuria: Blood in the urine may be present in some cases.
- Urinary retention: In severe cases, complete urinary retention may occur.

Causes and Risk Factors:
- Age: BPH is more common in older men, with prevalence increasing with age.
- Family history: of BPH or prostate-related conditions may increase the risk.
- Hormonal factors: Changes in hormone levels, particularly testosterone and dihydrotestosterone (DHT), play a role in prostate growth.
- Lifestyle factors: Obesity, sedentary lifestyle, and certain dietary factors may contribute to the development of BPH.
- Medical conditions: Diabetes and cardiovascular disease may be associated with an increased risk.

Epidemiology:
- BPH is highly prevalent among older men, with estimates suggesting that up to 50% of men over the age of 50 and 90% of men over the age of 80 may be affected.
- The prevalence of BPH varies by geographic region and ethnic group, with higher rates reported in Western countries.

Diagnosis:
- Medical History and Physical Examination: The APh will inquire about symptoms and perform a digital rectal examination (DRE) to assess prostate size and consistency.
- Urinary Flow Study: Measurement of urinary flow rate and post-void residual urine volume may be performed to assess bladder function.
- Prostate-Specific Antigen (PSA) Test: PSA levels may be measured to rule out prostate cancer and monitor disease progression.
- Transrectal Ultrasound (TRUS): TRUS may be used to visualize the prostate and assess its size and morphology.
- Cystoscopy: Cystoscopy is an invasive procedure involving the insertion of a flexible tube with a camera (cystoscope) into the urethra to evaluate the bladder and urethra.

Treatment:
- Watchful Waiting: For men with mild symptoms, periodic monitoring without active intervention may be appropriate.
- Medications:

    Alpha-blockers (e.g., tamsulosin, alfuzosin) and 5-alpha reductase inhibitors (e.g., finasteride, dutasteride) may be prescribed to relieve symptoms and reduce prostate size.

- Minimally Invasive Procedures:

    Procedures such as transurethral microwave therapy (TUMT), transurethral needle ablation (TUNA), and laser therapy may be used to reduce prostate tissue and relieve symptoms.

- Surgery:

    Transurethral resection of the prostate (TURP), laser prostatectomy, and open prostatectomy may be considered for men with severe symptoms or complications.

- Lifestyle Modifications:

    Lifestyle changes such as limiting fluid intake before bedtime, avoiding caffeine and alcohol, and maintaining a healthy weight may help alleviate symptoms.

11.5. Prostatitis

> ➢ *Prostatitis is inflammation of the prostate gland, typically causing pelvic pain, urinary symptoms, and sometimes sexual dysfunction.*
> ➢ *It can be acute or chronic, with various potential causes, including bacterial infection, pelvic trauma, or autoimmune issues.*
> ➢ *Treatment depends on the underlying cause and may involve antibiotics, anti-inflammatory medications, and lifestyle changes.*

Symptoms:
- Pain: pelvic pain, discomfort in the perineum (area between the anus and scrotum), genitals, lower abdomen, or lower back
- Urinary symptoms: urinary urgency, frequency, hesitancy, dysuria (painful urination), nocturia (frequent urination at night), and urinary retention
- Sexual dysfunction: erectile dysfunction, painful ejaculation, and decreased libido
- Flu-like symptoms: fever, chills, body aches, and fatigue
- Other symptoms: blood in the urine or semen, painful bowel movements, and discomfort while sitting

Causes and Risk Factors:
- Age: Prostatitis can occur at any age but is more common in men under 50.
- History of prostatitis: Previous episodes of prostatitis increase the risk of recurrent episodes.
- Urinary Tract Infections (UTIs): UTIs can sometimes spread to the prostate gland, leading to prostatitis.
- Sexual activity: Recent sexual activity, especially with multiple partners, may increase the risk.
- Catheterization: Having a urinary catheter in place can increase the risk of bacterial prostatitis.
- Certain medical conditions: Conditions that affect urinary flow or weaken the immune system, such as benign prostatic hyperplasia (BPH) or diabetes, may increase the risk.

Epidemiology:
- Prostatitis is a common condition, accounting for approximately 8% of urology clinic visits.

- Chronic prostatitis/chronic pelvic pain syndrome (CP/CPPS) is the most prevalent form, affecting about 2-10% of men worldwide.

Diagnosis:
- <u>Medical History and Physical Examination:</u> The APh will inquire about symptoms and perform a physical examination, including a digital rectal examination (DRE) to assess the prostate gland.
- <u>Urine Tests:</u> Urinalysis and urine culture may be performed to detect signs of infection and identify the causative organism.
- <u>Prostate-Specific Antigen (PSA) Test:</u> PSA levels may be measured to assess for prostate inflammation or infection.
- <u>Imaging Studies:</u> Transrectal ultrasound (TRUS) or magnetic resonance imaging (MRI) may be used to evaluate the prostate gland and rule out other conditions.
- <u>Prostate Biopsy:</u> In some cases, a prostate biopsy may be performed if cancer is suspected.

Treatment:
- <u>Antibiotics:</u> Antibiotic therapy is the mainstay of treatment for bacterial prostatitis. The choice of antibiotics depends on the type of prostatitis and the causative organism.
- <u>Alpha-blockers:</u> Alpha-blockers may be prescribed to relax the muscles of the prostate gland and improve urinary flow in cases of chronic prostatitis/chronic pelvic pain syndrome (CP/CPPS).
- <u>Pain Medications:</u> Nonsteroidal anti-inflammatory drugs (NSAIDs) or other pain medications may be recommended to alleviate discomfort.
- <u>Physical Therapy:</u> Pelvic floor physical therapy or relaxation techniques may be beneficial for managing pelvic pain and muscle tension.
- <u>Lifestyle Modifications:</u> Drinking plenty of fluids, avoiding caffeine and alcohol, and practicing good hygiene habits may help alleviate symptoms.

11.6. Urinary Incontinence

> ➤ *Urinary incontinence is the involuntary leakage of urine, often due to weakened pelvic floor muscles, nerve damage, or underlying medical conditions.*
> ➤ *It can range from occasional leaks to complete loss of bladder control, impacting daily life and causing embarrassment.*
> ➤ *Treatment options include pelvic floor exercises, lifestyle changes, medications, and, in some cases, surgery to improve bladder function and control.*

Symptoms:

- Stress incontinence: urine leakage occurring during activities such as coughing, sneezing, laughing, or exercising
- Urge incontinence: sudden and intense urge to urinate, followed by involuntary leakage of urine
- Overflow incontinence: inability to completely empty the bladder, leading to frequent or constant dribbling of urine
- Functional incontinence: difficulty reaching the bathroom due to physical or cognitive impairments, resulting in accidental leakage
- Mixed incontinence: combination of two or more types of urinary incontinence

Causes and Risk Factors:

- Age: Urinary incontinence becomes more common with age, particularly in postmenopausal women and older adults.
- Gender: Women are at higher risk of stress and mixed urinary incontinence due to factors such as pregnancy, childbirth, and menopause.
- Pregnancy and childbirth: Vaginal delivery and multiple pregnancies can weaken pelvic floor muscles and increase the risk of stress incontinence.
- Obesity: Excess weight can put pressure on the bladder and pelvic floor muscles, leading to urinary incontinence.
- Chronic conditions: Diabetes, neurological disorders, and prostate enlargement can affect bladder function and increase the risk of urinary incontinence.
- Medications: Diuretics, alpha-blockers, and sedatives can contribute to urinary incontinence.

- Smoking: Smoking is associated with chronic coughing, which can exacerbate stress incontinence.

Epidemiology:
- Urinary incontinence affects patients of all ages but is more common in older adults.
- Prevalence rates vary depending on the type of incontinence and population studied.
- Estimates suggest that around 25-45% of women and 10-30% of men experience urinary incontinence at some point in their lives.

Diagnosis:
- Medical History: The APh will inquire about symptoms, medical history, medications, and lifestyle factors.
- Physical Examination: to assess pelvic floor muscle strength, pelvic organ prolapse, and signs of infection
- Urinalysis: to rule out urinary tract infections or other underlying conditions
- Bladder Diary: Keeping a record of urinary habits, including frequency, volume, and leakage episodes, can provide valuable information for diagnosis.
- Diagnostic Tests: Additional tests such as urodynamic studies, cystoscopy, or imaging studies may be ordered in certain cases to evaluate bladder function and identify any structural abnormalities.

Treatment:
- Behavioral Therapies: Pelvic floor muscle exercises (Kegel exercises), bladder training, and biofeedback techniques can help improve bladder control and reduce symptoms.
- Lifestyle Modifications: Dietary changes (e.g., avoiding caffeine and acidic foods), weight loss, and smoking cessation may alleviate symptoms.
- Medications: Depending on the type of urinary incontinence, medications such as anticholinergics, beta-3 agonists, or topical estrogen therapy may be prescribed to manage symptoms.
- Medical Devices: In some cases, devices such as urethral inserts or pessaries may be recommended to support the bladder and reduce leakage.
- Surgery: Surgical interventions such as sling procedures, bladder neck suspension, or artificial urinary sphincter implantation may be

considered for severe cases of urinary incontinence that do not respond to conservative treatments.

11.7. Glomerulonephritis

> ➢ *Glomerulonephritis is inflammation of the glomeruli, the filtering units of the kidneys, leading to impaired kidney function and often causing blood or protein in the urine, swelling, and high blood pressure.*
> ➢ *It can result from various causes, including infections, autoimmune diseases, and certain medications.*
> ➢ *Treatment aims at managing symptoms, addressing the underlying cause, and preventing complications like kidney failure.*

Symptoms:
- Hematuria, which may appear pink, brown, or red
- Proteinuria, or excess protein in the urine, causing foamy urine
- Edema in the face, hands, abdomen, or legs, often noticed in the morning
- Hypertension
- Reduced urine output
- Fatigue and weakness
- Joint pain
- Fever

Causes and Risk Factors:
- Autoimmune diseases: Conditions such as lupus, vasculitis, and IgA nephropathy increase the risk.
- Infections: Streptococcal infections (such as strep throat) and viral infections (such as hepatitis B and C), can trigger glomerulonephritis.
- Diabetes: Uncontrolled diabetes increases the risk.
- Hypertension: damages the glomeruli over time
- Family history: of kidney disease or autoimmune conditions
- Exposure to toxins: Certain medications, toxins, or chemicals may cause glomerular injury.

Epidemiology:
- Glomerulonephritis can affect patients of any age, gender, or ethnicity.

- The incidence and prevalence vary depending on the underlying cause and geographic location.
- Chronic glomerulonephritis is a leading cause of chronic kidney disease and end-stage renal disease worldwide.

Diagnosis:
- Medical History and Physical Examination: The APh will evaluate symptoms, medical history, and physical signs such as edema and hypertension.
- Urinalysis: Presence of hematuria, proteinuria, and urinary sediment may suggest glomerular involvement.
- Blood Tests: Measurement of serum creatinine, blood urea nitrogen (BUN), electrolytes, and markers of inflammation.
- Imaging Studies: Ultrasound or CT scan of the kidneys may be performed to assess kidney size and structure.
- Kidney Biopsy: Definitive diagnosis often requires a kidney biopsy to examine the glomeruli under a microscope and determine the underlying cause.

Treatment:

Treatment varies depending on the underlying cause and severity of glomerulonephritis.

- Immunosuppressive Therapy: In autoimmune or immune-mediated forms of glomerulonephritis, corticosteroids and other immunosuppressive medications may be prescribed to suppress inflammation and immune activity.
- Blood Pressure Control: Management of hypertension with antihypertensive medications may reduce the risk of further kidney damage.
- Proteinuria Management: ACE inhibitors or angiotensin receptor blockers (ARBs) may be used to reduce proteinuria and slow the progression of kidney disease.
- Diuretics: to help reduce fluid retention and edema
- Dietary Changes: Restriction of sodium, protein, and potassium intake may be recommended to reduce the workload on the kidneys.
- Dialysis or Kidney Transplant: In cases of advanced kidney failure, dialysis or kidney transplantation may be necessary to replace lost kidney function.

11.8. Polycystic Kidney Disease

> ➢ *Polycystic kidney disease (PKD) is a genetic disorder characterized by the growth of numerous cysts in the kidneys, leading to kidney enlargement and eventual loss of function.*
>
> ➢ *It can cause symptoms such as flank pain, hypertension, and hematuria, with complications including kidney failure and cysts in other organs.*
>
> ➢ *Management focuses on symptom relief, blood pressure control, and supportive care, with potential need for dialysis or kidney transplant in advanced stages.*

Symptoms:
- Abdominal or flank pain: caused by the enlargement of the kidneys due to cyst growth
- Hematuria: often occurs due to cyst rupture or bleeding within the cysts
- Hypertension: can be a result of kidney damage or due to the activation of the renin-angiotensin-aldosterone system
- Urinary tract infections (UTIs): may occur due to obstruction caused by cysts
- Kidney Stones: formed by cysts obstructing the urinary tract
- Proteinuria: protein in the urine, indicating kidney damage
- Abdominal fullness or bloating: Enlarged kidneys can cause discomfort or a feeling of fullness in the abdomen.
- Flank masses: Large kidney cysts may be palpable as masses in the abdomen or flank region.
- Intracranial aneurysms: may lead to headaches, visual disturbances, or neurological deficits if they rupture

Causes and Risk Factors:
- Genetic mutation: PKD is primarily caused by mutations in the PKD1 or PKD2 genes, inherited in an autosomal dominant pattern.
- Family history: Having a first-degree relative with PKD increases the risk of developing the condition.
- Age: Symptoms typically manifest between the ages of 30 and 40, although they can occur at any age.
- Gender: PKD affects men and women equally.

- Race/Ethnicity: PKD occurs in all racial and ethnic groups, but prevalence rates may vary.

Epidemiology:
- PKD is one of the most common inherited kidney disorders, affecting approximately 1 in 500 to 1 in 1,000 patients worldwide.
- Autosomal Dominant PKD (ADPKD) is more common than Autosomal Recessive PKD (ARPKD).
- ADPKD accounts for approximately 90% of all PKD cases and usually presents in adulthood.
- ARPKD is rarer and typically presents in infancy or childhood.

Diagnosis:
- Imaging Studies: Ultrasound, CT scan, or MRI of the abdomen can visualize cysts in the kidneys and confirm the diagnosis.
- Genetic Testing: DNA analysis can identify mutations in the PKD1 or PKD2 genes for confirmation of the diagnosis and for genetic counseling.
- Laboratory Tests: Urinalysis, blood tests (e.g., serum creatinine, BUN), and imaging may be performed to assess kidney function and complications such as hypertension.

Treatment:
- Management of Complications: Treatment focuses on controlling symptoms and managing complications such as hypertension, UTIs, kidney stones, and pain.
- Blood Pressure Control: ACE inhibitors or ARBs may be used to lower blood pressure and slow the progression of kidney disease.
- Pain Management: Analgesics or other pain management strategies may be prescribed to alleviate abdominal or flank pain.
- Dialysis and Transplantation: In advanced stages of PKD with kidney failure, dialysis or kidney transplantation may be necessary.
- Genetic Counseling: Patients with PKD and their families may benefit from genetic counseling to understand inheritance patterns, risks, and family planning options.

11.9. Interstitial Cystitis

> ➢ *Interstitial cystitis (IC) is a chronic bladder condition characterized by pelvic pain, urinary urgency, and frequency, often with nocturia and pain during intercourse.*
> ➢ *Its exact cause is unknown, but theories include bladder lining defects, inflammation, or autoimmune factors.*
> ➢ *Treatment involves symptom management with medications, lifestyle changes, and sometimes bladder instillations or nerve stimulation therapies.*

Symptoms:
- Chronic pelvic pain: pain in the pelvic region, often described as pressure, discomfort, or tenderness, lasting more than six weeks
- Urgency and frequency: frequent, urgent need to urinate, often accompanied by small urine volumes
- Bladder pain: pain or discomfort in the bladder or lower abdomen, worsening as the bladder fills and improving after urination
- Dysuria: pain or burning sensation during urination
- Nocturia: increased frequency of urination at night
- Hematuria: This is less common.
- Painful sexual intercourse: discomfort or pain during sexual activity, particularly in women
- Symptoms worsened by certain foods or beverages: Some patients may experience symptom exacerbation after consuming certain foods or drinks, such as caffeine, alcohol, acidic foods, or artificial sweeteners.

Causes and Risk Factors:
- Gender: Interstitial cystitis is more common in women than in men.
- Age: Symptoms typically manifest in adulthood, with peak onset between the ages of 30 and 40.
- Other chronic pain conditions: patients with a history of other chronic pain disorders, such as fibromyalgia or irritable bowel syndrome (IBS), may be at higher risk.
- Pelvic trauma or surgery: Previous pelvic surgery, childbirth, or trauma to the pelvic region may increase the risk.
- Family history: may increase susceptibility to the condition.

- Autoimmune disorders: There may be a link between interstitial cystitis and autoimmune conditions such as lupus or Sjögren's syndrome.

Epidemiology:
- Prevalence: Interstitial cystitis is estimated to affect 2 to 6% of the general population in the United States, with varying prevalence rates worldwide.
- Diagnosis: The condition is often underdiagnosed or misdiagnosed due to overlapping symptoms with other urinary tract disorders.

Diagnosis:
- <u>Medical History and Physical Examination:</u> The APh will review the patient's medical history and conduct a physical examination to assess symptoms and rule out other potential causes.
- <u>Urinalysis and Urine Culture:</u> These tests may be performed to rule out urinary tract infections (UTIs) and other urinary abnormalities.
- <u>Cystoscopy:</u> A cystoscopy with bladder distention may be performed to visualize the bladder lining for signs of inflammation, hemorrhages, or ulcers.
- <u>Potassium Sensitivity Test:</u> Instillation of potassium chloride solution into the bladder during cystoscopy may reproduce symptoms in patients with interstitial cystitis.
- <u>Biopsy:</u> In some cases, a bladder biopsy may be performed to evaluate for signs of inflammation or other abnormalities.

Treatment:
- <u>Lifestyle Modifications:</u> Avoiding known triggers such as certain foods, beverages, and activities that worsen symptoms.
- <u>Bladder Training:</u> Techniques to gradually increase the intervals between urination and improve bladder capacity.
- <u>Physical Therapy:</u> Pelvic floor physical therapy may help alleviate pelvic pain and urinary symptoms.
- <u>Medications:</u>
  - Oral medications: Tricyclic antidepressants, antihistamines, pentosan polysulfate sodium (Elmiron), and other medications may be prescribed to manage symptoms.
  - Intravesical therapy: Instillation of medications directly into the bladder, such as dimethyl sulfoxide (DMSO) or lidocaine, may provide relief.

- Neuromodulation: Electrical nerve stimulation therapies, such as sacral neuromodulation for pudendal nerve stimulation, may be considered for refractory cases.
- Bladder Instillation: introduction of medications or solutions into the bladder via a catheter for symptom relief
- Surgical Options: In severe cases, surgical procedures such as bladder augmentation or urinary diversion may be considered.

11.10. Hydronephrosis

> ➢ *Hydronephrosis is a condition characterized by the swelling of the kidneys due to the buildup of urine, often caused by obstruction in the urinary tract, such as kidney stones or tumors.*
> ➢ *It can lead to symptoms like flank pain, urinary frequency, and fever, and if severe or left untreated, it may cause kidney damage or failure.*
> ➢ *Treatment aims to relieve the obstruction and address underlying causes through medications, surgery, or other interventions.*

Symptoms:
- Flank pain: pain or discomfort in the side or back, often on one side, where the affected kidney is located
- Abdominal pain: particularly in the area of the affected kidney
- Urinary symptoms: changes in urinary frequency, urgency, or pattern, including difficulty urinating
- Hematuria: may be visible or detected on urinalysis
- Nausea and vomiting: may occur in severe cases or if the underlying cause is related to a blockage
- Fever and chills

Causes and Risk Factors:
- Urinary tract obstruction: Conditions that obstruct or block the flow of urine from the kidneys to the bladder, such as kidney stones, tumors, or strictures, increase the risk of hydronephrosis.
- Urinary tract infections (UTIs): Recurrent or untreated UTIs can lead to inflammation and scarring of the urinary tract, potentially resulting in hydronephrosis.
- Congenital anomalies: Structural abnormalities present at birth, such as ureteropelvic junction (UPJ) obstruction or vesicoureteral reflux (VUR), may predispose patients to hydronephrosis.

- Kidney stones: can cause blockages within the urinary tract, leading to hydronephrosis
- Enlarged prostate: Benign prostatic hyperplasia (BPH) in men can compress the urethra and obstruct urine flow, contributing to hydronephrosis.

Epidemiology:

The prevalence of hydronephrosis varies depending on the underlying cause and population studied. It can affect patients of any age, from newborns to older adults.

Diagnosis:
- Imaging Studies: Ultrasound, CT scan, or MRI of the abdomen and pelvis can visualize the kidneys and urinary tract to identify signs of hydronephrosis and potential causes.
- Urinalysis: can detect signs of infection or blood in the urine, which may suggest underlying causes of hydronephrosis.
- Renal Function Tests: Blood tests such as serum creatinine and blood urea nitrogen (BUN) may be ordered to assess kidney function.

Treatment:
- Management of Underlying Cause: such as surgical removal of kidney stones or correction of urinary tract obstructions
- Pain Management: Analgesic medications may be prescribed to alleviate pain associated with hydronephrosis.
- Antibiotics: may be necessary to manage urinary tract infections associated with hydronephrosis
- Ureteral Stenting: Placement of a stent in the ureter can help relieve obstruction and restore normal urine flow.
- Percutaneous Nephrostomy: In cases of severe hydronephrosis or ureteral obstruction, a nephrostomy tube may be inserted through the skin into the kidney to drain urine.
- Surgical Intervention: Pyeloplasty or nephrectomy may be required for certain cases of hydronephrosis, particularly if conservative measures are ineffective.

11.11. Hematuria

> ➢ *Hematuria is the presence of blood in the urine, which can be visible or microscopic and may indicate underlying kidney or urinary tract problems such as infections, kidney stones, or tumors.*
> ➢ *Evaluation typically involves medical history, physical examination, urine tests, and imaging studies to determine the cause.*
> ➢ *Treatment is tailored to the underlying condition and may include medications, surgery, or lifestyle changes.*

Symptoms:

- Visible blood in urine: Hematuria may present as pink, red, or cola-colored urine.
- Microscopic hematuria: Blood may be detected in urine during laboratory analysis, even if not visible to the naked eye.
- Urinary symptoms: Patients with hematuria may experience other urinary symptoms such as pain or burning during urination, increased urinary frequency, or urgency.
- Abdominal or flank pain: may accompany hematuria
- Fever or chills: If hematuria is caused by a urinary tract infection (UTI) or kidney infection, patients may experience fever, chills, or other signs of infection.

Causes and Risk Factors:

- Age: Hematuria can occur at any age but is more common in older adults due to UTIs, kidney stones, or prostate enlargement (BPH).
- Gender: Men are at higher risk of hematuria due to conditions such as enlarged prostate (BPH), prostate cancer, or UTIs. In women, risk factors may include UTIs, kidney stones, or menstrual-related issues.
- Medical history: Previous history of kidney stones, UTIs, kidney disease, or certain cancers increases the risk.
- Medications: Some medications, such as blood thinners (anticoagulants) or certain antibiotics, may increase the risk of bleeding and hematuria.
- Family history: of kidney disease, kidney stones, or certain genetic conditions may cause increased risk
- Smoking: Tobacco use is associated with an increased risk of bladder cancer, which can cause hematuria.

Epidemiology:
- Prevalence: Hematuria is a common finding and can occur in patients of any age, race, or gender.
- Incidence: The incidence of hematuria varies depending on the underlying cause and population studied.

Diagnosis:
- Physical Examination: The APh may perform a physical examination to assess for signs of UTI, kidney stones, or other conditions.
- Urinalysis: Examination of a urine sample can detect the presence of blood and other abnormalities that may suggest the underlying cause.
- Imaging Studies: Imaging tests such as ultrasound, CT scan, or MRI may be ordered to visualize the urinary tract and identify potential causes.
- Cystoscopy: A cystoscope may be inserted into the urethra and bladder to visually inspect the urinary tract for abnormalities.
- Biopsy: In some cases, a biopsy of the bladder or kidneys may be obtained to further evaluate suspected underlying conditions such as cancer.

Treatment:
- Treatment of Underlying Cause:

    Management of hematuria involves addressing the underlying condition responsible for the bleeding. This may include antibiotics for urinary tract infections, medications for kidney stones, or surgical intervention for tumors or structural abnormalities.
- Symptomatic Relief: Pain medications or other supportive measures may be prescribed to alleviate discomfort.
- Monitoring: Regular follow-up with a healthcare provider may be recommended to monitor hematuria and assess response to treatment, as well as to screen for potential complications or recurrence.

11.12. Renal Artery Stenosis

> ➤ Renal artery stenosis is a narrowing of the arteries that supply blood to the kidneys, often due to atherosclerosis or fibromuscular dysplasia.
> ➤ It can lead to or have symptoms of hypertension, kidney dysfunction, fluid retention, and occasionally abdominal or flank pain.
> ➤ Treatment options range from medications to angioplasty or stenting to restore blood flow and prevent complications.

Symptoms:
- Hypertension: can be caused by renal artery stenosis and is often difficult to control with medication
- Decreased kidney function: Progressive narrowing of the renal artery can impair blood flow to the affected kidney, resulting in reduced kidney function.
- Fluid retention: leading to edema in the legs or other areas
- Abdominal or flank pain: particularly during physical activity or after eating
- Heart-related symptoms: Severe cases may contribute to chest pain or shortness of breath.

Causes and Risk Factors:
- Atherosclerosis: Hardening of the arteries is the most common cause of renal artery stenosis. Risk factors for atherosclerosis include smoking, hypertension, high cholesterol, diabetes, and older age.
- Fibromuscular dysplasia: abnormal growth or development of the walls of the renal arteries, leading to narrowing or blockage
- Family history: of renal artery stenosis or related conditions may cause increased risk.
- Smoking: Tobacco use is a significant risk factor for atherosclerosis and may increase the likelihood of developing renal artery stenosis.
- Hypertension: Chronic hypertension can contribute to the development or progression of renal artery stenosis.

Epidemiology:
- The prevalence of renal artery stenosis varies depending on the population studied and underlying risk factors.
- Atherosclerotic renal artery stenosis is more common in older adults, particularly those with other cardiovascular risk factors.

- Fibromuscular dysplasia is more commonly seen in younger patients, especially women.

Diagnosis:
- Imaging Studies: Imaging tests such as ultrasound, CT angiography, magnetic resonance angiography (MRA), or renal arteriography may be used to visualize the renal arteries and identify areas of stenosis.
- Renal Function Tests: Blood tests to assess kidney function, such as serum creatinine and estimated glomerular filtration rate (eGFR), may be performed.
- Blood Pressure Monitoring: Persistent or difficult-to-control hypertension may prompt further evaluation for renal artery stenosis.
- Angiography: Invasive procedures such as renal arteriography may be necessary for definitive diagnosis and treatment planning.

Treatment:
- Medications: Blood pressure medications, such as ACE inhibitors, ARBs, or diuretics, may be prescribed to help manage hypertension and reduce the risk of complications.
- Percutaneous Transluminal Renal Angioplasty (PTRA) with Stenting: This minimally invasive procedure involves inserting a catheter with a balloon into the narrowed renal artery to widen the blockage and placing a stent to help keep the artery open.
- Surgical Revascularization: Open surgery may be necessary to bypass or repair the narrowed or blocked portion of the renal artery.
- Lifestyle Modifications: Smoking cessation, adopting a healthy diet, regular exercise, and weight management may help reduce the risk of progression and complications.

11.13. Renal Cyst

> ➢ *Renal cysts are fluid-filled sacs that develop in the kidneys, often as a result of age-related changes or underlying kidney conditions.*
> ➢ *Most renal cysts are benign and asymptomatic, but larger cysts or those associated with polycystic kidney disease can lead to complications such as pain, hypertension, or kidney impairment.*
> ➢ *Treatment depends on the size, number, and symptoms of the cysts, ranging from monitoring to medical or surgical intervention.*

Symptoms:
- Most renal cysts are asymptomatic and are often discovered incidentally during imaging studies conducted for unrelated reasons.
- Large cysts may cause symptoms such as dull flank pain, abdominal discomfort, or a palpable mass in the abdomen.
- Rarely, complications such as hemorrhage into the cyst, infection (cyst infection), or rupture may occur, leading to symptoms such as fever, sudden onset of severe flank pain, or hematuria.

Causes and Risk Factors:
- Age: more common with advancing age
- Family history: There may be a genetic predisposition to developing renal cysts, especially in cases of autosomal dominant polycystic kidney disease (ADPKD).
- Other renal conditions: Patients with certain kidney disorders, such as ADPKD or medullary sponge kidney, may have an increased risk.
- Smoking: Tobacco use may be associated with an increased risk.

Epidemiology:
- Renal cysts are common and are often found incidentally on imaging studies.
- Simple renal cysts are more prevalent in older patients, with up to 50% of patients over the age of 50 having at least one cyst.
- Autosomal dominant polycystic kidney disease (ADPKD) is the most common hereditary kidney disorder, affecting approximately 1 in 400 to 1 in 1,000 patients worldwide.

Diagnosis:
- Imaging Studies: Renal cysts are typically identified using ultrasound, CT scan, or MRI. These imaging techniques can help differentiate between simple cysts and complex cystic lesions or solid masses.
- Laboratory Tests: Blood tests such as serum creatinine and blood urea nitrogen (BUN) may be performed to assess kidney function.
- Urinalysis: Urine analysis may be conducted to check for the presence of blood or protein in the urine, which may indicate underlying kidney problems.

Treatment:
- Observation: Simple renal cysts that are asymptomatic and do not cause complications often do not require treatment and may be monitored periodically with imaging studies.

- Symptomatic Relief: Pain may be managed with over-the-counter pain medications such as acetaminophen or nonsteroidal anti-inflammatory drugs (NSAIDs).
- Drainage or Aspiration: Large or symptomatic cysts may be drained or aspirated using a needle under ultrasound or CT guidance to provide temporary relief of symptoms.
- Sclerotherapy: involves injecting a sclerosing agent into the cyst to shrink it and prevent recurrence of fluid accumulation
- Surgery: Cyst decortication, laparoscopic cystectomy, or nephrectomy (partial or complete removal of the kidney) may be necessary for complex cysts, cysts causing significant symptoms, or suspected cancerous cysts.

11.14. Nephrotic Syndrome

> ➢ *Nephrotic syndrome is a kidney disorder characterized by the presence of protein in the urine (proteinuria), low blood protein levels (hypoalbuminemia), edema, and high cholesterol levels.*
>
> ➢ *It can result from various underlying causes, such as minimal change disease, focal segmental glomerulosclerosis, or membranous nephropathy.*
>
> ➢ *Treatment typically involves medications to reduce proteinuria, control blood pressure, and manage edema, along with addressing the underlying cause if possible.*

Symptoms:
- Massive proteinuria: excretion of large amounts of protein in the urine, leading to frothy or foamy urine
- Hypoalbuminemia: low levels of albumin in the blood, resulting in edema (swelling) particularly in the face, abdomen, and lower extremities
- Hyperlipidemia: elevated levels of cholesterol and triglycerides in the blood
- Edema: especially in the face, abdomen, and lower extremities
- Fatigue and weakness: due to loss of protein and fluid imbalance
- Decreased urine output

Causes and Risk Factors:
- Age: Nephrotic syndrome can occur at any age, but it is more common in children between 2 and 6 years of age and in adults between 30 and 50 years of age.
- Underlying conditions: Certain medical conditions, such as diabetes, lupus, amyloidosis, and certain infections (e.g., HIV, hepatitis B and C), increase the risk of developing nephrotic syndrome.
- Medications: Some medications, including nonsteroidal anti-inflammatory drugs (NSAIDs), certain antibiotics, and some drugs used to treat high blood pressure and cancer, may increase the risk of nephrotic syndrome.
- Genetics: Certain genetic disorders, such as Alport syndrome and Fabry disease, may predispose patients to nephrotic syndrome.

Epidemiology:
- Nephrotic syndrome is relatively rare, with an estimated incidence of 2-7 cases per 100,000 children and 16 cases per 100,000 adults per year.
- It can occur at any age but is more common in children than in adults.
- Certain types of nephrotic syndrome, such as minimal change disease, are more prevalent in children, while others, such as focal segmental glomerulosclerosis (FSGS) and membranous nephropathy, are more common in adults.

Diagnosis:
- Urinalysis: Urine dipstick testing may reveal significant proteinuria (3+ or 4+ protein).
- Blood Tests: Blood tests may show hypoalbuminemia (low serum albumin levels) and hyperlipidemia (elevated cholesterol and triglyceride levels).
- Kidney Biopsy: A kidney biopsy may be performed to determine the underlying cause of nephrotic syndrome and guide treatment decisions.
- Imaging Studies: Imaging tests such as ultrasound or CT scan may be used to assess the size and structure of the kidneys and rule out other kidney diseases.

Treatment:
- Corticosteroids: Initial treatment often involves corticosteroids (e.g., prednisone) to reduce inflammation and proteinuria. They are particularly effective in children with minimal change disease.

- **Immunosuppressive Therapy:** In cases of steroid-resistant nephrotic syndrome or relapse, immunosuppressive medications such as cyclophosphamide, cyclosporine, or mycophenolate mofetil may be used.
- **Diuretics:** may be prescribed to help reduce edema and fluid retention
- **Blood Pressure Control:** Angiotensin-converting enzyme (ACE) inhibitors or angiotensin II receptor blockers (ARBs) may be used to control blood pressure and reduce proteinuria.
- **Dietary Changes:** A low-sodium diet may help reduce edema.
- **Treatment of Underlying Conditions:** If nephrotic syndrome is secondary to an underlying condition (e.g., diabetes, lupus), treatment of the underlying disease is essential.

11.15. Nephritic syndrome

> ➤ *Nephritic syndrome refers to inflammation of the kidneys, leading to symptoms such as hematuria, proteinuria, hypertension, and fluid retention.*
> ➤ *It can result from various causes, including infections, autoimmune diseases, and certain medications.*
> ➤ *Treatment aims at managing symptoms, controlling inflammation, and addressing the underlying cause to prevent kidney damage and complications like kidney failure.*

Symptoms:
- Hematuria: may appear red or cola-colored
- Proteinuria: typically in smaller amounts compared to nephrotic syndrome
- Hypertension: may be a result of impaired kidney function
- Edema: usually less pronounced than in nephrotic syndrome
- Oliguria: reduced urine output or decreased urine production
- Azotemia: elevated levels of nitrogen-containing compounds such as urea and creatinine in the blood, indicating impaired kidney function
- Urinary casts: Microscopic examination of urine may reveal cellular casts, which are cylindrical structures formed from the proteins and cells that pass through the kidney tubules.

Causes and Risk Factors:
- Autoimmune disorders: Conditions such as lupus nephritis, IgA nephropathy, and anti-glomerular basement membrane (anti-GBM) disease increase the risk of developing nephritic syndrome.
- Infections: Certain infections, particularly bacterial infections such as streptococcal infections (post-streptococcal glomerulonephritis), can lead to nephritic syndrome.
- Genetic factors: Some forms of nephritic syndrome may have a genetic predisposition, such as Alport syndrome or familial IgA nephropathy.
- Environmental factors: Exposure to certain environmental toxins or medications may increase the risk of developing nephritic syndrome.

Epidemiology:
- The incidence and prevalence of nephritic syndrome vary depending on the underlying cause.
- Post-streptococcal glomerulonephritis, a common cause of nephritic syndrome in children, often occurs following a streptococcal infection, such as strep throat or impetigo.
- Other forms of nephritic syndrome, such as lupus nephritis or IgA nephropathy, may occur more frequently in adults and are often associated with autoimmune diseases.

Diagnosis:
- Urinalysis: Examination of urine may reveal hematuria (red blood cells in the urine) and proteinuria (although typically less than in nephrotic syndrome).
- Blood Tests: Blood tests may show elevated levels of creatinine and urea nitrogen, indicating impaired kidney function. Serologic tests may be performed to detect underlying autoimmune diseases or infections.
- Kidney Biopsy: A kidney biopsy may be performed to confirm the diagnosis and determine the underlying cause of nephritic syndrome. Histologic examination of kidney tissue can provide valuable information about the pattern of glomerular injury and guide treatment decisions.

Treatment:
- Treatment of Underlying Cause:
    Management of nephritic syndrome involves treating the underlying condition responsible for the kidney inflammation. This may include antibiotics for bacterial infections,

immunosuppressive therapy for autoimmune diseases, or supportive care for other causes.

- <u>Blood Pressure Control:</u>

    Controlling hypertension is important to help preserve kidney function and reduce the risk of complications. Medications such as angiotensin-converting enzyme (ACE) inhibitors or angiotensin II receptor blockers (ARBs): may be used to lower blood pressure and reduce proteinuria.

- <u>Fluid and Electrolyte Management:</u> Monitoring and managing fluid and electrolyte balance is essential, particularly in patients with oliguria or azotemia.

- <u>Symptom Management:</u> Symptomatic treatment may include measures to relieve edema, such as diuretics, and medications to control pain or discomfort.

11.16. Urinary Incontinence

➢ *Urinary incontinence is the involuntary leakage of urine, often due to weakened pelvic floor muscles, nerve damage, or underlying medical conditions.*

> ➢ *Urinary incontinence is the involuntary leakage of urine, often due to weakened pelvic floor muscles, nerve damage, or underlying medical conditions.*
>
> ➢ *It can range from occasional leaks to complete loss of bladder control, impacting daily life and causing embarrassment.*
>
> ➢ *Treatment options include pelvic floor exercises, lifestyle changes, medications, and, in some cases, surgery to improve bladder function and control.*

Symptoms:

- Stress incontinence: involuntary leakage of urine, which may occur during activities such as coughing, sneezing, laughing, or lifting heavy objects
- Urge incontinence: sudden, intense urge to urinate followed by leakage of urine before reaching the toilet
- Frequent urination or waking up multiple times during the night to urinate
- Difficulty initiating urination or incomplete emptying of the bladder
- Nocturnal enuresis in children or adults.

- Mixed incontinence: A combination of stress and urge incontinence symptoms.

Causes and Risk Factors:
- Age: Aging is a significant risk factor for urinary incontinence due to changes in bladder function, pelvic floor muscles, and hormonal levels.
- Gender: Women are more prone to urinary incontinence than men due to factors such as pregnancy, childbirth, and menopause.
- Pregnancy and childbirth: Vaginal childbirth, especially multiple deliveries or prolonged labor, can weaken pelvic floor muscles and damage nerves controlling bladder function.
- Menopause: Estrogen depletion during menopause can lead to changes in vaginal tissues and urinary tract function, increasing the risk of incontinence.
- Obesity: Excess body weight can put pressure on the bladder and pelvic floor muscles, leading to stress incontinence.
- Pelvic floor disorders: Conditions such as pelvic organ prolapse, cystocele, rectocele, or previous pelvic surgeries can contribute to urinary incontinence.
- Neurological conditions: Disorders affecting the nervous system, such as multiple sclerosis, Parkinson's disease, spinal cord injuries, or stroke, can disrupt bladder control and lead to urinary incontinence.
- Chronic cough: Persistent coughing due to conditions such as chronic obstructive pulmonary disease (COPD), asthma, or smoking can increase intra-abdominal pressure and trigger stress incontinence.

Epidemiology:

Urinary incontinence is a common condition affecting people of all ages, genders, and backgrounds.
- Its prevalence increases with age, with estimates suggesting that up to 30-40% of women over the age of 60 experience some form of urinary incontinence.
- However, urinary incontinence can also affect men, particularly those with prostate conditions or neurological disorders.
- The prevalence of urinary incontinence may vary depending on factors such as geographical location, cultural practices, and access to healthcare services.

Diagnosis:
- Medical history: The APP will inquire about symptoms, medical history, medications, lifestyle factors, and potential underlying causes of urinary incontinence.
- Physical examination: A pelvic exam may be performed to assess for signs of pelvic organ prolapse, pelvic floor muscle strength, and neurological function.
- Urinalysis: Urine testing may be conducted to check for signs of infection, blood, or other abnormalities.
- Bladder diary: Keeping a record of fluid intake, urinary frequency, urgency episodes, and episodes of incontinence over several days can help evaluate bladder function and identify patterns.
- Urodynamic testing: Specialized tests such as uroflowmetry, cystometry, or pressure flow studies may be performed to assess bladder and urethral function and diagnose specific types of urinary incontinence.
- Imaging studies: Imaging tests such as ultrasound, cystoscopy, or magnetic resonance imaging (MRI) may be used to evaluate the urinary tract and assess for structural abnormalities or other underlying conditions contributing to urinary incontinence.

Treatment:
- Behavioral therapies:

    Lifestyle modifications such as bladder training, scheduled voiding, fluid management, pelvic floor exercises (Kegel exercises), and dietary changes may help improve bladder control and reduce symptoms.
- Pelvic floor therapy:

    Physical therapy techniques such as biofeedback, electrical stimulation, or pelvic floor muscle training supervised by a specialized therapist can help strengthen pelvic floor muscles and improve bladder control.
- Medications:

    Medications such as anticholinergics, beta-3 adrenergic agonists, or tricyclic antidepressants may be prescribed to relax bladder muscles, reduce urinary urgency, or increase bladder capacity in individuals with overactive bladder or urge incontinence.

- Medical devices:

    Devices such as vaginal pessaries or urethral inserts may be used to support pelvic organs or prevent urine leakage in individuals with pelvic organ prolapse or stress incontinence.

- Interventional therapies:

    Procedures such as botulinum toxin injections into the bladder muscle, bulking agent injections into the urethra, or sacral neuromodulation may be considered for refractory cases of urinary incontinence.

- Surgery:

    Surgical interventions such as sling procedures, bladder neck suspension, artificial urinary sphincter placement, or sacral nerve stimulation may be recommended for severe cases of stress incontinence or pelvic organ prolapse that do not respond to conservative treatments.

11.17. Erectile Dysfunction

> ➢ *Erectile dysfunction (ED) is the inability to achieve or maintain an erection sufficient for sexual intercourse.*
>
> ➢ *It can result from various factors, including physical conditions like cardiovascular disease, diabetes, or hormonal imbalances, as well as psychological factors such as stress or anxiety.*
>
> ➢ *Treatment options include medications, lifestyle changes, therapy, or, in some cases, surgical interventions.*

Symptoms:
- Difficulty achieving an erection
- Difficulty maintaining an erection during sexual activity
- Reduced sexual desire or libido
- Premature ejaculation or delayed ejaculation
- Psychological distress or anxiety related to sexual performance

Causes and Risk Factors:
- Age: Aging is a significant risk factor for erectile dysfunction, with prevalence increasing with age due to changes in vascular health, hormonal levels, and overall health status.
- Chronic medical conditions: Conditions such as diabetes, hypertension, cardiovascular disease, obesity, metabolic syndrome,

or neurological disorders can impair blood flow, nerve function, or hormonal balance, contributing to erectile dysfunction.

- Lifestyle factors: Smoking, excessive alcohol consumption, substance abuse, sedentary lifestyle, poor nutrition, or lack of exercise can increase the risk of erectile dysfunction by affecting vascular health, hormonal levels, or psychological well-being.
- Medications: Certain medications such as antihypertensives, antidepressants, antipsychotics, diuretics, hormone therapy, or chemotherapy drugs may cause or exacerbate erectile dysfunction as a side effect.
- Psychological factors: Stress, anxiety, depression, performance anxiety, relationship problems, or past trauma can contribute to erectile dysfunction by affecting sexual arousal, libido, or confidence.
- Hormonal imbalances: Low testosterone levels or imbalances in other hormones such as thyroid hormones or cortisol may affect sexual function and contribute to erectile dysfunction.
- Pelvic or genital trauma: Injuries or surgeries affecting the pelvic area or genital region may damage nerves, blood vessels, or tissues involved in the erectile process, leading to erectile dysfunction.

Epidemiology:

- Erectile dysfunction is a common condition affecting men of all ages, although its prevalence increases with age. Estimates suggest that up to 30 million men in the United States are affected by erectile dysfunction to some extent.
- The prevalence of erectile dysfunction may vary depending on factors such as geographical location, cultural practices, access to healthcare services, and underlying health conditions.
- While erectile dysfunction is more common in older men, it can also affect younger men, particularly those with underlying medical or psychological factors.

Diagnosis:

- <u>Medical History:</u> The APh will inquire about symptoms, medical history, medications, lifestyle factors, sexual history, and potential underlying causes of erectile dysfunction.
- <u>Physical Examination:</u> to assess for signs of underlying medical conditions such as hypertension, diabetes, cardiovascular disease, or hormonal imbalances

- Laboratory Tests: to measure levels of hormones such as testosterone, thyroid hormones, or prolactin, as well as markers of cardiovascular health such as lipid profiles or glucose levels
- Psychological Evaluation: A mental health assessment may be conducted to evaluate for symptoms of anxiety, depression, stress, or relationship issues contributing to erectile dysfunction.
- Erectile function tests: Specialized tests such as penile Doppler ultrasound, nocturnal penile tumescence (NPT) testing, or intracavernosal injection tests may be performed to assess penile blood flow, vascular function, or nocturnal erections.

Treatment:
- Lifestyle Modifications:

    Making lifestyle changes such as smoking cessation, reducing alcohol consumption, improving diet and nutrition, increasing physical activity, and managing stress may help improve erectile function and overall sexual health.

- Medications:

    Oral medications such as phosphodiesterase type 5 (PDE5) inhibitors (e.g., sildenafil, tadalafil, vardenafil) are commonly prescribed as first-line treatment for erectile dysfunction and work by enhancing blood flow to the penis to facilitate erections.

- Hormone Therapy:

    Hormone replacement therapy (e.g., testosterone replacement therapy) may be recommended for men with low testosterone levels (hypogonadism) contributing to erectile dysfunction.

- Psychotherapy:

    Counseling, cognitive-behavioral therapy (CBT), or sex therapy may be beneficial for addressing psychological factors such as anxiety, depression, or relationship issues affecting erectile function.

- Vacuum Erection Devices:

    Mechanical devices such as vacuum erection devices (VEDs) can be used to create a vacuum around the penis, drawing blood into the erectile tissues and facilitating an erection.

- Penile Injections:

    Intracavernosal injections of medications such as alprostadil may be used to stimulate penile blood flow and produce erections in men who do not respond to oral medications.

- Penile Implants:

    Surgical placement of penile implants (penile prosthesis) may be considered for men with severe erectile dysfunction refractory to other treatments, allowing for on-demand erections through manual manipulation of the implanted device.

11.18. Overactive Bladder

> ➤ *Overactive bladder (OAB) is a condition characterized by frequent, sudden urges to urinate, often accompanied by urinary incontinence or nocturia.*
>
> ➤ *It may result from bladder muscle contractions or nerve dysfunction and can significantly impact quality of life.*
>
> ➤ *Treatment typically involves lifestyle changes, bladder training, medications, and in some cases, medical procedures to alleviate symptoms and improve bladder control.*

Symptoms:
- Urgency: sudden, intense urge to urinate that is difficult to control
- Frequency: increased urinary frequency, often defined as urinating *more than eight times* in a 24-hour period
- Nocturia: waking up multiple times during the night to urinate, disrupting sleep patterns
- Urge incontinence: leakage of urine associated with the sudden urge to urinate, which may result in accidents if a restroom is not reached in time

Causes and Risk Factors:
- Age: OAB becomes more common with advancing age, particularly in individuals over 65 years old.
- Gender: Women are more likely to experience OAB than men, possibly due to factors such as childbirth, hormonal changes, and pelvic floor muscle weakness.
- Obesity: Excess body weight can put pressure on the bladder and exacerbate OAB symptoms.
- Neurological conditions: Conditions affecting the nervous system, such as multiple sclerosis, Parkinson's disease, spinal cord injury, or stroke, can disrupt bladder function and increase the risk of OAB.

- Bladder conditions: Bladder infections, bladder stones, bladder cancer, or bladder inflammation can irritate the bladder and contribute to OAB symptoms.
- Medications: Certain medications such as diuretics, anticholinergics, antidepressants, sedatives, or antipsychotics may increase the risk of OAB or exacerbate symptoms.
- Pelvic floor disorders: Pelvic organ prolapse, pelvic surgery, or pelvic floor muscle weakness can affect bladder control and contribute to OAB symptoms.

Epidemiology:
- OAB is a common urinary disorder that affects millions of people worldwide. Its prevalence increases with age, with estimates suggesting that up to 30-40% of adults over the age of 65 experience OAB symptoms.
- While OAB can occur at any age, it is more prevalent in older adults, particularly women.
- The exact prevalence of OAB may vary depending on factors such as geographical location, cultural practices, access to healthcare services, and underlying health conditions.

Diagnosis:
- Medical History: The APh will inquire about symptoms, medical history, medications, lifestyle factors, urinary habits, fluid intake, and potential contributing factors to OAB.
- Physical Examination: to assess for signs of pelvic floor muscle weakness, neurological conditions, or other underlying conditions contributing to OAB
- Urinalysis: to check for signs of infection, blood, or other abnormalities
- Bladder Diary: Keeping a record of fluid intake, urinary frequency, urgency episodes, and episodes of incontinence over several days can help evaluate bladder function and identify patterns.
- Urodynamic Testing: Specialized tests such as cystometry or pressure flow studies may be performed to assess bladder function, bladder capacity, and detrusor muscle activity.
- Post-Void Residual (PVR) Measurement: Ultrasound or catheterization may be used to measure the amount of urine remaining in the bladder after voiding to assess bladder emptying.

Treatment:

- Lifestyle Modifications: Bladder training, scheduled voiding, pelvic floor exercises (Kegel exercises), fluid management, and dietary changes may help improve bladder control and reduce OAB symptoms.

- Bladder Medications:

    Anticholinergics (e.g., oxybutynin, tolterodine, solifenacin) or beta-3 adrenergic agonists (e.g., mirabegron) may be prescribed to relax bladder muscles, reduce urinary urgency, and decrease bladder contractions.

- Neuromodulation Therapy:

    Sacral nerve stimulation (intermittent or continuous) or percutaneous tibial nerve stimulation (PTNS) may be used to modulate nerve activity and improve bladder control in individuals with refractory OAB symptoms.

- Botox Injections:

    Botulinum toxin injections into the bladder muscle may be considered for individuals with severe OAB symptoms who do not respond to other treatments, temporarily paralyzing bladder muscles and reducing urge incontinence episodes.

- Percutaneous Posterior Tibial Nerve Stimulation (PPTNS):

    A thin needle electrode is inserted near the ankle to deliver electrical stimulation to the tibial nerve, modulating bladder function and reducing OAB symptoms.

- Surgical Interventions:

    Surgical procedures such as bladder augmentation, urinary diversion, or urinary diversion may be considered for individuals with severe OAB symptoms refractory to conservative treatments, although these interventions are generally reserved for rare cases.

References

- Levey, A. S., Becker, C., & et al. (2015). KDIGO 2015 Clinical Practice Guideline Update for the diagnosis, evaluation, prevention, and treatment of Chronic Kidney Disease-Mineral and Bone Disorder (CKD-MBD). Kidney International Supplements, 7(1), 1-59.

- Kellum, J. A., Lameire, N., & et al. (2013). Diagnosis, evaluation, and management of acute kidney injury: A KDIGO summary (Part 1). Critical Care, 17(1), 204.

- Khan, S. R., Pearle, M. S., & et al. (2016). Kidney stones. Nature Reviews Disease Primers, 2(1), 16008.
- McVary, K. T., Roehrborn, C. G., & et al. (2011). Update on AUA guideline on the management of benign prostatic hyperplasia. Journal of Urology, 185(5), 1793-1803.
- Nickel, J. C., & Shoskes, D. A. (2012). Phenotypic approach to the management of chronic prostatitis/chronic pelvic pain syndrome. Current Urology Reports, 13(4), 307-313.
- Gormley, E. A., Lightner, D. J., & et al. (2012). Diagnosis and treatment of overactive bladder (non-neurogenic) in adults: AUA/SUFU guideline. Journal of Urology, 188(6), 2455-2463.
- Floege, J., Barbour, S. J., & et al. (2019). Management and treatment of glomerular diseases (part 1): Conclusions from a Kidney Disease: Improving Global Outcomes (KDIGO) Controversies Conference. Kidney International, 95(2), 268-280.
- Torres, V. E., Harris, P. C., & et al. (2007). Polycystic kidney disease: Genes, proteins, animal models, disease mechanisms and therapeutic opportunities. Journal of Internal Medicine, 261(1), 17-31.
- Hanno, P. M., Erickson, D., & et al. (2015). Diagnosis and treatment of interstitial cystitis/bladder pain syndrome: AUA guideline amendment. Journal of Urology, 193(5), 1545-1553.
- Fernbach, S. K., Maizels, M., & et al. (1993). Pediatric renal ultrasonography: Pearls, pitfalls, and pictorial review. American Journal of Roentgenology, 160(5), 1057-1066.
- Davis, R., Jones, J. S., & et al. (2012). Diagnosis, evaluation and follow-up of asymptomatic microhematuria (AMH) in adults: AUA guideline. Journal of Urology, 188(6), 2473-2481.
- Wheatley, K., Ives, N., & et al. (2009). Revascularization versus medical therapy for renal-artery stenosis. New England Journal of Medicine, 361(20), 1953-1962.
- Kitiyakara, C., & Kopp, J. B. (2016). Egf receptors, metformin, and nephrotic syndrome. New England Journal of Medicine, 374(10), 979-980.
- Barbour, S. J., Cattran, D. C., & et al. (2012). The rationale and scope of the new classification of systemic lupus erythematosus nephritis. Kidney International, 87(4), 789-796.

Chapter 12: Dermatologic Disorders

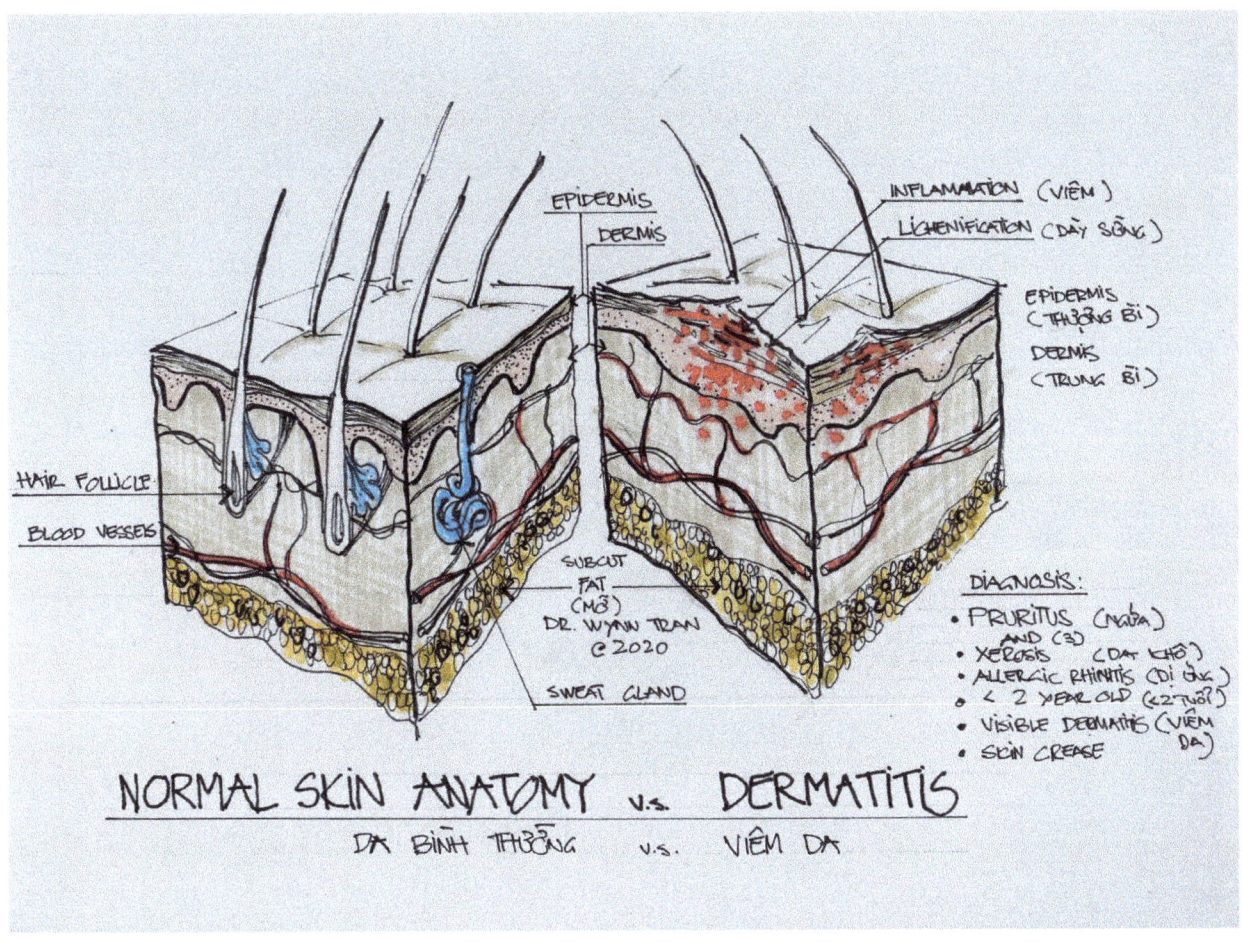

The APh should be familiar with the presentation, diagnosis, and management of these common dermatologist disorders to provide appropriate care and referral to the dermatologist when necessary.

12.1. Acne Vulgaris

> ➢ *Acne vulgaris is a common skin condition characterized by the formation of pimples, blackheads, and whiteheads, typically on the face, neck, chest, and back.*
>
> ➢ *It results from clogged hair follicles due to excess oil production, bacteria, and inflammation, and can lead to scarring if left untreated.*
>
> ➢ *Treatment options include topical medications, oral antibiotics, retinoids, and in severe cases, isotretinoin or other systemic therapies, along with lifestyle modifications and skincare routines.*

Symptoms:

- Lesions may appear on the face, neck, chest, back, and shoulders.
    - Comedones: non-inflammatory lesions characterized by clogged pores, appearing as blackheads or whiteheads
    - Inflammatory Lesions: papules, pustules, nodules, and cysts, which are red, swollen, and tender
- Scarring: Severe acne lesions can lead to permanent scarring.

Causes and Risk Factors:

- Hormonal changes: particularly during puberty, menstruation, pregnancy, or hormonal disorders, can trigger acne
- Family history
- Excessive oil production: overproduction of sebum by the sebaceous glands
- Clogged pores: accumulation of dead skin cells and bacteria within hair follicles
- Bacterial infection: *Propionibacterium acnes* (*P. acnes*) bacteria can contribute to inflammation and acne lesions.
- Environmental factors: exposure to pollutants, humidity, and certain cosmetics or skincare products
- Dietary factors: High-glycemic-index foods and dairy products may exacerbate acne in some patients.

Epidemiology:

- Acne is one of the most common skin conditions worldwide, affecting patients of all ages but most commonly adolescents and young adults.
- Prevalence peaks during puberty, with up to 85% of adolescents experiencing acne to some degree.

- While acne tends to improve with age, it can persist into adulthood and may affect approximately 10-20% of adults, particularly women.

Diagnosis:

Diagnosis is primarily clinical, based on the characteristic appearance of acne lesions. Severity can be assessed using standardized grading scales, such as the Global Acne Grading System (see below) or the Acne Severity Index (ASI). Differential diagnosis may include other skin conditions with similar features, such as rosacea, folliculitis, or perioral dermatitis.

Global Acne Grading System (GAGS) Score	
Lesion Type	Points
<ul><li>Comedones (open or closed)</li><li>Papules</li><li>Pustules</li><li>Nodules</li></ul>	1 2 3 4
Body Area	Factor
<ul><li>Face</li><li>Chest</li><li>Back</li><li>Shoulders</li></ul>	Factor of 2 Factor of 3 Factor of 3 Factor of 2

- Calculating the Score: For each body area, count the number of each type of lesion and multiply by their respective factors. Sum the scores from all areas to get the total GAGS score.
- Interpretation:
    - 0-18: Mild Acne.
    - 19-30: Moderate Acne.
    - 31-38: Severe Acne.
    - 39 and above: Very Severe Acne.

Treatment:

- Topical Agents: benzoyl peroxide, retinoids, topical antibiotics, and/or azelaic acid.
- Oral Medications: oral antibiotics (e.g., tetracyclines), hormonal therapies (e.g., combined oral contraceptives, spironolactone), and/or oral isotretinoin (for severe or refractory cases).
- Procedures: chemical peels, laser therapy, microdermabrasion, and/or extraction of comedones or cysts.

- **Lifestyle Modifications:** gentle cleansing, avoiding harsh skincare products, and adopting a healthy diet may help manage acne.

Isotretinoin and iPledge Program for severe acne:

- Isotretinoin is a highly effective medication derived from vitamin A, used to treat severe or cystic acne that has not responded to other treatments. Isotrenioin is usually given in conjunction with the iPledge program. The medication reduces the production of sebum, helping to prevent the formation of acne.

- The treatment often produces long-term or permanent results after a single course of 4 to 6 months. However, isotretinoin can cause a range of side effects, from mild (e.g., dry skin) to severe.

- The iPledge program is a federally mandated risk management program in the United States, designed to prevent the exposure of isotretinoin to pregnant women due to the high risk of fetal birth defects associated with the drug.

12.2. Atopic Dermatitis

> ➤ *Atopic dermatitis, or eczema, is a chronic inflammatory skin condition characterized by itching, redness, and scaling, often occurring in areas with thin skin such as the face, neck, and flexor surfaces.*
>
> ➤ *It results from a combination of genetic, environmental, and immune factors.*
>
> ➤ *Management involves moisturizers, topical corticosteroids, immunomodulators, and avoiding triggers to alleviate symptoms and prevent flare-ups.*

Symptoms:

- Pruritus: itchy skin, which can be severe and disruptive, leading to scratching and excoriation.
- Erythema: redness and inflammation of the skin, often accompanied by papules, vesicles, or crusting.
- Dry skin: Skin may appear dry, rough, and scaly, especially in chronic cases.
- Lichenification: thickening and hardening of the skin, often due to chronic scratching or rubbing.
- Excoriations: Scratched areas of skin may become raw, weepy, or crusty.

- Distribution: Common areas affected include flexural surfaces (e.g., elbows, knees), face, neck, and hands, although involvement can vary widely.

Causes and Risk Factors:
- Genetics: Family history of atopic dermatitis, asthma, or allergic rhinitis increases the risk.
- Immune dysregulation: Abnormal immune responses and defects in skin barrier function contribute to the development of eczema.
- Environmental factors: Exposure to irritants, allergens, harsh soaps, detergents, or dry weather can exacerbate symptoms.
- Age: Atopic dermatitis often begins in infancy or childhood, but it can persist into adulthood or develop later in life.
- Medical History: Patients with a history of allergic conditions are more likely to develop eczema.
- Stress: Psychological stress or emotional factors may exacerbate symptoms in some patients.

Epidemiology:
- Atopic dermatitis is a common chronic inflammatory skin condition, affecting patients of all ages worldwide.
- It often begins in infancy, with approximately 60% of cases presenting during the first year of life.
- The prevalence of atopic dermatitis has been increasing over recent decades, particularly in industrialized countries.
- While many children outgrow the condition, some patients may experience persistent or recurrent symptoms into adulthood.

Diagnosis:
- <u>Clinical Evaluation:</u> Diagnosis is primarily based on the characteristic appearance and distribution of skin lesions, along with a history of itching and rash.
- <u>Exclusion of Other Conditions:</u> Other skin conditions with similar features, such as contact dermatitis or psoriasis, should be ruled out.
- <u>Skin Patch Testing:</u> to identify potential allergens contributing to eczema flare-ups.

Treatment:
- <u>Emollients and Moisturizers:</u> Regular use of emollients helps to hydrate the skin and restore the skin barrier.

- **Topical Corticosteroids:** Corticosteroid creams or ointments are commonly used to reduce inflammation and itching during flare-ups.
- **Topical Calcineurin Inhibitors:** Tacrolimus and pimecrolimus are alternative options for managing eczema, particularly in sensitive areas.
- **Topical Phosphodiesterase-4 (PDE-4) Inhibitor:** Crisaborole is a newer topical medication that inhibits PDE-4 and reduces inflammation.
- **Antihistamines:** Oral antihistamines may help alleviate itching and improve sleep quality in patients with eczema.
- **Phototherapy:** Narrowband UVB phototherapy or ultraviolet A (UVA) phototherapy may be recommended for patients with moderate to severe eczema.
- **Systemic Immunomodulators:** Systemic medications such as oral corticosteroids, cyclosporine, methotrexate, or dupilumab may be prescribed for severe, refractory cases.

Lifestyle Modifications:
- Avoid triggers: Identifying and avoiding triggers such as harsh soaps, irritants, allergens, and environmental factors can help prevent flare-ups.
- Skin care practices: Gentle skin care practices, including avoiding hot baths, using mild soap, and patting the skin dry, can help minimize irritation.
- Stress management: Stress reduction techniques such as relaxation exercises, meditation, or counseling may be beneficial for some patients.

12.3. Contact Dermatitis

> *Contact dermatitis is a skin condition caused by direct contact with an irritant or allergen, resulting in redness, itching, and sometimes blistering or rash formation.*
>
> *It can be classified as irritant or allergic, with triggers ranging from soaps and cosmetics to plants and metals.*
>
> *Treatment involves identifying and avoiding the offending substance, along with topical corticosteroids and soothing agents to alleviate symptoms.*

Symptoms:
- Rash: red, itchy, or swollen skin at the site of contact with the offending substance.
- Blistering: formation of blisters or bumps on the skin, which may ooze or crust over.
- Burning or stinging: often accompanying irritation and discomfort
- Dry, flaky, cracked skin: especially in chronic cases.
- Inflammation: leading to warmth, tenderness, and sometimes pain of the affected area.
- Localized Swelling: due to fluid accumulation, particularly in severe reactions.

Causes and Risk Factors:
- Allergens: Exposure to allergens such as certain metals, latex, fragrances, preservatives, or plants can trigger allergic contact dermatitis.
- Irritants: Contact with irritants such as soaps, detergents, solvents, or chemicals in cosmetics or personal care products can cause irritant contact dermatitis.
- Occupational exposure: Certain occupations, such as healthcare workers, hairdressers, cleaners, and construction workers, have a higher risk of contact dermatitis due to frequent exposure to irritants or allergens.
- Atopic or sensitive skin: Patients with a history of atopic dermatitis or other allergic conditions may be more prone.
- Genetic predisposition: Genetic factors may influence a patient's susceptibility to contact dermatitis.
- Medical history: Previous episodes of contact dermatitis increase the risk of recurrence upon re-exposure to the offending substance.

Epidemiology:
- Contact dermatitis is a common inflammatory skin condition, affecting patients of all ages and demographics.
- The prevalence of contact dermatitis varies depending on factors such as geographical location, occupation, and environmental exposures.
- Occupational contact dermatitis is particularly prevalent among certain industries, with an estimated prevalence ranging from 20% to 50% among certain occupational groups.

Diagnosis:
- Clinical Evaluation: Diagnosis is based on the characteristic appearance of the rash, along with a thorough history of recent exposures.
- Patch Testing: to identify specific allergens or irritants responsible for the dermatitis.
- Skin Biopsy: to rule out other potential causes of the rash.

Treatment:
- Avoidance: The primary treatment for contact dermatitis involves identifying and avoiding the triggering substances or allergens.
- Topical Corticosteroids: Topical corticosteroid creams or ointments are commonly used to reduce inflammation and relieve itching.
- Topical Calcineurin Inhibitors: Calcineurin inhibitors such as tacrolimus or pimecrolimus may be prescribed for patients who do not respond to or cannot tolerate corticosteroids.
- Emollients: Moisturizing creams or ointments can help soothe and hydrate the skin, reducing dryness and preventing further irritation.
- Antihistamines: Oral antihistamines may be used to alleviate itching and discomfort, particularly in cases of allergic contact dermatitis.
- Cool Compresses: Applying cool, wet compresses to the affected area can provide relief from itching and inflammation.
- Barrier Protection: In occupational settings, barrier creams or gloves may be used to protect the skin from exposure to irritants or allergens.

12.4. Psoriasis

> ➢ *Psoriasis is a chronic autoimmune skin disorder characterized by the rapid buildup of skin cells, leading to thick, red patches covered with silvery scales.*
>
> ➢ *It often occurs on the elbows, knees, scalp, and lower back and may cause itching, pain, or burning.*
>
> ➢ *Treatment options include topical medications, phototherapy, systemic medications, and biologic agents to manage symptoms and control flare-ups.*

Symptoms:
- Red, raised, and inflamed skin: Psoriasis typically presents as red patches of skin covered with silvery scales. These patches are often itchy and may be painful.
- Thickened or pitted nails: Psoriasis can affect the nails, causing changes such as pitting, thickening, or separation from the nail bed.
- Joint pain and swelling: Some patients may develop psoriatic arthritis, characterized by joint pain, stiffness, and swelling.
- Dry, cracked skin: Psoriasis patches may become dry, cracked, and prone to bleeding, particularly in areas of friction or trauma.

Causes and Risk Factors:
- Genetic predisposition: Family history plays a significant role in psoriasis, with patients having a family member with psoriasis being at higher risk.
- Environmental triggers: Stress, skin injury (Koebner phenomenon), infections, and certain medications can trigger or exacerbate psoriasis symptoms.
- Immune system dysregulation: Psoriasis is considered an autoimmune condition, where the immune system mistakenly attacks healthy skin cells, leading to inflammation and rapid skin cell turnover.
- Lifestyle factors: Smoking, obesity, and excessive alcohol consumption have been associated with an increased risk of psoriasis development and worsening symptoms.

Epidemiology:
- Psoriasis affects approximately 2-3% of the global population, with prevalence varying by geographic region and ethnicity.
- It can occur at any age but most commonly manifests in early adulthood, between the ages of 15 and 35.
- Psoriasis affects both sexes equally and can occur in patients of any racial or ethnic background.

Workup and Diagnosis:
- <u>Clinical Examination:</u> Diagnosis of psoriasis is primarily based on clinical presentation, including the appearance and distribution of skin lesions.
- <u>Skin Biopsy:</u> In some cases, a skin biopsy may be performed to confirm the diagnosis and rule out other skin conditions that may mimic psoriasis.

- Assessment of Severity: The severity of psoriasis can be assessed using various scoring systems, such as the Psoriasis Area and Severity Index (PASI), which takes into account the extent and severity of skin involvement, as well as the impact on quality of life.

Psoriasis Score (PASI)

The Psoriasis Area and Severity Index (PASI) is a tool used to measure the severity and extent of psoriasis, considering the area of the body affected and the severity of lesions based on redness, thickness, and scaling.

A total PASI score ranges from **0 to 72**, where higher scores indicate more severe psoriasis.

Treatment:

- Topical Treatments: Corticosteroids, vitamin D analogs, retinoids, and calcineurin inhibitors are commonly used topical medications to reduce inflammation and promote skin healing.
- Phototherapy: Ultraviolet (UV) light therapy, including narrow-band UVB and PUVA (psoralen plus UVA), can help to improve psoriasis symptoms by slowing down skin turnover and reducing inflammation.
- Systemic Medications: For moderate to severe psoriasis that is not adequately controlled with topical treatments and phototherapy, systemic medications such as methotrexate, cyclosporine, acitretin, or biologic agents (e.g., TNF inhibitors, IL-17 inhibitors) may be prescribed.
- Lifestyle Modifications: Avoiding triggers such as stress, skin injury, smoking, and excessive alcohol consumption may help to reduce psoriasis flare-ups and improve overall disease management.

12.5. Seborrheic Dermatitis

> ➢ *Seborrheic dermatitis is a common inflammatory skin condition characterized by red, itchy, and flaky patches, typically affecting areas with high oil production such as the scalp, face, and chest.*
> ➢ *It may be associated with a yeast called Malassezia, hormonal changes, or other factors.*
> ➢ *Treatment involves medicated shampoos, topical antifungal or corticosteroid creams, and lifestyle modifications to manage symptoms and prevent recurrence.*

Symptoms:
- Redness and scaling: Seborrheic dermatitis typically presents as red, inflamed skin covered with greasy or yellowish scales. Common areas affected include the scalp, face, and trunk.
- Itching: The affected areas may be itchy, and scratching can worsen inflammation and scaling.
- Dandruff: Seborrheic dermatitis of the scalp often manifests as dandruff, with flaking and scaling of the scalp skin.
- Cradle cap: In infants, seborrheic dermatitis may present as thick, yellowish, greasy scales on the scalp, known as cradle cap.
- Oily skin: Seborrheic dermatitis may be associated with oily or greasy skin in affected areas.

Causes and Risk Factors:
- Malassezia yeast: Overgrowth of the fungus *Malassezia* on the skin is believed to play a significant role in the development of seborrheic dermatitis.
- Hormonal changes such as those occurring during puberty, pregnancy, or with certain medical conditions, may contribute to seborrheic dermatitis.
- Certain neurological conditions, such as Parkinson's disease or stroke, may predispose patients to seborrheic dermatitis.
- Immune System Dysfunction: Conditions that weaken the immune system, such as HIV/AIDS or autoimmune disorders, may increase the risk of seborrheic dermatitis.
- Environmental Factors: Cold, dry weather and stress may exacerbate symptoms of seborrheic dermatitis.

Epidemiology:
- Seborrheic dermatitis is a common skin condition that can affect patients of all ages, from infants to older adults.
- It tends to be more prevalent in infants (as cradle cap) and in adults between the ages of 30 and 60 years.
- Men are more commonly affected than women.

Diagnosis:
- <u>Clinical Examination:</u> Diagnosis of seborrheic dermatitis is typically based on clinical presentation, including the appearance and distribution of skin lesions.

- **Differential Diagnosis:** Seborrheic dermatitis should be differentiated from other skin conditions that may present with similar symptoms, such as psoriasis, eczema, or fungal infections.
- **Scalp Examination:** may reveal characteristic signs of seborrheic dermatitis, such as dandruff or yellowish, greasy scale

Treatment:

- **Topical Antifungals:** Antifungal agents, such as ketoconazole or selenium sulfide, are commonly used to reduce fungal overgrowth and inflammation in seborrheic dermatitis.
- **Topical Steroids:** Low-potency corticosteroid creams or lotions may be prescribed to reduce inflammation and itching associated with seborrheic dermatitis.
- **Medicated Shampoos:** Shampoos containing antifungal agents, coal tar, salicylic acid, or zinc pyrithione can help to control seborrheic dermatitis of the scalp.
- **Emollients:** Moisturizing creams may be recommended to soothe dry, irritated skin and prevent further flares.
- **Lifestyle Modifications:** Avoiding triggers such as harsh soaps, cold weather, stress, and excessive use of hair products may help to reduce symptoms of seborrheic dermatitis.

12.6. Rosacea

> - *Rosacea is a chronic inflammatory skin condition characterized by facial redness, visible blood vessels, and sometimes papules and pustules resembling acne.*
> - *Triggers may include sun exposure, heat, spicy foods, alcohol, and stress.*
> - *Treatment typically involves topical or oral medications, laser therapy, and lifestyle modifications to reduce symptoms and flare-ups.*

Symptoms:

- Facial redness: Persistent redness, often in the central part of the face, is a hallmark symptom of rosacea.
- Flushing: Rosacea may be accompanied by frequent flushing or blushing episodes, which can be triggered by various factors such as hot drinks, spicy foods, alcohol, sunlight, or emotional stress.

- Small red bumps (papules) and pus-filled lesions (pustules) resembling acne may develop on the face, particularly in the central facial region.
- Telangiectasia may appear on the surface of the skin, particularly on the cheeks, nose, and chin.
- Ocular symptoms: Some patients with rosacea may experience eye symptoms such as dryness, burning, itching, or irritation.

Causes and Risk Factors:
- Fair skin: Rosacea is more common in patients with fair skin and tends to affect those of northern European descent.
- Family history: may increase a patient's risk
- Gender: Although rosacea can affect patients of any gender, it tends to be more common in women, while men may experience more severe forms of the condition.
- Age: Rosacea typically manifests in adulthood, with onset usually occurring between the ages of 30 and 50 years.
- Various triggers such as sun exposure, hot or spicy foods, alcohol consumption, emotional stress, and certain medications may exacerbate symptoms of rosacea.

Epidemiology:
- Rosacea is a common chronic skin condition, affecting millions of patients worldwide.
- It tends to be more prevalent in patients with fair skin and is less common in patients with darker skin tones.
- The prevalence of rosacea may vary depending on geographical location and ethnicity, with higher rates reported in northern European populations.

Diagnosis:
- Clinical Examination: Diagnosis of rosacea is primarily based on clinical evaluation of the skin and associated symptoms.
- Subtypes: Rosacea can manifest in different subtypes, including erythematotelangiectatic rosacea (characterized by facial redness and visible blood vessels), papulopustular rosacea (with papules and pustules), phymatous rosacea (thickening of the skin, particularly on the nose), and ocular rosacea (involving the eyes).
- Differential Diagnosis: Rosacea should be differentiated from other skin conditions that may present with similar symptoms, such as acne, lupus, or allergic reactions.

Treatment:

- Topical Therapies: Metronidazole, azelaic acid, or ivermectin may be prescribed to reduce redness and inflammation associated with rosacea.

- Oral Antibiotics: Doxycycline, minocycline, or tetracycline may be used to control inflammatory lesions in rosacea.

- Laser Therapy: Laser or intense pulsed light (IPL) therapy may be recommended to reduce facial redness, telangiectasia, or visible blood vessels in rosacea.

- Avoidance of Triggers: Identifying and avoiding triggers that exacerbate rosacea symptoms, such as sun exposure, spicy foods, alcohol, and certain skincare products, is an important aspect of management.

- Skincare: Gentle skincare practices, including the use of mild cleansers and moisturizers, and sun protection measures can help to soothe and protect sensitive skin affected by rosacea.

12.7. Dermatophytosis

> ➤ *Dermatophytosis, commonly known as ringworm, is a fungal infection of the skin, hair, or nails, resulting in red, scaly patches or circular lesions with raised borders.*
>
> ➤ *It spreads through direct contact with infected people, animals, or contaminated objects and can affect various body parts.*
>
> ➤ *Treatment involves topical or oral antifungal medications to eradicate the fungus and prevent recurrence.*

Symptoms:

- Skin lesions: Dermatophytosis typically presents with circular, red, scaly lesions on the skin, often with raised borders and central clearing.

- Itching: Affected areas may be accompanied by itching, burning, or discomfort.

- Hair and nail involvement: Fungal infections can also affect the scalp or nails, causing hair loss, scalp scaling, or thickened, discolored nails.

- Secondary infections: Scratching of affected areas may lead to secondary bacterial infections.

Causes and Risk Factors:
- Warm and moist environments: Fungi thrive in warm, moist environments, making patients who frequent such environments more susceptible to infection.
- Close contact: Sharing personal items such as towels, clothing, or sports equipment with an infected patient can increase the risk of transmission.
- Compromised immunity: Immunocompromised patients, such as those with HIV/AIDS or diabetes, are more susceptible to fungal infections.
- Poor hygiene: Inadequate hygiene practices, such as wearing tight-fitting clothing or not properly drying off after swimming, can increase the risk of infection.
- Age: Children and elderly patients may be more prone to fungal infections due to factors such as immature or weakened immune systems.

Epidemiology:
- Dermatophytosis is a common fungal infection worldwide, affecting patients of all ages and demographics.
- The prevalence of fungal infections may vary depending on geographical location, climate, and socio-economic factors.
- Certain populations, such as athletes, patients living in crowded or communal settings, and those with pre-existing skin conditions, may be at higher risk of dermatophytosis.

Diagnosis:
- Clinical Examination: Diagnosis of dermatophytosis is primarily based on clinical evaluation of the skin lesions, including their appearance, location, and distribution.
- KOH Examination: Microscopic examination of skin scrapings or nail clippings using potassium hydroxide (KOH) preparation can help visualize fungal elements such as hyphae or spores.
- Fungal Culture: Culturing of skin or nail samples on specific media may be performed to identify the causative fungus and guide treatment, particularly in cases of diagnostic uncertainty or treatment resistance.

Treatment:
- Topical Antifungals: Most cases of dermatophytosis can be effectively treated with topical antifungal medications such as clotrimazole,

terbinafine, or miconazole, applied to the affected areas for several weeks.

- Oral Antifungals: In severe or widespread infections, oral antifungal medications such as terbinafine, fluconazole, or itraconazole may be prescribed for a specified duration.
- Maintaining Hygiene: Good hygiene practices, including keeping the affected areas clean, dry, and well-ventilated, can help prevent the spread and recurrence of fungal infections.
- Avoiding Contamination: Avoid sharing personal items such as towels, clothing, or footwear, and practice proper foot hygiene, especially in communal bathing areas or locker rooms, to reduce the risk of transmission.

12.8. Scabies

> ➤ *Scabies is a contagious skin infestation caused by the Sarcoptes scabiei mite, resulting in intense itching, especially at night, and a characteristic rash with small red bumps and linear burrows.*
>
> ➤ *It spreads through close contact and can affect anyone, leading to discomfort and secondary infections if left untreated.*
>
> ➤ *Treatment typically involves topical medications like permethrin or oral medications like ivermectin to kill the mites and relieve symptoms.*

Symptoms:

- Itching: Intense itching, often worse at night, is the hallmark symptom of scabies. Itching is caused by the body's allergic reaction to the mites, their eggs, and their waste.
- Skin rash: The itching is accompanied by a pimple-like rash, typically appearing in the folds of the skin, such as between the fingers, wrists, elbows, armpits, waist, buttocks, and genital area.
- Tracks or burrows: In some cases, thin, irregular tracks or burrows may be visible on the skin surface. These are caused by the mites tunneling beneath the skin to lay eggs.
- Secondary infections: Excessive scratching may lead to skin damage and secondary bacterial infections.

Causes and Risk Factors:

- Close contact: Direct, prolonged skin-to-skin contact with an infested patient, such as during sexual activity, sharing of clothing or

bedding, or close family contact, increases the risk of scabies transmission.
- Crowded living conditions: Environments such as nursing homes, childcare facilities, prisons, or refugee camps, where close contact is common, facilitate the spread of scabies.
- Weakened immune system: Patients with weakened immune systems, such as those with HIV/AIDS, cancer, or certain medications (e.g., corticosteroids), may be more susceptible to scabies infestation and complications.
- Poor hygiene: Poor personal hygiene and inadequate sanitation may contribute to the spread of scabies in some settings.
- Age: Scabies can affect patients of all ages, but it is more common in children and the elderly due to factors such as close contact in schools or nursing homes.

Epidemiology:
- Scabies is a global health issue, affecting millions of patients worldwide, particularly in resource-limited settings.
- Outbreaks of scabies may occur in institutions such as nursing homes, hospitals, childcare facilities, and prisons.
- The prevalence of scabies varies depending on factors such as geographical location, socio-economic status, and living conditions.

Diagnosis:
- Clinical Evaluation: Diagnosis of scabies is primarily based on clinical examination of the skin rash and symptoms. The characteristic appearance of the rash, along with itching, is highly suggestive of scabies.
- Skin Scraping: Skin scraping may be performed to identify mites, eggs, or fecal matter under a microscope. This involves scraping the skin with a scalpel blade or blunt edge and examining the collected material.
- Burrow Ink Test: The burrow ink test involves applying ink to a suspected burrow and wiping it away with an alcohol swab. The ink may reveal the presence of a hidden burrow.

Treatment:
- Topical Scabicides:

    The primary treatment for scabies is the application of topical scabicidal medications, such as permethrin cream or lotion, sulfur ointment, or benzyl benzoate lotion, to the entire body

from the neck down. These medications kill the mites and their eggs.
- **Oral Medications:** In some cases, oral medications such as ivermectin may be prescribed for severe or resistant cases of scabies.
- **Treating Close Contacts:** Close contacts of patients with scabies should also be treated, even if they are asymptomatic, to prevent reinfestation and further spread of the mites.
- **Environmental Measures:** Washing or dry-cleaning infested clothing, bedding, and towels in hot water and vacuuming carpets and furniture can help eliminate mites from the environment and reduce the risk of reinfestation.

12.9. Impetigo

> ➤ *Impetigo is a contagious bacterial skin infection commonly caused by Staphylococcus aureus or Streptococcus pyogenes, leading to red sores that rupture and form honey-colored crusts.*
>
> ➤ *It often affects children and spreads through direct contact or contaminated objects, with treatment involving topical or oral antibiotics to clear the infection and prevent spread.*
>
> ➤ *Good hygiene practices and proper wound care are essential for prevention.*

Symptoms:
- Skin lesions: Impetigo typically presents as red sores or blisters on the face, hands, arms, or other exposed areas of the body.
- Fluid-filled blisters: The sores may rupture, leaving behind honey-colored crusts or scabs.
- Itching: The affected area may be itchy.
- Spread: Impetigo lesions can spread rapidly and may be contagious.

Causes and Risk Factors:
- Close contact: Impetigo is highly contagious and spreads through close contact with infected patients or contaminated objects.
- Age: Children, particularly those between 2 and 6 years old, are more susceptible to impetigo due to their close contact in schools and daycare settings.
- Warm, humid environments: Impetigo is more common in warm, humid climates.

- Skin trauma or irritation: Skin injuries, insect bites, or pre-existing skin conditions may increase the risk of impetigo.
- Poor hygiene: may contribute to the spread of impetigo

Epidemiology:
- Impetigo is a common bacterial skin infection, especially among children.
- It can occur sporadically or in outbreaks, particularly in settings with close contact, such as schools or daycare centers.
- Impetigo can affect patients of any age but is more common in children.

Diagnosis:
- Clinical Examination: Diagnosis of impetigo is primarily based on clinical examination of the skin lesions. The characteristic appearance of honey-colored crusts or blisters, along with a history of close contact or risk factors, is suggestive of impetigo.
- Culture: In some cases, a bacterial culture of the skin lesions may be performed to identify the causative bacteria and guide antibiotic therapy.

Treatment:
- Topical Antibiotics: Mild cases of impetigo may be treated with topical antibiotics, such as mupirocin ointment or fusidic acid cream, applied directly to the affected area several times a day for about a week.
- Oral Antibiotics: In cases of widespread or severe impetigo, oral antibiotics such as oral cephalexin, dicloxacillin, or erythromycin may be prescribed for about 7-10 days.
- Hygiene Measures: Keeping the affected area clean and dry, washing hands regularly, and avoiding scratching or picking at the lesions can help prevent the spread of impetigo and promote healing.
- Avoiding Close Contact: Infected patients should avoid close contact with others, particularly children, until the lesions have healed or for at least 24 hours after starting antibiotic treatment.
- Environmental Cleaning: Household surfaces, clothing, and towels should be regularly cleaned and disinfected to prevent the spread of impetigo.

12.10. Warts

> ➢ Warts are benign skin growths caused by human papillomavirus (HPV) infection, presenting as rough, raised bumps on the skin's surface.
>
> ➢ They can occur anywhere on the body and spread through direct contact or contact with contaminated surfaces.
>
> ➢ Treatment options include topical medications, cryotherapy, laser therapy, or surgical removal to eliminate warts and prevent recurrence.

Symptoms:

- Skin growths: Warts typically appear as small, rough, raised bumps on the skin. They may have a grainy texture and can vary in color, including flesh-colored, white, pink, or brown.
- Pain or discomfort: Warts may cause pain or discomfort, particularly if they develop on weight-bearing areas like the soles of the feet (plantar warts) or on the hands.
- Clustering: Warts may occur singly or in clusters.
- Location: Warts can develop on any part of the body, including the hands, feet, fingers, toes, knees, elbows, and genitals.

Causes and Risk Factors:

- Viral infection: Warts are caused by infection with the human papillomavirus (HPV), which can be transmitted through direct contact with an infected person or contaminated surfaces.
- Weakened immune system: patients with weakened immune systems, such as those with HIV/AIDS or undergoing immunosuppressive therapy, may be more susceptible to developing warts.
- Skin trauma: Skin injuries or cuts may provide entry points for the HPV virus, increasing the risk of developing warts.
- Age: Children and young adults are more prone to developing warts, although they can occur at any age.
- Occupation or activities: Frequent exposure to moist environments (e.g., swimming pools, communal showers) or shared surfaces (e.g., gym equipment) may increase the risk of contracting HPV and developing warts.

Epidemiology:

- Warts are common skin infections caused by HPV.

- They can affect patients of all ages, but are more prevalent in children and adolescents.
- The prevalence of warts varies depending on factors such as age, gender, and geographical location.

Diagnosis:
- Clinical Examination: Diagnosis of warts is typically based on clinical examination of the skin lesions. The characteristic appearance of raised, rough bumps on the skin, along with a history of risk factors or exposure to HPV, is suggestive of warts.
- Dermoscopy: Dermoscopic examination may aid in the diagnosis of warts by revealing characteristic features such as thrombosed capillaries (black dots) and finger-like projections (pseudo-hair).
- Skin Biopsy: In rare cases where the diagnosis is uncertain or there are atypical features, a skin biopsy may be performed to confirm the diagnosis and rule out other skin conditions.

Treatment:
- Topical Treatments:

    Over-the-counter (OTC) topical treatments containing salicylic acid or formaldehyde may be applied directly to the wart to help dissolve the wart tissue and stimulate immune responses against the virus.
- Cryotherapy: Freezing the wart with liquid nitrogen to destroy the affected tissue is commonly performed by healthcare professionals in a clinical setting.
- Electrosurgery or Curettage: physically removing the wart using a sharp instrument (curette) or burning it off with an electric current
- Laser Therapy: destroys the wart tissue by targeting it with a high-intensity laser beam
- Immunotherapy:

    Immunotherapy involves stimulating the body's immune response to attack and eliminate the wart virus. It may involve the use of medications such as imiquimod or intralesional injections of antigens.
- Surgical Excision: Surgically removing the wart under local anesthesia may be considered for large or stubborn warts that do not respond to other treatments.

Prevention:
- Avoiding contact: Avoiding direct contact with warts and contaminated surfaces can help reduce the risk of transmission.
- Good hygiene practices: Washing hands regularly and keeping the skin clean and dry, can help prevent the spread of warts.
- Avoiding sharing personal items: Avoid sharing towels, socks, shoes, or other personal items with patients who have warts.
- Boosting immunity: Regular exercise, balanced diet, and adequate sleep to maintain a healthy immune system may help reduce the risk of developing warts.

12.11. Molluscum Contagiosum

> *Molluscum contagiosum is a viral skin infection caused by the poxvirus, characterized by small, flesh-colored or pearly bumps with a central indentation.*
>
> *It spreads through direct skin-to-skin contact and can affect any part of the body, particularly in children and immunocompromised individuals.*
>
> *Treatment may involve cryotherapy, topical medications, or in some cases, the condition resolves on its own without intervention.*

Symptoms:
- Skin lesions: Molluscum contagiosum presents as small, flesh-colored, dome-shaped papules or nodules on the skin.
- Central dimple: Each lesion typically has a central dimple or indentation, giving it a characteristic appearance resembling a pearl.
- Grouping: The lesions may occur singly or in clusters, and they can vary in size from a pinhead to a pencil eraser.
- Locations: Molluscum lesions can develop on any part of the body, but they are commonly found on the face, neck, armpits, arms, hands, and genital area.
- Itching: In some cases, molluscum lesions may cause mild itching or irritation, especially if they become inflamed or secondary bacterial infection occurs.

Causes and Risk Factors:
- Direct skin-to-skin contact: Molluscum contagiosum is highly contagious and can spread through direct contact with infected patients or contaminated surfaces.

- Children and adolescents: Molluscum contagiosum is more common in children and adolescents, particularly those who participate in activities that involve close contact or sharing of personal items (e.g., sports, daycare settings).
- Weakened immune system: Patients with weakened immune systems, such as those with HIV/AIDS or undergoing immunosuppressive therapy, may be more susceptible to developing widespread or persistent molluscum lesions.
- Environmental factors: Warm and humid climates may facilitate the spread of molluscum contagiosum.
- Medical Conditions: Patients with atopic dermatitis (eczema) or other skin conditions with compromised skin barrier function may be at increased risk of developing molluscum contagiosum lesions.

Epidemiology:
- Molluscum contagiosum is a common viral skin infection caused by the molluscum contagiosum virus (MCV).
- It can affect patients of all ages but is most commonly seen in children and adolescents.
- The prevalence of molluscum contagiosum varies geographically and among different populations.

Diagnosis:
- Clinical Examination: Diagnosis of molluscum contagiosum is usually based on the characteristic appearance of the skin lesions during a clinical examination.
- Visual Inspection: The APh may visually inspect the skin lesions to look for the typical features of molluscum, including the central dimple and smooth, dome-shaped appearance.
- Differential Diagnosis: Molluscum contagiosum lesions may resemble other skin conditions such as warts, chickenpox, or milia, so a thorough differential diagnosis may be necessary.

Treatment:
- Observation: In many cases, molluscum contagiosum lesions may resolve spontaneously over time without specific treatment, particularly in healthy patients with intact immune function.
- Physical Removal: The APh may recommend physical removal of patient lesions through techniques such as cryotherapy (freezing), curettage (scraping), or laser therapy.

- **Topical Treatments:** Imiquimod cream or podophyllotoxin solution may be applied directly to the lesions to stimulate immune responses or destroy the virus.
- **Antiviral Therapy:** Cidofovir or cantharidin may be prescribed to treat extensive or persistent molluscum contagiosum infections.
- **Preventive Measures:** To prevent the spread of molluscum contagiosum, patients should avoid direct skin-to-skin contact with infected patients and refrain from sharing personal items such as towels, clothing, or razors.
- **Good Hygiene:** Practicing good hygiene, such as washing hands regularly and keeping the skin clean and dry, can help reduce the risk of spreading molluscum contagiosum.

Complications:

- Molluscum contagiosum lesions are generally benign and asymptomatic, but complications such as secondary bacterial infection or scarring may occur in some cases, particularly if lesions are scratched or manipulated.
- Patients with weakened immune systems may be at increased risk of developing widespread or persistent molluscum contagiosum lesions, which may require more aggressive treatment approaches.

12.12. Tinea Versicolor

> ➤ *Tinea versicolor is a common fungal infection of the skin caused by Malassezia yeast, resulting in patches of discolored skin that may be lighter or darker than the surrounding skin.*
>
> ➤ *It typically affects areas with high oil production, such as the chest, back, and upper arms, and is more common in warm, humid climates.*
>
> ➤ *Treatment involves antifungal medications, topical creams, or medicated shampoos to eliminate the yeast and restore normal skin pigmentation.*

Symptoms:

- Skin discoloration: Tinea versicolor typically presents as small, flat, round, or oval-shaped patches of skin that may be lighter or darker than the surrounding skin.
- Scaling: The affected areas often have fine scales or mild flaking, which may be more noticeable after sun exposure or sweating.

- Locations: Tinea versicolor commonly affects areas of the body with a high density of sebaceous glands, such as the chest, back, shoulders, and upper arms. However, it can also occur on the neck, face, abdomen, and groin.
- Asymptomatic: In many cases, tinea versicolor is asymptomatic or causes minimal itching or discomfort. However, some patients may experience mild itching or irritation.

Causes and Risk Factors:
- Warm and humid climate: Tinea versicolor is more common in regions with warm, humid climates, where fungal growth is favored.
- Excessive sweating: Profuse sweating, particularly in hot and humid conditions, can create an environment conducive to fungal overgrowth and the development of tinea versicolor.
- Oily skin: patients with naturally oily or greasy skin may be more prone to developing tinea versicolor due to increased sebum production, which can promote fungal colonization.
- Immunocompromised state: patients with weakened immune systems, such as those with HIV/AIDS, organ transplant recipients, or patients on immunosuppressive therapy, may have an increased risk of tinea versicolor.
- Adolescents and young adults: Tinea versicolor commonly occurs during adolescence and young adulthood, possibly due to hormonal changes and increased sebaceous gland activity during this period.

Epidemiology:
- Tinea versicolor is a common fungal skin infection caused by the yeast *Malassezia furfur* (formerly known as *Pityrosporum ovale* or *Pityrosporum orbiculare*).
- It is prevalent worldwide and affects patients of all ages, races, and genders.
- The incidence of tinea versicolor may vary depending on geographic location, climate, and other environmental factors.

Diagnosis:
- Clinical Examination: Diagnosis of tinea versicolor is primarily based on the characteristic appearance of the skin lesions during a clinical examination.
- Wood's Lamp Examination: A Wood's lamp, which emits ultraviolet (UV) light, may be used to visualize fluorescence patterns on the affected skin. In tinea versicolor, affected areas may appear yellow-green or coppery under Wood's lamp illumination.

- Skin Scraping: In some cases, a skin scraping or fungal culture may be performed to confirm the presence of Malassezia yeast on the skin.

Treatment:
- Antifungal Medications:

    Topical antifungal agents such as ketoconazole, terbinafine, or ciclopirox are commonly used to treat tinea versicolor. These medications may be applied as creams, lotions, or shampoos, depending on the location and extent of the infection.

- Oral Antifungal Therapy: In cases of extensive or recurrent tinea versicolor, oral antifungal medications such as fluconazole or itraconazole may be prescribed.
- Maintenance Therapy: To prevent recurrence, patients with a history of tinea versicolor may benefit from periodic use of antifungal shampoos or creams as maintenance therapy.
- Good Hygiene Practices: Regular bathing, thorough drying of the skin, and wearing breathable clothing, can help reduce the risk of tinea versicolor recurrence.
- Avoidance of Predisposing Factors: Minimizing exposure to factors that promote fungal growth, such as excessive sweating, occlusive clothing, and prolonged use of oily or greasy skincare products, may help prevent tinea versicolor.

Complications:
- Tinea versicolor is typically a benign condition and does not cause serious health problems. However, it can have cosmetic implications, particularly if the lesions are extensive or occur on visible areas of the body.
- Recurrence of tinea versicolor is common, especially in patients predisposed to fungal infections or those living in warm, humid climates.
- Long-term complications or sequelae of tinea versicolor are rare, but secondary bacterial or fungal infections may occur in some cases, particularly if the affected skin is scratched or irritated.

12.13. Urticaria

> ➢ *Urticaria, also known as hives, is a skin condition characterized by itchy, raised welts or wheals that appear suddenly and can change shape and location within minutes to hours.*
> ➢ *It is often triggered by allergic reactions to food, medication, insect stings, or other substances, but can also result from non-allergic factors like stress or temperature changes.*
> ➢ *Treatment involves identifying and avoiding triggers, antihistamines to relieve itching, and in severe cases, corticosteroids or other medications to suppress the immune response.*

Symptoms:
- Raised, red or pink welts or bumps on the skin that may vary in size and shape
- Itching, which may be mild to severe and can interfere with daily activities
- Swelling of the affected area, particularly around the eyes, lips, face, throat, or hands
- Burning or stinging sensation on the skin
- Blanched or pale centers in the welts (called wheals)
- The welts may come and go within hours, often moving to different areas of the body.

Causes and Risk Factors:
- Allergies: Urticaria can be triggered by allergic reactions to certain foods, medications, insect stings, latex, or other allergens.
- Medications: Some medications, particularly antibiotics, pain relievers (such as aspirin or NSAIDs), and certain blood pressure medications, can cause urticaria as a side effect.
- Infections: Viral or bacterial infections, such as the common cold, strep throat, or hepatitis, may trigger acute urticaria.
- Physical triggers: Certain physical stimuli, such as pressure (dermatographism), cold (cold urticaria), heat, sunlight (solar urticaria), exercise (exercise-induced urticaria), or friction, may induce urticaria in susceptible patients.
- Stress: Emotional stress or anxiety may exacerbate or trigger episodes of urticaria in some patients.

- Underlying conditions: Chronic urticaria may be associated with underlying conditions such as autoimmune disorders, thyroid disease, or chronic infections.

Epidemiology:
- Urticaria is a common skin condition that can affect patients of all ages, genders, and ethnicities.
- Acute urticaria is more common in children and young adults and often resolves spontaneously within a few hours to days.
- Chronic urticaria, defined as hives lasting for six weeks or longer, affects approximately 1-3% of the population and can persist for months or years.

Diagnosis:
- <u>Clinical Examination:</u> Diagnosis of urticaria is usually based on a thorough medical history and physical examination.
- <u>Recent Exposures:</u> A healthcare provider may ask about recent exposures to potential triggers, such as foods, medications, or environmental allergens.
- <u>Tests:</u>
  - In some cases, allergy testing, blood tests, or skin prick tests may be performed to identify specific allergens or underlying conditions.
  - If chronic urticaria is suspected, additional tests such as thyroid function tests or autoimmune markers may be ordered to evaluate for underlying causes.

Treatment:
- <u>Avoidance of triggers:</u> Identifying and avoiding known triggers, such as certain foods, medications, or environmental allergens, can help prevent recurrent episodes of urticaria.
- <u>Antihistamines:</u>

    Oral antihistamines, such as loratadine, cetirizine, or fexofenadine, are typically the first-line treatment for relieving itching and reducing the frequency and severity of urticaria episodes. In some cases, higher doses or combination therapy with different antihistamines may be necessary.

- <u>Corticosteroids:</u>

    Short courses of oral corticosteroids may be prescribed for severe or refractory cases of urticaria to reduce inflammation and suppress immune responses. However, long-term use of corticosteroids is generally not recommended due to potential side effects.

- Topical treatments: Topical corticosteroid creams or ointments may be used to relieve itching and inflammation associated with localized urticaria.
- Other medications: In cases of chronic urticaria that do not respond to conventional treatments, additional medications such as leukotriene receptor antagonists, omalizumab (anti-IgE therapy), or immunosuppressants may be considered.
- Emergency treatment: Severe allergic reactions or anaphylaxis may require prompt treatment with epinephrine (adrenaline) and emergency medical care.

12.14. Seborrheic Keratosis

> *Seborrheic keratosis is a common noncancerous skin growth characterized by waxy, wart-like lesions that range in color from tan to black and often have a stuck-on appearance.*
> *They typically occur in older adults on areas exposed to the sun, such as the face, chest, back, or shoulders.*
> *Treatment is generally unnecessary unless they cause irritation or cosmetic concerns, in which case they can be removed surgically or with cryotherapy.*

Symptoms:
- Raised bumps or growths on the skin, typically tan, brown, black, or flesh-colored
- Round or oval-shaped lesions with a waxy, scaly, or crusty surface
- Lesions may vary in size, ranging from a few millimeters to several centimeters in diameter
- Often appear singly or in clusters on areas of the body exposed to the sun, such as the face, neck, chest, back, or scalp
- Lesions are usually painless but may occasionally become itchy or irritated

Causes and Risk Factors:
- Age: Seborrheic keratoses are more common in older adults, typically appearing after the age of 40.

- Sun exposure: Chronic sun exposure is a significant risk factor for the development of seborrheic keratoses, particularly on sun-exposed areas of the skin.
- Family history: may increase the risk
- Skin type: Patients with fair skin are more prone to developing seborrheic keratoses.
- Hormonal changes: Pregnancy, hormonal therapy, or conditions such as Addison's disease may be associated with an increased risk of developing seborrheic keratoses.

Epidemiology:
- Seborrheic keratoses are common benign skin growths that affect patients of all races and ethnicities.
- Prevalence increases with age, with the majority of cases occurring in patients over 40 years old.
- They are more common in adults but can also occur in younger patients, particularly those with a family history of seborrheic keratoses.

Diagnosis:
- Clinical Examination:
    - Diagnosis of seborrheic keratoses is usually based on clinical examination and observation of characteristic skin lesions.
    - The APh may perform a physical examination to evaluate the appearance, texture, and distribution of the skin growths.
- Skin Biopsy: to confirm the diagnosis and rule out other skin conditions, particularly if the lesions are atypical or suspicious for skin cancer

Treatment:
- Observation: In many cases, seborrheic keratoses are harmless and do not require treatment unless they become symptomatic or cosmetically bothersome.
- Cryotherapy: using liquid nitrogen to freeze and destroy the lesion
- Curettage and desiccation: Scraping off the lesion followed by cauterization (burning) of the base is another common method of removal for patient lesions.
- Electrosurgery: High-frequency electrical current is used to burn and remove seborrheic keratoses.
- Laser therapy: to target and destroy the pigment in seborrheic keratoses, causing them to darken and flake off

- Topical treatments: Certain topical medications, such as hydrogen peroxide, tretinoin, or topical acids, may be applied to patient lesions to help remove them over time.
- Combination therapy: Combining different treatment modalities, such as cryotherapy with curettage or laser therapy, may be more effective for removing multiple or large seborrheic keratoses.

12.15. Actinic Keratosis

> *Actinic keratosis is a precancerous skin lesion caused by prolonged sun exposure, appearing as dry, scaly patches or rough, crusty bumps.*
>
> *It commonly occurs on sun-exposed areas such as the face, scalp, hands, and arms, and if left untreated, it can progress to squamous cell carcinoma.*
>
> *Treatment options include cryotherapy, topical medications, photodynamic therapy, or surgical removal to prevent progression to skin cancer.*

Symptoms:
- Rough, scaly, or crusty skin patches
- Flat or slightly raised lesions with a reddish, brown, or flesh-colored appearance
- Itching, burning, or tenderness in the affected area
- Lesions may vary in size, ranging from a few millimeters to several centimeters in diameter.
- Lesions commonly appear on sun-exposed areas of the body, such as the face, scalp, ears, neck, arms, and hands.

Causes and Risk Factors:
- Sun exposure: Prolonged or excessive exposure to UV radiation from the sun, particularly without adequate sun protection, is the primary risk factor for developing actinic keratoses.
- Fair skin: Patients with fair or light-colored skin are more susceptible to UV damage and have a higher risk of developing AK.
- Age: Actinic keratoses are more common in older adults, with the risk increasing with age.
- Gender: Men have a higher prevalence of actinic keratoses compared to women, possibly due to greater sun exposure and less use of sun protection measures.

- History of sunburns: Previous episodes of sunburn, especially during childhood or adolescence, increase the risk of developing AK later in life.
- Immunosuppression: Conditions or medications that weaken the immune system, such as organ transplantation or immunosuppressive drugs, may increase the risk of AK.
- Occupational exposure: Certain occupations with outdoor work, such as farming, construction, or landscaping, may increase the risk of AK due to prolonged sun exposure.

Epidemiology:
- Actinic keratoses are common skin lesions that affect millions of patients worldwide.
- The prevalence of AK increases with age, with estimates suggesting that up to 40% of patients over the age of 60 may have at least one actinic keratosis.
- AK is more common in regions with high levels of UV radiation, such as sunny climates and areas closer to the equator.

Diagnosis:
- <u>Clinical Examination:</u> Diagnosis of actinic keratosis is usually based on visual inspection of the skin.
- <u>Dermoscopy:</u> Dermoscopy may be used to evaluate the characteristics of skin lesions and aid in the diagnosis of actinic keratoses.
- <u>Skin Biopsy:</u> to confirm the diagnosis of actinic keratosis and rule out other skin conditions or skin cancer

Treatment:
- <u>Cryotherapy:</u> Using liquid nitrogen to freeze and destroy the lesions is a common treatment for actinic keratoses.
- <u>Topical Medications:</u>
    - Topical fluorouracil (5-FU): A chemotherapy cream applied to the affected area to selectively target and kill abnormal skin cells.
    - Imiquimod cream: A topical immune response modifier that stimulates the body's immune system to attack and eliminate AK cells.
    - Diclofenac gel: A non-steroidal anti-inflammatory gel that helps reduce inflammation and promote regression of actinic keratoses.

- - Ingenol mebutate gel: A topical medication derived from a plant extract that causes cell death in AK lesions.
- **Photodynamic Therapy (PDT):** PDT involves applying a photosensitizing agent to the skin followed by exposure to a specific wavelength of light, which activates the medication and destroys AK cells.
- **Surgical excision:** may be necessary for larger or persistent lesions
- **Laser therapy:** to selectively target and destroy AK cells while minimizing damage to surrounding healthy tissue
- **Chemical peels:** Acids or other chemical agents may help remove actinic keratoses and improve skin texture and appearance.

12.16. Folliculitis

> *Folliculitis is a common skin condition characterized by inflammation of hair follicles, resulting in red, pus-filled bumps or pustules that may be itchy or painful.*
>
> *It can occur anywhere on the body and is often caused by bacteria, fungi, or irritation from shaving or tight clothing.*
>
> *Treatment involves topical or oral antibiotics, antifungal medications, warm compresses, and avoiding potential triggers to reduce symptoms and prevent recurrence.*

Symptoms:
- Red, itchy, or tender bumps or pustules around hair follicles
- Small, pus-filled blisters or whiteheads at the base of hair shafts
- Pain or discomfort in affected areas, particularly when touched or rubbed
- Swelling, redness, or tenderness of the skin surrounding the affected follicles
- Occasionally, folliculitis may cause crusting, scaling, or scarring of the skin

Causes and Risk Factors:
- Bacterial infection: *Staphylococcus aureus* is the most common bacteria responsible for folliculitis, particularly in cases associated with shaving or friction.

- Fungal infection: Yeast or fungal infections, such as those caused by *Candida* or *dermatophytes*, can lead to folliculitis, especially in warm and humid environments.
- Viral infection: Herpes simplex virus (HSV) or varicella-zoster virus (VZV) infections may cause viral folliculitis, characterized by clusters of red, painful lesions.
- Trauma or irritation: Friction from tight clothing, shaving, waxing, or use of occlusive skincare products can irritate hair follicles and predispose to folliculitis.
- Immunocompromised state: Patients with weakened immune systems, such as those with HIV/AIDS, diabetes, or undergoing immunosuppressive therapy, are at higher risk of developing folliculitis.
- Hot tub or pool exposure: *Pseudomonas aeruginosa*, a bacteria commonly found in water environments, can cause hot tub folliculitis or "hot tub rash."
- Occlusive skincare products: Heavy or greasy skincare products, such as oils or moisturizers, can clog hair follicles and contribute to folliculitis development.

Epidemiology:
- Folliculitis is a common skin condition that can affect patients of all ages, genders, and ethnicities.
- The prevalence of folliculitis varies depending on the underlying cause and environmental factors.
- Certain populations, such as athletes, military personnel, or patients living in tropical climates, may have a higher incidence of folliculitis due to increased exposure to risk factors.

Diagnosis:
- <u>Clinical Examination:</u> Diagnosis of folliculitis is usually based on the appearance and distribution of skin lesions.
- <u>Medical History:</u> The APh may inquire about recent activities, such as shaving, swimming, or exposure to potential sources of infection.
- <u>Skin Culture:</u> In cases of suspected bacterial or fungal folliculitis, a skin culture or swab may be performed to identify the causative organism and guide treatment.

Treatment:
- <u>Topical Antimicrobials:</u> Mild cases of folliculitis may respond to over-the-counter topical treatments containing antibacterial or antifungal agents, such as benzoyl peroxide, mupirocin, or clotrimazole.

- Warm Compresses: Applying warm compresses to affected areas can help soothe discomfort, reduce inflammation, and promote drainage of pus from the follicles.
- Avoidance of Irritants: Avoiding shaving, wearing tight clothing, or using harsh skincare products can help prevent further irritation and promote healing of folliculitis lesions.
- Oral Antibiotics: In cases of severe or recurrent bacterial folliculitis, oral antibiotics such as dicloxacillin, cephalexin, or trimethoprim-sulfamethoxazole may be prescribed.
- Antifungal Medications: For fungal folliculitis, oral or topical antifungal medications may be necessary to eradicate the infection.
- Antiviral Medications: In cases of viral folliculitis caused by herpes simplex or varicella-zoster virus, antiviral medications such as acyclovir or valacyclovir may be prescribed.
- Steroid Creams: Topical corticosteroids may help reduce inflammation and itching associated with folliculitis, particularly in cases of eosinophilic folliculitis or folliculitis decalvans.
- Drainage or Incision: Large, painful, or recurrent folliculitis lesions may require drainage or incision to remove pus and promote healing.

12.17. Cellulitis

> ➤ *Cellulitis is a bacterial skin infection characterized by redness, swelling, warmth, and tenderness in the affected area.*
> ➤ *It occurs when bacteria enter the skin through a break or crack, leading to inflammation of the deeper layers.*
> ➤ *Prompt treatment with antibiotics is crucial to prevent complications such as abscess formation or bloodstream infection.*

Symptoms:
- Red, swollen, warm, and tender skin
- Fever and chills
- Pain and discomfort
- May progress to blisters and skin abscesses

Causes and Risk Factors:
- Typically caused by *Staphylococcus aureus* and *Streptococcus pyogenes*

- Risk factors include: skin injuries, chronic skin conditions, weakened immune system, chronic edema in the arms or legs, obesity, and history of cellulitis.

Diagnosis:

- Clinical Examination: The APh should observe the characteristic appearance of inflamed skin.
- Blood Tests: to assess the severity of infection and rule out systemic involvement

Treatment:

- First-Line Antibiotics:
    - Cephalexin, a first-generation cephalosporin, is often considered a first-line oral antibiotic for uncomplicated cellulitis.
    - Dicloxacillin, a penicillinase-resistant penicillin, is another first-line option for cellulitis, particularly in areas where MSSA is prevalent.
    - Clindamycin is an alternative option for cellulitis, especially when MRSA is suspected or in patients with penicillin allergies.
- Second-Line Antibiotics:
    - Trimethoprim-sulfamethoxazole (TMP-SMX) is effective against both *Staphylococcus aureus* (including MRSA) and *Streptococcus pyogenes*.
    - Doxycycline is another alternative for cellulitis, particularly when MRSA coverage is needed.

12.18. Skin Abscess

> ➤ A skin abscess is a localized collection of pus within the skin, typically caused by a bacterial infection, often Staphylococcus aureus.
> ➤ It presents as a painful, swollen, and tender mass with redness and warmth, sometimes accompanied by fever.
> ➤ Treatment involves incision and drainage of the abscess, along with antibiotics if the infection is severe or widespread.

Symptoms:

- Pain, redness, swelling, and warmth at the site
- A visible, palpable, and fluctuant lump or induration

Causes and Risk Factors:
- The primary cause of skin abscesses is the infection of the skin and underlying tissues with bacteria, predominantly *Staphylococcus aureus*.
- Weakened immune system
- Skin conditions that cause breaks in the skin, such as eczema or acne
- Close contact environments
- Poor hygiene
- Previous abscess

Diagnosis:

Diagnosis is based on clinical examination. The APh should observe the characteristic appearance of a localized, pus-filled pocket induration.

Treatment:

The evidence-based treatment of skin abscesses involves a combination of incision and drainage (I&D) along with appropriate antibiotic therapy.

- <u>Incision and Drainage (I&D):</u>

    I&D is the cornerstone of treatment for skin abscesses. It involves making an incision to drain the accumulated pus and debris from the abscess cavity.

- <u>Antibiotic Therapy:</u>
    - Antibiotics are not routinely required for uncomplicated skin abscesses after adequate I&D. However, they may be considered in certain cases.
    - Antibiotic therapy should be targeted based on culture and sensitivity results if available or guided by local resistance patterns.

- <u>Pain Management:</u>
    - Pain management is an essential aspect of abscess treatment. Local anesthesia should be administered before I&D to minimize discomfort.
    - Nonsteroidal anti-inflammatory drugs (NSAIDs) or acetaminophen can be used for post-procedural pain management.

12.19. Pruritus

> ➤ *Pruritus, commonly known as itching, is an unpleasant sensation that prompts the desire to scratch the skin, resulting from various causes such as dry skin, allergies, skin conditions, or systemic diseases.*
>
> ➤ *It can be acute or chronic, significantly impacting quality of life.*
>
> ➤ *Management involves identifying and treating the underlying cause, along with moisturizers, antihistamines, corticosteroids, or other medications to relieve itching.*

Symptoms:
- Itchy skin, which may be localized to specific areas or widespread across the body
- Redness, inflammation, or rash in the affected area, particularly with persistent scratching
- Dry or scaly skin, especially in chronic cases of pruritus
- Secondary skin changes, such as excoriations (skin abrasions), thickening, or lichenification (hardening and thickening of the skin)

Causes and Risk Factors:
- Skin conditions: Eczema, psoriasis, dermatitis, or scabies, can cause itching as a primary symptom.
- Allergies: Foods, medications, insect bites, or environmental allergens may trigger itching.
- Dry skin, particularly in cold or dry climates, can lead to itching.
- Irritants: Exposure to harsh soaps, detergents, or chemicals may cause itching.
- Systemic diseases: Underlying medical conditions such as kidney disease, liver disease, thyroid disorders, diabetes, or certain cancers may be associated with pruritus.
- Neurological disorders: Nerve-related conditions, such as neuropathy or multiple sclerosis, may cause itching.
- Medications: Opioids, antifungal drugs, certain antibiotics, and chemotherapy agents, can cause itching as a side effect.
- Pregnancy: Hormonal changes during pregnancy may lead to itching, particularly in the abdomen and breasts.

Epidemiology:
- Pruritus is a common symptom that can affect patients of all ages, genders, and ethnicities.

- Itching may occur acutely due to transient causes or chronically as a result of underlying medical conditions.
- The prevalence of chronic pruritus increases with age, particularly in older adults.

Diagnosis:
- Medical History: The APh will take a detailed medical history to identify potential triggers, duration, and pattern of itching.
- Physical Examination: Examination of the skin and other body systems can help identify signs of underlying skin conditions or systemic diseases.
- Laboratory Tests: Blood tests, skin biopsies, or allergy testing may be performed to diagnose underlying medical conditions contributing to pruritus.
- Patch Testing: to identify specific allergens causing allergic contact dermatitis
- Skin Scrapings: Microscopic examination of skin scrapings may be performed to detect the presence of parasites or fungal infections.

Treatment:
- Addressing Underlying Causes: Treatment of underlying medical conditions, such as eczema, psoriasis, or liver disease, is essential to relieve itching.
- Topical Treatments: Moisturizing creams, lotions, or ointments can help hydrate and soothe dry, itchy skin.
- Antihistamines: Oral antihistamines, such as cetirizine, loratadine, or diphenhydramine, can help relieve itching associated with allergies or allergic skin conditions.
- Topical Corticosteroids: Prescription-strength corticosteroid creams or ointments may be used to reduce inflammation and itching in localized areas.
- Antipruritic Medications: Topical or oral medications, such as menthol, calamine lotion, capsaicin cream, or gabapentin, may help alleviate itching.
- Phototherapy: Light therapy using ultraviolet (UV) light may be beneficial for certain types of chronic pruritus, such as prurigo nodularis or chronic urticaria.
- Systemic Medications: In severe or refractory cases of pruritus, systemic medications such as oral corticosteroids, immunosuppressants, or biologics may be prescribed.

- Behavioral Interventions: Stress-reduction techniques, relaxation exercises, or cognitive-behavioral therapy (CBT) may help manage itching associated with psychological stress or anxiety.

12.20. Inversa Acne

> *Inverse acne, also known as hidradenitis suppurativa (HS), is a chronic inflammatory skin condition characterized by painful, recurrent nodules, abscesses, and sinus tracts, typically occurring in areas with skin-to-skin contact such as the armpits, groin, and buttocks.*
>
> *It often leads to scarring and can significantly impact quality of life.*
>
> *Treatment involves medications, topical therapies, antibiotics, immunomodulators, and in severe cases, surgical interventions.*

Symptoms:
- Painful, tender, and inflamed nodules or boils in the affected areas
- Formation of abscesses, cysts, or pus-filled lesions that may rupture and drain foul-smelling fluid
- Formation of sinus tracts or tunnels beneath the skin surface, leading to recurrent flare-ups and scarring
- Itching, burning, or discomfort in the affected areas, particularly during flare-ups
- Thickened, scarred skin with hypertrophic or keloid-like lesions in chronic cases

Causes and Risk Factors:
- Genetics: Family history of hidradenitis suppurativa is a significant risk factor, suggesting a genetic predisposition to the condition
- Gender: HS is more common in women than men, with a female-to-male ratio of approximately 3:1.
- Age: Onset typically occurs after puberty, although HS can develop at any age, with peak incidence in the third and fourth decades of life.
- Obesity: Excess weight or obesity is strongly associated with HS, likely due to increased friction and occlusion of skin folds.
- Smoking: Cigarette smoking is a known risk factor for HS, with smokers having a higher prevalence and severity of the condition compared to non-smokers.

- Hormonal factors: Hormonal fluctuations, such as those occurring during puberty, menstruation, or pregnancy, may exacerbate symptoms of HS.
- Environmental factors: Heat, humidity, and sweating can trigger flare-ups of hidradenitis suppurativa, particularly in areas with occluded or irritated skin.

Epidemiology:
- Hidradenitis suppurativa is a relatively common chronic skin condition, although its exact prevalence varies depending on the population studied and diagnostic criteria used.
- Prevalence estimates range from 0.05% to 4% of the general population, with higher rates reported in certain subgroups, such as patients with obesity or a family history of HS.
- HS affects patients of all races and ethnicities, although it may be underdiagnosed or misdiagnosed in certain populations.
- The condition can have a significant impact on quality of life, causing pain, discomfort, and psychological distress due to its chronic and relapsing nature.

Diagnosis:
- <u>Clinical Examination:</u> Diagnosis of hidradenitis suppurativa is typically based on the characteristic clinical features, including the presence of inflamed nodules, abscesses, sinus tracts, and scarring in typical anatomical locations.
- <u>Medical History:</u> A detailed medical history may reveal risk factors such as obesity, smoking, or family history of HS.
- <u>Differential Diagnosis:</u> Hidradenitis suppurativa should be differentiated from other conditions that present with similar symptoms, such as acne vulgaris, folliculitis, pilonidal cysts, or cutaneous abscesses.
- <u>Imaging Studies:</u> Ultrasound or magnetic resonance imaging (MRI) may be performed to evaluate the extent of involvement and identify sinus tracts or deep-seated lesions.

Treatment:
- <u>Topical Treatments:</u> Topical antibiotics, antiseptics, or corticosteroids may be prescribed for mild cases of hidradenitis suppurativa to reduce inflammation and prevent bacterial colonization.
- <u>Systemic Medications:</u> Oral antibiotics, such as tetracycline, clindamycin, or rifampicin, are commonly used for moderate to

severe cases of HS to suppress inflammation and control bacterial overgrowth.

- <u>Biologic Therapies:</u> Adalimumab or infliximab may be prescribed for severe or refractory cases of HS to target specific inflammatory pathways involved in the disease.
- <u>Intralesional Injections:</u> Injections of corticosteroids or other anti-inflammatory medications may be administered directly into patient lesions to reduce inflammation and promote healing.
- <u>Surgical Interventions:</u> Surgical drainage, debridement, or excision of affected areas may be necessary for large, painful, or recurrent lesions.
- <u>Laser Therapy:</u> Laser treatments such as carbon dioxide (CO_2) laser or Nd:YAG laser may be used to reduce inflammation, destroy sinus tracts, and improve scarring in hidradenitis suppurativa.
- <u>Lifestyle Modifications:</u> Weight loss, smoking cessation, and avoiding tight-fitting clothing or shaving in affected areas can help reduce friction and irritation, thereby minimizing flare-ups of HS.

12.21. Lichen Planus

> *Lichen planus (LP) is a chronic inflammatory condition affecting the skin, hair, nails, and mucous membranes, marked by itchy, purplish-red bumps and white lacy patches.*
>
> *It's associated with genetic factors, hepatitis C, certain medications, and possibly dental materials. Lichen planus is common in middle-aged adults and affects about 1-2% of the global population.*
>
> *Diagnosis LP involves physical examination, skin biopsy, and sometimes blood tests, with treatment aimed at symptom relief.*

Symptoms:

- Itchy rash: The most common symptom is a rash that itches severely. It often appears on the inner wrists, legs, torso, or genitals.
- Lacy white patches: on mucous membranes, such as the inside of the mouth or vagina
- Painful sores: in the mouth or vagina
- Hair loss and scalp rash: can lead to scarring
- Nail damage: Nails may become thin, ridge, split, or in severe cases, the patient may lose the nail entirely.

Causes and Risk Factors:
- Genetic predisposition: There may be a genetic component, as lichen planus is sometimes seen in families.
- Hepatitis C infection: There's an association between lichen planus and chronic hepatitis C virus infection.
- Certain medications: Drugs containing arsenic, bismuth, or gold, and certain heart disease and high blood pressure medications can trigger lichen planus.
- Dental materials: Some cases of oral lichen planus are believed to be triggered by amalgam fillings in the teeth.

Epidemiology:
- Age: Lichen planus can occur at any age but is most commonly seen in middle-aged adults.
- Gender: It tends to affect more women than men.
- Global Prevalence: The condition is seen worldwide, with varying prevalence rates, often affecting about 1-2% of the population.

Skin Findings:
- Purple, flat-topped bumps: The hallmark of lichen planus are shiny, flat-topped bumps that are purplish in color.
- Wickham's striae: Fine, white lines may be seen on the surface of the bumps.
- Symmetrical pattern: The rash often appears in a symmetrical pattern on both sides of the body.

Diagnosis:
- <u>Physical Examination:</u> Diagnosis is typically made based on the appearance of the skin or mucous membranes.
- <u>Biopsy:</u> may be performed to confirm the diagnosis, especially in atypical cases
- <u>Blood Tests:</u> While not diagnostic, blood tests may be used to rule out hepatitis C or other conditions.
- <u>Patch Testing:</u> may be recommended if a drug reaction is suspected

Treatment:
- <u>Managing Symptoms:</u> This is the main focus of treatment and may be done with topical corticosteroids or oral medications to suppress the immune system and antihistamines for itching. Light therapy may also be used in some cases.

- **Infection Management:** Since lichen planus can be associated with hepatitis C, managing this underlying infection can also be part of the treatment strategy.
- **Supportive Care:** Regular monitoring and supportive care are essential, especially for cases affecting the mucous membranes, to prevent complications such as scarring.

12.22. Cutaneous Lupus

> ➢ *Cutaneous lupus erythematosus manifests as skin lesions, ranging from the "butterfly" rash across the cheeks to discoid rashes and photosensitivity, primarily triggered by sunlight.*
>
> ➢ *It's more prevalent in women and certain ethnic groups, with genetic and environmental factors as key risk elements.*
>
> ➢ *Treatment focuses on managing symptoms through medications like antimalarials and lifestyle adjustments like sun avoidance.*

Symptoms:
- Photosensitivity: Exposure to too much sunlight can cause skin lesions or exacerbate existing ones.
- Discoid rash: thick, red, scaly patches that can cause scarring and hair loss when they occur on the scalp
- Subacute cutaneous lupus: Presents as sores or lesions in sun-exposed areas, typically not scarring but may cause skin discoloration.
- Acute cutaneous lupus: Characterized by the classic "butterfly" rash across the cheeks and nose, which is a hallmark of systemic lupus but can occur in cutaneous lupus without other systemic symptoms.

Causes and Risk Factors:
- Genetic predisposition: A family history of lupus or other autoimmune diseases can increase risk.
- Environmental triggers: Sunlight, infections, and certain medications can trigger lupus skin symptoms.
- Hormonal influences: Lupus is more common in women than men, suggesting hormonal factors may play a role.
- Smoking: can exacerbate skin symptoms and may interfere with the effectiveness of treatment

Epidemiology:
- Prevalence: Cutaneous lupus is a subset of lupus erythematosus; lupus affects approximately 20 to 150 per 100,000 people worldwide.
- Age and Gender: Most commonly diagnosed in people of childbearing age, lupus is significantly more prevalent in women.
- Ethnicity: Higher incidence and severity have been observed in African American, Hispanic, Asian, and Native American populations compared to Caucasians.

Skin Findings:
- Discoid lesions: Circular, raised, scaly patches that may scar and cause pigment changes.
- Malar rash: The "butterfly" rash is erythematous and may be mildly scaly, sparing the nasolabial folds.
- Photosensitivity: skin reaction or worsening of the rash after sun exposure

Diagnosis:
- Physical Examination: The APh should perform an assessment of the skin lesions and their pattern.
- Skin Biopsy: A biopsy of the lesion can confirm the diagnosis by showing characteristic changes under the microscope.
- Blood Tests: While not diagnostic for cutaneous lupus alone, antinuclear antibody (ANA) tests may be positive and help in diagnosing systemic involvement.
- Direct Immunofluorescence: can show deposition of immune complexes in the skin, confirming lupus skin disease

Treatment:
- Managing Symptoms: Treatment strategies may include topical corticosteroids, antimalarial drugs (hydroxychloroquine), and avoiding sun exposure to manage symptoms and prevent new lesions from forming.
- Supportive Care: Monitoring for potential progression to systemic lupus erythematosus is also crucial for patients with cutaneous lupus.

12.23. Oral Lesions

> ➤ Oral lesions encompass a wide range of conditions affecting the mouth, from benign sores and ulcers to malignant cancers, with symptoms including pain, visible changes in mouth tissue, and discomfort.
>
> ➤ Risk factors include tobacco use, alcohol consumption, HPV infection, poor oral hygiene, and nutritional deficiencies.
>
> ➤ Treatment varies from symptomatic care for benign conditions to more aggressive interventions for malignancies, emphasizing the importance of preventive care and regular dental check-ups.

Symptoms:

- Pain or discomfort in the mouth, which may be constant or occur only when eating or drinking
- Visible changes in the mouth tissue, such as sores, ulcers, white patches (leukoplakia), red patches (erythroplakia), or mixed red and white patches
- Bleeding or numbness in the mouth without any apparent cause
- Swelling of the gums, tongue, or other areas inside the mouth

Causes and Risk Factors:

- Tobacco use: Smoking or chewing tobacco significantly increases the risk of oral lesions.
- Alcohol consumption: Heavy drinking is another major risk factor, especially when combined with tobacco use.
- Human Papillomavirus (HPV): Certain strains of HPV, particularly HPV-16, are associated with oral cancers and lesions.
- Poor oral hygiene and ill-fitting dentures can lead to lesions or exacerbate existing conditions.
- Nutritional deficiencies, such as vitamin B12, iron, and folate, can cause oral ulcers and other lesions.

Epidemiology:

- The prevalence of oral lesions varies widely, depending on the specific condition, geographical location, and population demographics. Conditions like oral lichen planus, candidiasis, and leukoplakia are relatively common in the general population.
- Oral cancer, a severe form of oral lesion, has a higher incidence in men than women and is more common in older individuals.

Mucosal Findings:
- Ulcers: painful sores that may bleed easily
- White or red patches: Leukoplakia presents as white patches, while erythroplakia is characterized by red, velvety patches.
- Masses or lumps in the oral cavity or throat
- Color changes in the mouth, such as dark pigments or unusually pale areas

Diagnosis:
- <u>Clinical Examination:</u> may also be performed by a dentist, focusing on the history and physical appearance of the lesion
- <u>Skin Biopsy:</u> often necessary to rule out malignancy and determine the exact nature of the lesion
- <u>Imaging Tests:</u> X-rays, CT scans, or MRIs may be used to assess the extent of lesions suspected to be malignant.
- <u>Blood Tests:</u> help identify underlying systemic conditions that may present with oral lesions, such as vitamin deficiencies or anemia

Treatment:

Treatment varies significantly based on the type of lesion, underlying cause, and potential for malignancy. It can range from monitoring and symptomatic care for benign lesions to surgical removal, radiation, and chemotherapy for cancerous lesions.

Preventive measures include maintaining good oral hygiene, avoiding tobacco and excessive alcohol, and regular dental check-ups.

12.24. Vitiligo

> ➢ *Vitiligo is a chronic autoimmune condition characterized by the loss of skin pigmentation, resulting in white patches on various parts of the body due to the destruction of melanocytes.*
> ➢ *It can affect any skin area and is often symmetrical.*
> ➢ *Treatment options include topical steroids, phototherapy, and, in some cases, surgical interventions to restore color or reduce the appearance of patches.*

Symptoms:

The hallmark symptom of vitiligo is the development of depigmented patches on the skin.

- Appear gradually: Vitiligo patches often start small and may expand over time.
- Affect any body part: Vitiligo can occur on any area of the body, including the face, hands, feet, arms, and genitalia.
- Symmetric distribution: Patches may appear symmetrically on both sides of the body.
- Progressive: The condition can be progressive, with new patches developing over time.
- Hair and mucous membrane involvement: Vitiligo can also affect hair, resulting in white or gray hair, and mucous membranes.

Diagnosis:

Diagnosing vitiligo is typically based on clinical evaluation, although additional tests may be performed to confirm the diagnosis.

- Physical Examination: The APh should examine the skin to assess the extent and distribution of depigmented patches. It is important to distinguish vitiligo from similar skin conditions such as tinea.
- Wood's Lamp Examination: A Wood's lamp (ultraviolet light) may be used to highlight depigmented areas, making them more visible.
- Biopsy (Optional): In some cases, a skin biopsy may be performed to confirm the absence of melanocytes in the affected area. This can help rule out other conditions.

Biopsy Considerations:

A punch biopsy for vitiligo involves removing a small sample of skin from an affected area. The sample is then examined under a microscope to confirm the absence of melanocytes. Biopsy is typically reserved for cases where the diagnosis is uncertain or when other skin conditions need to be ruled out.

Treatment:

- Potent Topical Corticosteroids: These may help reduce inflammation and repigment the skin.
- Topical Calcineurin Inhibitors: non-steroidal creams (e.g., tacrolimus, pimecrolimus) for sensitive areas or when long-term steroid use is not suitable
- Psoralen Plus Ultraviolet A (PUVA) Therapy: a combination of psoralen (a light-sensitizing medication) and UVA light exposure
- Narrowband Ultraviolet B (NB-UVB) Therapy: exposure to UVB light of a specific wavelength
- Excimer Laser: targeted UVB light therapy for smaller areas

- **Microskin or Tattooing:** camouflaging depigmented areas with skin-colored tattoos
- **Oral Medications:** Some oral medications may be used, such as corticosteroids, psoralen, or Janus kinase inhibitors (e.g., ruxolitinib).

12.25. Alopecia

> ➢ *Alopecia encompasses a range of conditions causing hair loss, from genetic factors in androgenetic alopecia to autoimmune causes in alopecia areata, and stress-related in telogen effluvium.*
>
> ➢ *Symptoms vary from thinning hair to complete baldness, with diagnosis typically involving clinical examination, blood tests, and sometimes scalp biopsy.*
>
> ➢ *Treatment options range from topical treatments and medications to address underlying causes, to surgical options for more permanent solutions.*

Symptoms:
- Hair thinning: Gradual thinning on top of the head is the most common form, affecting both sexes.
- Patchy bald spots: Circular bald spots, usually affecting the scalp, but can occur in beards and eyebrows.
- Sudden loosening of hair: A handful of hair might come out when combing or washing your hair, typically after a physical or emotional shock.
- Full-body hair loss: Some medical treatments, like chemotherapy, can cause hair loss all over the body.
- Scaling patches: Scalp infections can lead to scaly patches and hair loss.

Causes and Risk Factors:
- Family History/Genetics
- Age
- Significant Stress
- Nutritional Deficiencies
- Medical Conditions: such as lupus, diabetes, and thyroid disorders
- Hormonal Changes
- Medications and Supplements

Epidemiology:
- Androgenetic Alopecia: Affects approximately 50% of men by the age of 50 and 50% of women by the age of 70.
- Alopecia Areata: Affects about 0.1%–0.2% of the population at some point in their lifetime.
- Telogen Effluvium and Anagen Effluvium: Prevalence is difficult to estimate due to underreporting and the transient nature of these conditions.

Skin Findings:
- Androgenetic alopecia: miniaturization of hair follicles, with reduced hair diameter and length
- Alopecia areata: smooth, round patches of complete hair loss, sometimes with exclamation point hairs at the periphery
- Telogen effluvium: diffuse thinning of hair across the scalp without obvious patches
- Scarring alopecias: loss of hair follicles, replaced by scar tissue.

Diagnosis:
- <u>Clinical Examination:</u> including scalp examination and history
- <u>Pull Test:</u> to see how easily hair comes out
- <u>Blood Tests:</u> to uncover medical conditions related to hair loss
- <u>Scalp Biopsy:</u> to look for the underlying cause of hair loss
- <u>Dermoscopy:</u> examining hair follicles with a handheld microscope

Treatment:
- <u>Androgenetic Alopecia:</u> minoxidil, finasteride (men only), and hair transplant surgery
- <u>Alopecia Areata:</u> corticosteroids (topical, intralesional, or oral), topical immunotherapy, and JAK inhibitors
- <u>Telogen Effluvium:</u> addressing the underlying cause (e.g., stress, nutritional deficiencies) and time.
- <u>Scarring Alopecias:</u> anti-inflammatory medications, antibiotics, or antifungals depending on the cause, and sometimes surgical removal of scarred areas
- <u>Supportive Care:</u> psychological support, cosmetic options like wigs or hairpieces, and education about the condition

12.26. Burn

> ➤ *Burns are injuries to skin and subcutaneous tissues caused by heat, chemicals, electricity, or radiation, ranging from mild (first-degree) to severe (third and fourth-degree) with symptoms like pain, redness, and blistering.*
> ➤ *Risk factors include exposure to open flames, hot liquids, chemicals, and excessive sun.*
> ➤ *Treatment varies by severity, from cooling and bandaging for minor burns to surgical intervention and rehabilitation for more severe injuries.*

Symptoms:
- Pain: Varies with the severity of the burn; some severe burns may damage nerves and be less painful initially.
- Redness and swelling: common in all types of burns
- Blisters: may develop hours after the initial injury, especially in second-degree burns
- Charred or white skin: appears in third-degree burns
- Shock symptoms: such as pale complexion, weakness, and cool, clammy skin, indicating a more severe condition

Causes and Risk Factors:
- Exposure to open flames: common in household and workplace accidents
- Scalding from hot liquids or steam: a risk in kitchens and bathrooms
- Electrical burns: from exposed wires, outlets, or lightning strikes
- Chemical burns: from strong acids, alkalis, or other corrosive materials
- Sunburn: from prolonged exposure to ultraviolet rays without protection
- Radiation burns: from therapeutic radiation exposure or sunlamps

Skin Findings:
- Depends on severity of burn
- Redness, edema, inflammation, pain, and blisters
- Sometimes numbness due to nerve damage

Types:
- First-Degree Burns (Superficial Burns): Affect only the epidermis.

- Second-Degree Burns (Partial Thickness Burns): Extend into the dermis.
- Third-Degree Burns (Full Thickness Burns): Penetrate the full thickness of the skin, damaging the tissue beneath.
- Fourth-Degree Burns: Extend beyond the skin into muscles, ligaments, tendons, nerves, blood vessels, and bones.

Diagnosis:
- <u>Visual Examination:</u> the primary method for assessing burn depth and extent
- <u>Patient History:</u> Information on how the burn occurred can provide crucial details for treatment.
- <u>Diagnostic Tests:</u> May include blood tests, imaging tests (like X-rays for electrical burns), and in severe cases, a biopsy.

Estimate Burn Area by Rule of 9:

The "Rule of Nines" is a method used by medical professionals to estimate the total body surface area (TBSA) affected by a burn.
- Head and Neck: 9%
- Each Upper Limb (Arm): 9%
- Each Lower Limb (Leg): 18%
- The Front of the Torso: 18%
- The Back of the Torso: 18%
- Perineum (Genital Area): 1%

- For children and infants, the percentages are adjusted to account for their differing body proportions, notably with a larger head and neck area and smaller limb areas.
- This rule helps determine the extent of burn injury and guide initial fluid resuscitation and treatment decisions for burn patients. It is not directly related to prescribing topical medications but is a crucial tool in burn care.

Treatment:
- <u>First Aid:</u> involves cooling the burn, covering it with sterile, non-adhesive bandages, and taking pain relievers
- <u>Medical Treatment for Severe Burns:</u> may include IV fluids to prevent dehydration, antibiotics to prevent infection, tetanus shots, and pain medication
- <u>Wound Care:</u> Cleaning and dressing changes promotes healing and prevents infection.

- **Surgical Treatment:** skin grafts, debridement (removal of dead tissue), or reconstructive surgery for severe burns
- **Rehabilitation:** Physical therapy to maintain mobility and prevent scarring and contractures.
- **Preventive Measures:** Smoke alarms in buildings, safe handling of flammable materials, using sunscreen, and wearing protective clothing when handling chemicals or working with fire are essential preventive strategies.

12.27. Corticosteroid Prescribed Consideration

> ➤ *Corticosteroids are potent anti-inflammatory medications prescribed for various conditions such as asthma, allergies, arthritis, and skin disorders.*
>
> ➤ *Considerations include potential side effects like weight gain, increased blood sugar, and immune suppression, requiring careful monitoring, short-term use when possible, and tapering to minimize risks.*

12.27.1 Prescription Guidelines for the APh:

- Diagnosis and Assessment:
  - Begin by accurately diagnosing the patient's skin condition through a thorough history and physical examination.
  - Take into account any underlying medical conditions or allergies that may impact the choice of medication.
- Selection of Topical Medication:
  - Choose the appropriate type of topical medication based on the diagnosis (e.g., corticosteroids, antibiotics, antifungals, emollients).
  - Consider the potency of the medication based on the severity and location of the condition (e.g., low-potency corticosteroids for sensitive areas, high-potency corticosteroids for thicker skin).
- Education and Counseling:
  - Ensure the patient understands how to apply the medication, the frequency of application, and the expected duration of treatment.
  - Discuss potential side effects and when to seek medical attention.
  - Provide written instructions if needed.

- Prescription Details:
  - Specify the medication, including its generic and brand name, strength, and formulation (e.g., cream, ointment, lotion, gel).
  - Indicate the frequency of application (e.g., once or twice daily) and the duration of treatment.
  - Include any additional instructions or precautions (e.g., avoid sun exposure for photosensitizing medications).
- Monitoring and Follow-Up:
  - Schedule follow-up appointments to assess treatment progress, monitor for side effects, and adjust treatment if necessary.
  - Document the patient's response to treatment in the medical record.
- Combination Therapy:
  - In some cases, combining different topical medications may be more effective (e.g., using a corticosteroid with an emollient).
  - Ensure the patient understands how to apply each medication in combination.
- Safety Precautions:
  - Caution patients about potential side effects, including skin thinning, irritation, or allergic reactions.
  - Recommend appropriate sun protection if needed.
- Special Populations:
  - Tailor medication strength and application guidelines for pediatric and elderly patients as needed.
- Documentation:
  - Thoroughly document the diagnosis, treatment plan, and patient education in the medical record.
- Review of Medication List:
  - Ensure that the patient's medication list is up to date, considering potential drug interactions with topical medications.

12.27.2. Topical Steroid Classifications

Topical corticosteroids come in different types and classifications based on their potency and are categorized into several classes.
- Class 7 (Least Potent):
  - Hydrocortisone (over-the-counter creams)

- Class 6:
  - Alclometasone
  - Desonide
  - Hydrocortisone valerate
- Class 5:
  - Fluocinolone acetonide
  - Mometasone furoate
  - Triamcinolone acetonide
- Class 4:
  - Betamethasone valerate
  - Fluocinonide
  - Triamcinolone acetonide
- Class 3:
  - Betamethasone dipropionate
  - Desoximetasone
- Class 2:
  - Amcinonide
  - Betamethasone dipropionate augmented (with salicylic acid)
  - Diflorasone diacetate
- Class 1 (Most Potent):
  - Clobetasol propionate
  - Halobetasol propionate

Prolonged or inappropriate use of high-potency corticosteroids can lead to side effects, including skin thinning, stretch marks, and increased risk of skin infections.

12.27.3. Systemic corticosteroid

Systemic corticosteroids are potent anti-inflammatory medications used to treat a variety of medical conditions.

- <u>Dosage and Duration:</u> The dose and duration of systemic corticosteroid therapy depend on the condition being treated, its severity, and individual patient factors. Treatment typically starts with a high dose to induce remission, followed by a gradual tapering regimen to minimize side effects.
- <u>Conversion Equivalents:</u> When switching between different corticosteroid preparations or routes of administration, it's essential

to consider their relative potency. The following are approximate equivalent doses for commonly used systemic corticosteroids:
- Prednisone: 5 mg
- Prednisolone: 5 mg
- Methylprednisolone: 4 mg
- Dexamethasone: 0.75 mg
- Hydrocortisone: 20 mg

- Side Effects Monitoring: Long-term use of systemic corticosteroids can lead to various adverse effects, including weight gain, hypertension, diabetes, osteoporosis, and immunosuppression. Patients should be closely monitored for these side effects, and preventive measures or alternative treatments may be considered as needed.

- Tapering Regimen: Abrupt discontinuation of systemic corticosteroids can result in adrenal insufficiency or exacerbation of the underlying condition. Tapering the dose gradually over weeks to months allows the adrenal glands to resume normal cortisol production.

12.28. Description of Skin Lesions

Skin Lesions	Definitions	Examples
Macule	A macule is a small, flat, and discolored spot on the skin, typically less than 1 centimeter in diameter	A freckle is a common example of a macule
Papule	A papule is a raised, solid bump on the skin, measuring less than 1 centimeter in diameter	Acne pimples often start as papules
Plaque	A plaque is a flat-topped, raised lesion with a well-defined border, usually greater than 1 centimeter in diameter	Psoriasis can result in the formation of plaques on the skin

Nodule	A nodule is a palpable, firm, and elevated lesion, typically measuring between 1 and 2 centimeters in diameter	Lipomas are nodules composed of fatty tissue
Vesicle	A vesicle is a small, fluid-filled blister, less than 1 centimeter in diameter	Herpes simplex virus (HSV) can cause vesicles during an outbreak
Bulla	A bulla is a large, fluid-filled blister, typically greater than 1 centimeter in diameter	Second-degree burns can result in bullae formation
Pustule	A pustule is a small, elevated lesion containing pus	Pimples are common pustules associated with acne
Wheal	A wheal is a raised, edematous, and often pruritic (itchy) area of the skin, typically resulting from an allergic reaction or insect bite	Hives (urticaria) are characterized by wheals
Erosion	Erosion refers to the loss of the epidermal layer of skin, resulting in a moist, shallow depression	An open blister can lead to skin erosion
Ulcer	An ulcer is a deeper loss of skin that extends into the dermis, often with a concave appearance	Venous leg ulcers are a common type of skin ulcer
Scale	Scales are dry, flaky, and often adherent skin fragments that may be white, silver, or gray	Psoriasis plaques are covered in scales
Crust	Crusts are dried serum, blood, or pus on the surface of a skin lesion	Impetigo can result in yellow-brown crusts
Fissure	A fissure is a linear crack or slit-like opening in the skin	Anal fissures can cause discomfort and bleeding

Excoriations	Excoriations are linear or punctate erosions resulting from scratching or rubbing of the skin	Prurigo nodules can develop from repeated excoriation
Petechiae	Petechiae are small, red or purple, pinpoint spots on the skin caused by tiny hemorrhages in the capillaries	Petechiae may be associated with certain bleeding disorders

References

- Zaenglein, A. L., Pathy, A. L., & et al. (2016). Guidelines of care for the management of acne vulgaris. Journal of the American Academy of Dermatology, 74(5), 945-973.
- Eichenfield, L. F., Tom, W. L., & et al. (2014). Guidelines of care for the management of atopic dermatitis: Section 1. Diagnosis and assessment of atopic dermatitis. Journal of the American Academy of Dermatology, 70(2), 338-351.
- Jacob, S. E., Goldenberg, A., & et al. (2015). Systematic review of published trials: Long-term safety of topical corticosteroids and topical calcineurin inhibitors in pediatric patients with atopic dermatitis. BMC Pediatrics, 15(1), 1-12.
- Menter, A., Gottlieb, A., & et al. (2008). Guidelines of care for the management of psoriasis and psoriatic arthritis: Section 1. Overview of psoriasis and guidelines of care for the treatment of psoriasis with biologics. Journal of the American Academy of Dermatology, 58(5), 826-850.
- Gupta, A. K., Nicol, K., & et al. (2016). New insights into dandruff and seborrheic dermatitis: Malassezia yeasts as predisposing factors and symptom-triggering allergens. Journal of Drugs in Dermatology, 15(8), 982-985.
- Gallo, R. L., Granstein, R. D., & et al. (2018). Standard classification and pathophysiology of rosacea: The 2017 update by the National Rosacea Society Expert Committee. Journal of the American Academy of Dermatology, 78(1), 148-155.
- Elewski, B. E. (2014). Tinea capitis: A current perspective. Journal of the American Academy of Dermatology, 70(6), 1103-1111.
- Engelman, D., Fuller, L. C., & et al. (2019). Consensus criteria for the diagnosis of scabies: A Delphi study of international experts. PLoS Neglected Tropical Diseases, 13(9), e0007623.
- Hartman-Adams, H., Banvard, C., & et al. (2014). Diagnosis and management of impetigo. Pediatric Annals, 43(9), e220-e225.
- Kwok, C. S., Gibbs, S., & et al. (2014). Topical treatments for cutaneous warts. Cochrane Database of Systematic Reviews, 2014(9), CD001781.
- Silverberg, N. B. (2016). A pediatric approach to molluscum contagiosum. Cutis, 97(5), 336-340.
- Gupta, A. K., Chaudhry, M., & et al. (2016). Selenium sulfide shampoo for the treatment of tinea versicolor: A review. Journal of Dermatological Treatment, 27(2), 149-153.
- Kaplan, A. P., & Greaves, M. (2009). Pathogenesis of chronic urticaria. Clinical and Experimental Allergy, 39(6), 777-787.
- Schwartz, R. A., & Bridges, T. M. (2017). Seborrheic keratosis. Journal of the American Academy of Dermatology, 77(4), 609-618.

- Werner, R. N., Stockfleth, E., & et al. (2013). Evidence- and consensus-based (S3) guidelines for the treatment of actinic keratosis—International League of Dermatological Societies in cooperation with the European Dermatology Forum—Short version. Journal of the European Academy of Dermatology and Venereology, 27(12), 1584-1595.
- Marples, R. R. (2004). Management of superficial folliculitis. American Journal of Clinical Dermatology, 5(5), 339-344.
- Weisshaar, E., & Dalgard, F. (2009). Epidemiology of itch: Adding to the burden of skin morbidity. Acta Dermato-Venereologica, 89(4), 339-350.
- Kromann, C. B., Ibler, K. S., & et al. (2014). The prevalence of inverse recurrent suppuration: A community-based study of possible hidradenitis suppurativa. Dermatology, 228(2), 154-158.

Chapter 13: Pediatric Disorders

Reviewed by
Tanya Thuy Nguyen, MD, FAAP

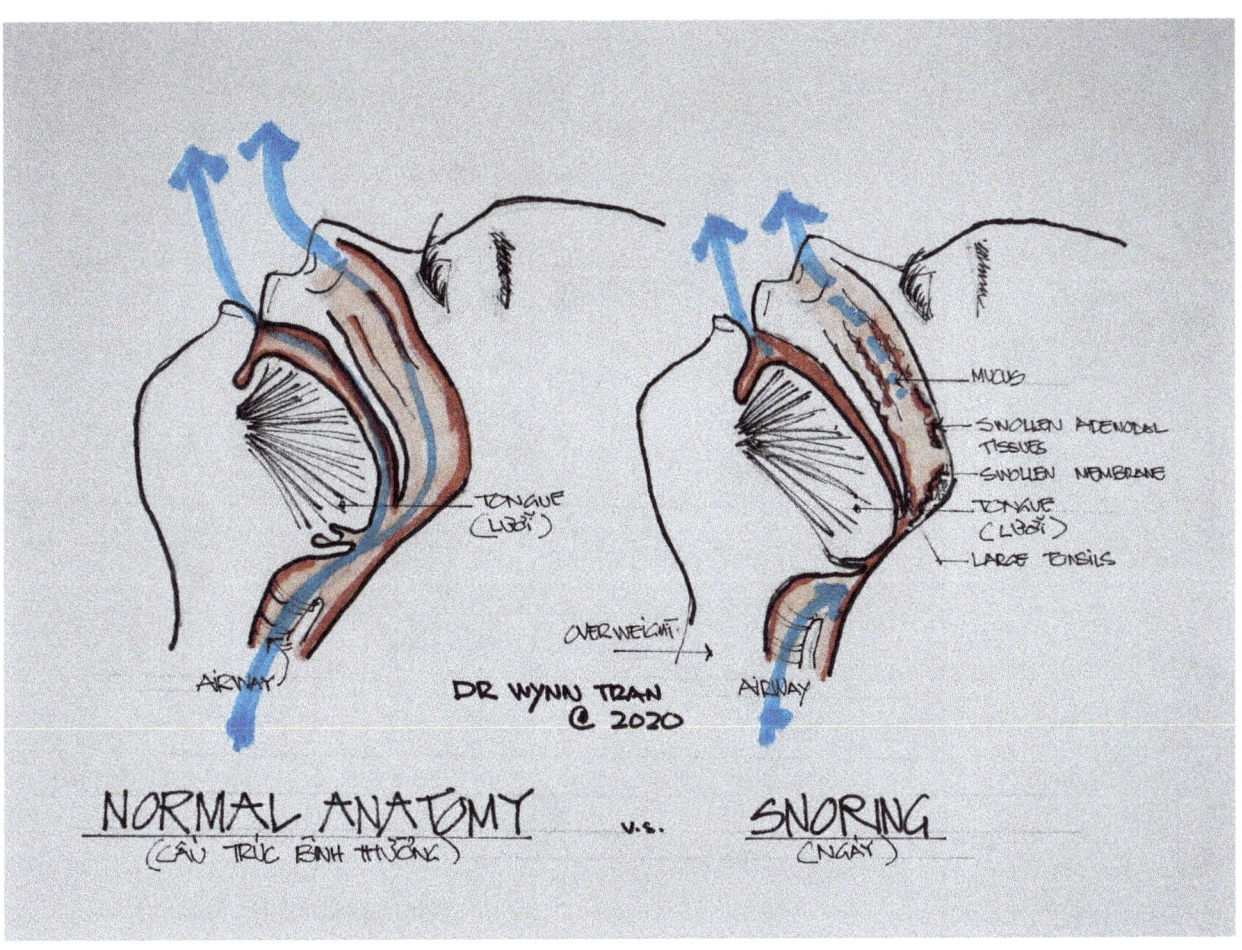

The APh should be familiar with the presentation, diagnosis, and management of these common pediatric conditions to provide appropriate care and referral to the pediatrician or pediatric specialists when necessary.

13.1. Upper Respiratory Infections

> ➤ *Upper respiratory infections (URIs) are common viral infections affecting the nose, throat, and sinuses, often causing symptoms like nasal congestion, sore throat, coughing, and mild fever.*
>
> ➤ *They spread through respiratory droplets and typically resolve on their own within a week.*
>
> ➤ *Treatment is focused on symptom relief, rest, hydration, and occasionally over-the-counter medications to alleviate discomfort.*

Symptoms:
- Runny or stuffy nose
- Sneezing
- Coughing
- Sore throat
- Mild fever
- Fatigue
- Headache
- Mild body aches
- Loss of appetite

Causes and Risk factors:
- Exposure to viruses: URIs are highly contagious and spread through respiratory droplets when an infected person coughs or sneezes.
- Age: Children, especially those under the age of six, are more susceptible to URIs due to their developing immune systems and increased exposure in daycare or school environments.
- Season: URIs are more common during colder months, typically fall and winter.

Diagnosis:

In most cases, the diagnosis of a common cold is based on the child's symptoms and a physical examination. Laboratory tests are usually not necessary unless complications are suspected.

Treatment:
- Rest: Ensure the child gets plenty of rest to help their body fight off the infection.

- **Hydration:** Encourage the child to drink fluids such as water, clear broth, or herbal tea to stay hydrated.
- **Saline Nasal Drops:** Use saline nasal drops to help relieve nasal congestion in infants and young children.
- **Humidifier:** Using a cool-mist humidifier in the child's room can help ease congestion and soothe a sore throat.
- **Over-The-Counter Medications:** Acetaminophen or ibuprofen may help reduce fever and relieve discomfort.
- **Avoiding Irritants:** Keep the child away from cigarette smoke and other respiratory irritants.
- **Antibiotics:** Antibiotics are not effective against viral infections like the common cold and should not be prescribed unless there is a bacterial complication such as a secondary bacterial infection.

Prevention:
- Hand hygiene: Encourage frequent handwashing with soap and water, especially after coughing, sneezing, or blowing the nose.
- Avoid close contact: Teach children to avoid close contact with sick patients, and keep them home from school or daycare when they are ill.
- Vaccination: Ensure the child is up-to-date on vaccinations, including the annual influenza vaccine.

13.2. Otitis Media

> ➤ *Otitis media (OM) is a common childhood ear infection, typically caused by bacteria or viruses, leading to ear pain, fever, and sometimes fluid or pus drainage from the ear.*
>
> ➤ *It often follows upper respiratory infections and can result in temporary hearing loss, but most cases resolve on their own without antibiotics.*
>
> ➤ *Treatment involves pain management, rest, and possibly antibiotics if severe or recurrent.*

Symptoms:
- Ear pain or discomfort, especially when lying down
- Tugging or pulling at the ear
- Difficulty sleeping
- Irritability or fussiness

- Fluid drainage from the ear (if the eardrum ruptures)
- Decreased hearing or hearing loss
- Fever
- Headache
- Loss of appetite

Causes and Risk factors:
- Age: Children under the age of 2 are at higher risk due to the anatomy of their eustachian tubes, which are shorter and more horizontal than in older children and adults.
- Exposure to infections: Being in close contact with other children, especially in daycare settings, increases the risk of exposure to respiratory viruses and bacteria that can cause OM.
- Allergies: Children with allergies are more prone to inflammation of the eustachian tubes, which can increase the risk of OM.
- Bottle feeding while lying down: Feeding infants while lying down can lead to the reflux of milk into the eustachian tubes, increasing the risk of infection.
- Exposure to tobacco smoke: Secondhand smoke can irritate the mucous membranes of the nose and throat, making children more susceptible to OM.

Epidemiology:

OM is one of the most common childhood illnesses worldwide, with the highest incidence occurring in children under the age of 2. It is estimated that over 80% of children will experience at least one episode of OM by the age of 3.

Diagnosis:

OM is typically diagnosed based on the child's symptoms and a physical examination of the ear by a healthcare provider. The provider may use an otoscope to visualize the eardrum and assess for signs of inflammation, fluid behind the eardrum, or a bulging eardrum.

Treatment:
- <u>Pain Relief:</u> Acetaminophen or ibuprofen can help alleviate ear pain and reduce fever.
- <u>Observation:</u> In some cases, particularly in mild cases of OM, the APh may recommend observation without the immediate use of antibiotics, as many cases of OM will resolve on their own within a few days.

- **Antibiotics:** If the child has severe symptoms or if the infection is suspected to be bacterial, antibiotics such as amoxicillin are commonly prescribed.
- **Ear Drops:** Antibiotic ear drops may be prescribed for children with recurrent or persistent OM, or for cases where oral antibiotics are not effective.
- **Ear Tube Placement:** In cases of recurrent or chronic OM, particularly if there is persistent fluid buildup or hearing loss, a pediatric otolaryngologist (ear, nose, and throat specialist) may recommend the placement of tympanostomy tubes (ear tubes) to help drain fluid from the middle ear and prevent future infections.

13.3. Asthma

> ➤ *Asthma in children is a chronic respiratory condition characterized by inflammation and narrowing of the airways.*
>
> ➤ *Symptoms such as wheezing, coughing, chest tightness, and shortness of breath, often triggered by allergens, respiratory infections, exercise, or environmental factors may occur.*
>
> ➤ *Management involves medications such as bronchodilators and inhaled corticosteroids to control symptoms, along with avoiding triggers, monitoring lung function, and having an asthma action plan to prevent exacerbations and promote quality of life.*

Symptoms:
- Wheezing: high-pitched whistling sound when breathing out
- Shortness of breath: difficulty breathing, especially during physical activity or at night
- Coughing: often worse at night or early morning, and may be triggered by cold air, exercise, or exposure to allergens
- Chest tightness: Children may describe a feeling of pressure or discomfort in their chest.
- Rapid breathing: increased respiratory rate during asthma exacerbations
- Fatigue: feeling tired or weak due to the extra effort required to breathe

Causes and Risk factors:
- Family history: Children with a family history of asthma or allergic conditions are at higher risk.

- Allergies: Sensitivity to allergens such as pollen, dust mites, pet dander, or mold can trigger asthma symptoms.
- Respiratory infections: Viral respiratory infections, especially those affecting the upper respiratory tract, can exacerbate asthma symptoms.
- Environmental factors: Exposure to tobacco smoke, air pollution, or other environmental pollutants can increase the risk of developing asthma.
- Obesity: Being overweight or obese is associated with an increased risk of asthma.
- Premature birth: Premature infants are at higher risk of developing asthma due to underdeveloped lungs.

Epidemiology:

Asthma is one of the most common chronic conditions in childhood, affecting approximately 9-10% of children in the United States. The prevalence of asthma has been increasing in recent decades, particularly in urban areas and among socioeconomically disadvantaged populations.

Diagnosis:

- Medical History: The APh will ask about the child's symptoms, family history of asthma or allergies, and any triggers that worsen symptoms.
- Physical Examination: The provider will listen to the child's lungs with a stethoscope and may look for signs of wheezing or other respiratory abnormalities.
- Lung Function Tests: Spirometry and peak flow measurement are commonly used to assess lung function and airflow obstruction.
- Allergy Testing: Skin prick testing or blood tests may be performed to identify specific allergens that trigger asthma symptoms.

Treatment:

- Controller Medications: Inhaled corticosteroids (e.g., fluticasone, budesonide) are the mainstay of asthma treatment and are used to reduce airway inflammation and prevent asthma exacerbations.
- Quick-Relief Medications: Short-acting beta-agonists (e.g., albuterol) are used as rescue medications to quickly relieve asthma symptoms during acute exacerbations.
- Allergy Management: Avoidance of triggers such as allergens or irritants can help prevent asthma attacks. Allergy medications or immunotherapy may also be recommended for children with allergic asthma.

- **Asthma Action Plan:** A written asthma action plan developed in collaboration with the child's healthcare provider helps parents and caregivers understand how to manage asthma symptoms and when to seek medical attention.
- **Monitoring:** Regular follow-up is important to monitor asthma control, adjust medication dosages as needed, and address any concerns or questions.

13.4. Allergic Rhinitis

> ➤ *Allergic rhinitis in children is an immune-mediated reaction to allergens, resulting in symptoms like sneezing, nasal congestion, itching, and watery eyes.*
>
> ➤ *It is commonly triggered by pollen, dust mites, pet dander, or mold spores and may impair sleep, school performance, and overall quality of life.*
>
> ➤ *Treatment involves allergen avoidance, antihistamines, intranasal corticosteroids, and allergy shots to alleviate symptoms and reduce allergic reactions.*

Symptoms:
- Sneezing
- Runny or stuffy nose
- Itchy nose, throat, or eyes
- Watery eyes
- Nasal congestion
- Coughing
- Fatigue or irritability due to disrupted sleep

Causes and Risk Factors:
- Family history: Children with a family history of allergic rhinitis or other allergic conditions are at higher risk.
- Environmental factors: Exposure to allergens such as pollen, dust mites, pet dander, mold, or air pollution can trigger allergic rhinitis.
- Age: Allergic rhinitis can develop at any age but is more common in school-age children and adolescents.
- Season: Depending on the type of allergen, symptoms may worsen during specific seasons, such as spring (pollen allergies) or winter (indoor allergens).

- Other allergic conditions: Children with asthma or atopic dermatitis are more likely to develop allergic rhinitis.

Epidemiology:

Allergic rhinitis is one of the most common chronic conditions in childhood, affecting approximately 10-20% of children worldwide. The prevalence of allergic rhinitis has been increasing in recent decades, particularly in urban areas and among socioeconomically disadvantaged populations. Seasonal allergic rhinitis tends to be more common in the spring and fall when pollen levels are higher.

Diagnosis:

- Medical History: The APh will ask about the child's symptoms, family history of allergic rhinitis or other allergic conditions, and any triggers that worsen symptoms.
- Physical Examination: The provider will examine the child's nose, throat, and eyes for signs of inflammation or allergic reactions.
- Allergy Testing: Skin prick testing or blood tests may be performed to identify specific allergens that trigger allergic rhinitis.
- Nasal Endoscopy: In some cases, nasal endoscopy may be performed to evaluate the nasal passages for signs of inflammation or obstruction.

Treatment:

- Allergen Avoidance: Identifying and avoiding triggers such as pollen, dust mites, pet dander, or mold can help reduce allergic rhinitis symptoms.
- Nasal Saline Irrigation: Rinsing the nasal passages with saline solution can help reduce nasal congestion and remove allergens.
- Antihistamines: Oral or nasal antihistamines are commonly used to relieve sneezing, itching, and runny nose associated with allergic rhinitis.
- Intranasal Corticosteroids: Prescription of over-the-counter nasal corticosteroid sprays are effective at reducing nasal inflammation and congestion in children with allergic rhinitis.
- Decongestants: Oral decongestants may be used for short-term relief of nasal congestion, but prolonged use can lead to rebound congestion and should be avoided.
- Immunotherapy: Allergy shots or sublingual immunotherapy may be recommended for children with severe allergic rhinitis who do not respond to other treatments.

Prevention:
- Reduce exposure to allergens: Keep windows closed during high pollen seasons, use air purifiers or filters, and regularly clean bedding to reduce exposure to dust mites and pet dander.
- Practice good hygiene: Encourage hand washing and avoid touching the face, especially after being outdoors.
- Monitor pollen counts: Check local pollen forecasts and try to limit outdoor activities on high pollen days.
- Consider allergy medications: Starting allergy medications before allergy season begins can help prevent symptoms from occurring or reduce their severity.

13.5. Dermatitis

> ➤ *Dermatitis, commonly known as eczema in children, is a chronic inflammatory skin condition characterized by dry, itchy, red, and inflamed patches.*
> ➤ *It often develops in infancy or early childhood and may be triggered by factors like genetics, allergens, irritants, or immune system dysregulation.*
> ➤ *Management involves moisturizers, topical corticosteroids, avoiding triggers, and identifying and treating underlying factors to control symptoms and prevent flare-ups.*

Symptoms:
- Itchy, red, or inflamed skin
- Dry, scaly, or cracked skin
- Rash, often with small bumps or blisters
- Thickened or leathery skin
- Discolored patches of skin
- Irritability or sleep disturbances due to itching
- Secondary infections due to scratching

Causes and Risk Factors:
- Family history: Children with a family history of eczema, asthma, or allergic rhinitis are at higher risk.
- Atopic predisposition: Eczema is commonly associated with other allergic conditions such as asthma and hay fever.

- Environmental factors: Exposure to irritants (e.g., harsh soaps, detergents, wool clothing), allergens (e.g., dust mites, pet dander, pollen), or dry conditions can trigger or exacerbate eczema symptoms.
- Immune system dysfunction: Abnormal immune responses may contribute to the development of eczema.
- Skin barrier dysfunction: Impaired skin barrier function, which may be due to genetic factors or environmental factors, can increase susceptibility to eczema.

Epidemiology:

Eczema is one of the most common skin conditions in children, affecting up to 20% of infants and young children. The prevalence of eczema has been increasing in recent decades, particularly in urban areas and developed countries. Eczema often begins in infancy, with symptoms typically improving as children get older. However, some children may continue to experience eczema into adulthood.

Diagnosis:

- Medical History: The APh will ask about the child's symptoms, family history of eczema or other allergic conditions, and any triggers that worsen symptoms.
- Physical Examination: The provider will examine the child's skin for signs of eczema, such as redness, inflammation, rash, or dryness.
- Skin Prick Testing or Allergy Testing: In some cases, allergy testing may be performed to identify specific allergens that trigger eczema flare-ups.
- Patch Testing: Patch testing may be recommended if contact dermatitis is suspected as a trigger for eczema symptoms.

Treatment:

- Moisturizers: Regular use of emollients or moisturizers helps to hydrate the skin and restore the skin barrier function.
- Topical Corticosteroids: Prescription or over-the-counter corticosteroid creams or ointments are used to reduce inflammation and itching during eczema flare-ups.
- Topical Calcineurin Inhibitors: Non-steroidal creams or ointments such as tacrolimus or pimecrolimus may be prescribed for children with moderate to severe eczema or for areas where corticosteroids cannot be used.

- **Avoidance of Triggers:** Identifying and avoiding triggers such as harsh soaps, detergents, fragrances, or allergens can help prevent eczema flare-ups.
- **Wet Wrap Therapy:** Wet wraps applied over moisturizers or topical medications can help hydrate the skin and reduce inflammation during severe eczema flare-ups.
- **Antihistamines:** Oral antihistamines may be used to relieve itching and improve sleep quality in children with eczema.
- **Immunomodulators:** In some cases, systemic immunomodulators such as cyclosporine or azathioprine may be prescribed for children with severe eczema that does not respond to other treatments.

Prevention:
- Maintain skin hydration: Use mild, fragrance-free moisturizers regularly to keep the skin hydrated and prevent dryness.
- Avoid irritants: Use gentle, hypoallergenic skincare products and avoid harsh soaps, detergents, or fabrics that may irritate the skin.
- Identify and avoid triggers: Keep a diary to identify triggers that worsen eczema symptoms and take steps to avoid them.
- Manage stress: Stress can exacerbate eczema symptoms, so finding stress-relief techniques such as mindfulness or relaxation exercises may be helpful for children with eczema.

13.6. Urinary Tract Infections

> ➤ *Urinary tract infections (UTIs) in children are bacterial infections affecting the kidneys, bladder, or urethra.*
> ➤ *Symptoms like fever, pain or burning during urination, abdominal pain, and increased urinary frequency may occur.*
> ➤ *Diagnosis involves urine tests, and treatment typically includes antibiotics tailored to the specific bacteria causing the infection, along with fluid intake and hygiene measures to prevent recurrence.*

Symptoms:
- Frequent urination
- Pain or burning sensation during urination
- Urgency to urinate
- Bedwetting or daytime accidents (in toilet-trained children)
- Foul-smelling or cloudy urine

- Abdominal or back pain
- Fever
- Irritability or fussiness (in infants)
- Poor feeding or decreased appetite (in infants)
- Vomiting or diarrhea (less common)

Causes and Risk Factors:

- Gender: Girls are more susceptible to UTIs than boys, especially during infancy and early childhood.
- Anatomical abnormalities: Structural abnormalities in the urinary tract, such as vesicoureteral reflux (VUR), ureteropelvic junction (UPJ) obstruction, or posterior urethral valves, increase the risk of UTIs.
- Urinary stasis: Conditions that prevent complete bladder emptying, such as constipation or dysfunctional voiding, can lead to urinary stasis and increase the risk of UTIs.
- Catheterization: Indwelling urinary catheters or instrumentation of the urinary tract increase the risk of UTIs.
- Immune system disorders: Children with conditions that weaken the immune system, such as diabetes or immunodeficiency disorders, are at higher risk of UTIs.
- Urinary retention: Incomplete bladder emptying due to neurogenic bladder dysfunction or bladder outlet obstruction can lead to UTIs.
- Poor toilet hygiene: Inadequate wiping technique or improper hygiene practices can introduce bacteria into the urinary tract and increase the risk of UTIs.

Epidemiology:

UTIs are common in children, with an estimated 8% of girls and 2% of boys experiencing at least one UTI by the age of 7 years. The incidence of UTIs is highest during infancy and early childhood, with a peak incidence between 2 months and 2 years of age. Recurrent UTIs are also common in children, particularly in those with underlying risk factors such as VUR or anatomical abnormalities.

Diagnosis:

- <u>Urinalysis:</u> A urine dipstick test or microscopic examination of urine can detect the presence of white blood cells, red blood cells, or bacteria in the urine, suggestive of a UTI.
- <u>Urine Culture:</u> to identify the specific bacteria causing the UTI and determine the appropriate antibiotic treatment

- Imaging Studies: Renal ultrasound, voiding cystourethrogram (VCUG), or dimercaptosuccinic acid (DMSA) scan may be performed to evaluate for structural abnormalities or VUR in children with recurrent UTIs or atypical presentations.
- Clinical Evaluation: The APh will perform a physical examination and evaluate the child's symptoms, including fever, abdominal or back pain, and urinary symptoms.

Treatment:

- Antibiotics: Oral antibiotics are the mainstay of treatment for UTIs in children.
    - The choice of antibiotic depends on the child's age, the severity of symptoms, and the results of urine culture and sensitivity testing. Commonly prescribed oral antibiotics include Amoxicillin-clavulanate, Trimethoprim-sulfamethoxazole (TMP-SMX), and Cephalexin.
    - Treatment duration can vary from 7 to 14 days. The APh should educate the child and parents to ensure the child completes the entire course of antibiotics to fully eradicate the infection and prevent resistance.
- Hydration: Encourage adequate fluid intake to help flush bacteria from the urinary tract and prevent dehydration.
- Symptomatic Relief: Over-the-counter pain relievers such as acetaminophen or ibuprofen may be used to alleviate fever, pain, or discomfort associated with UTIs.
- Follow-up: Children with UTIs should be followed up with their healthcare provider to monitor response to treatment, ensure resolution of symptoms, and assess for recurrence or complications.

13.7. Febrile Seizures

> ➤ *Febrile seizures in children are convulsions that occur during a fever, often between 6 months and 5 years old, typically lasting less than 5 minutes and rarely causing long-term complications.*
>
> ➤ *They may be frightening but usually do not indicate a serious underlying condition.*
>
> ➤ *Management involves fever control and reassurance, with further evaluation if seizure characteristics or associated symptoms raise concerns.*

Symptoms:
- Seizure activity during or shortly after a fever
- Loss of consciousness
- Muscle twitching or jerking movements
- Stiffening of the body
- Rolling or turning of the eyes
- Involuntary urination or defecation (less common)
- Postictal confusion or sleepiness

Causes and Risk Factors:
- Age: Febrile seizures most commonly occur in children between the ages of 6 months and 5 years, with a peak incidence between 12 and 18 months.
- Family history: Children with a family history of febrile seizures or epilepsy are at higher risk of experiencing febrile seizures themselves.
- Fever triggers: Rapidly rising body temperature, particularly due to viral infections such as influenza or upper respiratory tract infections, can trigger febrile seizures.
- Developmental delays: Children with developmental delays or neurological disorders may have an increased risk of febrile seizures.
- Previous febrile seizures: Children who have experienced one febrile seizure are at higher risk of recurrence with subsequent febrile illnesses.

Epidemiology:

Febrile seizures are the most common type of seizures in children, occurring in approximately 2-5% of children between the ages of 6 months and 5 years. Febrile seizures are more common in boys than girls and tend to occur during the first 24 hours of fever, particularly with rapid temperature elevation.

Diagnosis:
- <u>Clinical Evaluation:</u> The diagnosis of febrile seizures is based on a thorough clinical history and physical examination. The APh will assess the child's symptoms, including the presence of fever and seizure activity.
- <u>Laboratory Tests:</u> Complete blood count (CBC) and blood cultures may be performed to evaluate for underlying infection or systemic illness contributing to the fever.

- Imaging Studies: Brain magnetic resonance imaging (MRI) or computed tomography (CT) may be indicated if there are concerns about structural brain abnormalities or other underlying neurological conditions.

Treatment:

- Management of Fever:

    The primary goal of treatment for febrile seizures is to manage the underlying fever. Fever-reducing medications such as acetaminophen (Tylenol) or ibuprofen (Advil, Motrin) may be used to lower the child's body temperature.

- Seizure Management:

    During a febrile seizure, it is important to ensure the safety of the child and protect them from injury. Place the child on a soft surface away from any hazards and gently roll them onto their side to prevent choking. Do not restrain the child's movements or put anything in their mouth.

- Medical Evaluation:

    Children who experience febrile seizures should be evaluated by a healthcare provider to determine the underlying cause of the fever and assess for any complications. Further management and follow-up care will depend on the child's clinical condition and any underlying medical issues.

13.8. Bronchitis

> *Bronchitis in children is an inflammation of the bronchial tubes, typically caused by viral infections, leading to coughing, wheezing, chest discomfort, and sometimes fever.*
>
> *It is often self-limiting and resolves within a few weeks without specific treatment.*
>
> *Management focusing on symptom relief, hydration, rest, and monitoring for complications such as pneumonia.*

Symptoms:

- Cough, which may produce clear, yellow, green, or sometimes blood-tinged mucus
- Wheezing or difficulty breathing
- Chest congestion or tightness

- Sore throat
- Runny or stuffy nose
- Mild fever
- Fatigue or irritability
- Decreased appetite
- Muscle aches

Causes and Risk Factors:

- Exposure to respiratory viruses: Viral infections are the most common cause of acute bronchitis in children. Children who are in close contact with patients who have respiratory infections, such as colds or flu, are at higher risk.
- Age: Young children, particularly those under the age of 5, are more susceptible to bronchitis due to their developing immune systems and smaller airways.
- Exposure to irritants: Exposure to tobacco smoke, air pollution, or other environmental irritants can increase the risk of bronchitis in children.
- Underlying respiratory conditions: Asthma or cystic fibrosis may cause higher risk of developing bronchitis.

Epidemiology:

Bronchitis is a common respiratory condition in children, especially during the colder months of the year when respiratory viruses are more prevalent. It is estimated that acute bronchitis accounts for a significant number of pediatric outpatient visits and missed school days each year.

Diagnosis:

- <u>Clinical Evaluation:</u> The diagnosis of bronchitis in children is based on a thorough clinical history and physical examination. The APh will assess the child's symptoms, including cough, fever, and respiratory distress.
- <u>Chest Auscultation:</u> Listening to the child's lungs with a stethoscope may reveal wheezing or crackles, which are common findings in bronchitis.
- <u>Laboratory Tests:</u> In most cases, blood tests or imaging studies are not necessary for diagnosing bronchitis. However, if there are concerns about a bacterial infection or other underlying condition, the healthcare provider may order additional tests.

Treatment:
- Supportive Care: The primary treatment for acute bronchitis in children is supportive care to relieve symptoms and help the child feel more comfortable. This may include rest, adequate hydration, and over-the-counter medications such as acetaminophen or ibuprofen to reduce fever and alleviate discomfort.
- Humidification: Using a cool mist humidifier or taking steamy showers can help loosen mucus and ease chest congestion.
- Cough Management: Cough suppressants are generally not recommended for children, especially those under the age of 6, as they can have side effects and may not be effective. However, honey can be given to children over the age of 1 to help soothe cough symptoms.
- Avoiding Irritants: It is important to minimize exposure to tobacco smoke and other respiratory irritants that can exacerbate bronchitis symptoms.
- Antibiotics: Antibiotics are not usually recommended for acute bronchitis, as it is typically caused by viral infections. However, if the healthcare provider suspects a bacterial infection or if symptoms persist or worsen, they may prescribe antibiotics.

13.9. Croup

> ➢ Croup is a common childhood respiratory condition caused by viral infections, characterized by a barking cough, stridor, hoarseness, and respiratory distress.
> ➢ It primarily affects infants and young children, typically resolves within a few days.
> ➢ Management involves humidified air, hydration, and sometimes oral corticosteroids or nebulized epinephrine for severe cases.

Symptoms:
- Barking cough: Croup typically begins with a harsh, barking cough that may resemble the sound of a seal or a dog.
- Stridor: A high-pitched or musical sound heard when the child breathes in, which can be particularly noticeable when the child is crying or agitated.
- Hoarseness: The child's voice may become hoarse or raspy.

- **Difficulty breathing:** In severe cases, the child may have difficulty breathing or may exhibit retractions (visible pulling in of the chest wall) with each breath.
- **Fever:** Some children with croup may develop a low-grade fever.

Causes and Risk Factors:
- **Age:** Croup is most common in children between the ages of 6 months and 3 years, although it can occur in older children as well.
- **Season:** Croup tends to occur more frequently during the fall and winter months, coinciding with the peak season for viral respiratory infections.
- **Exposure to respiratory viruses:** Croup is often caused by viral infections, particularly the parainfluenza virus. Children who are in close contact with patients who have respiratory infections are at higher risk.
- **Medical history:** Children who have had croup in the past may be more susceptible to recurrent episodes.

Epidemiology:

Croup is a common respiratory condition in children, particularly in those under the age of 5. It is estimated that croup accounts for a significant number of pediatric emergency department visits and hospitalizations each year, especially during the fall and winter months when viral respiratory infections are more prevalent.

Diagnosis:
- <u>Clinical Evaluation:</u> The diagnosis of croup is based on a thorough clinical history and physical examination. The APh will assess the child's symptoms, including the characteristic barking cough, stridor, and hoarseness.
- <u>Assessment of Respiratory Distress:</u> The provider will evaluate the child's breathing, looking for signs of respiratory distress such as retractions, nasal flaring, and increased work of breathing.
- <u>Additional Tests:</u> In most cases, imaging studies or laboratory tests are not necessary for diagnosing croup. However, if the child's symptoms are severe or if there are concerns about complications, the healthcare provider may order a chest X-ray or other tests.

Treatment:
- <u>Humidified Air:</u> Breathing in humidified air from a cool mist humidifier or a steamy bathroom can help soothe the child's airways and reduce inflammation.

- **Encouraging Fluids:** can help prevent dehydration and keep the airways moist
- **Corticosteroids:** Oral or inhaled corticosteroids, such as dexamethasone or budesonide, are commonly used to reduce airway inflammation and improve symptoms in children with moderate to severe croup.
- **Nebulized Epinephrine:** may be used in severe cases of croup to quickly reduce airway swelling and improve breathing
- **Observation:** In most cases, children with mild croup can be managed at home with supportive care and close observation. However, children with severe symptoms or signs of respiratory distress may require hospitalization for further evaluation and treatment.

13.10. Constipation

> *Constipation in children involves infrequent bowel movements, hard stools, and difficulty passing stool, often leading to abdominal pain or discomfort.*
>
> *Causes may include dietary factors, dehydration, lack of physical activity, or underlying medical conditions.*
>
> *Management typically involves dietary changes, increased fluid intake, fiber supplementation, and behavioral modifications to promote regular bowel movements.*

Symptoms:
- Infrequent bowel movements: Children with constipation typically have bowel movements less frequently than usual.
- Difficulty passing stool: Children may experience pain or straining during bowel movements.
- Hard or dry stools: Stools may be hard, dry, or difficult to pass.
- Abdominal pain or discomfort: Children with constipation may complain of abdominal pain or discomfort.
- Stool withholding: Some children may withhold stool, leading to fecal impaction or soiling (encopresis).
- Loss of appetite or irritability: Constipated children may experience loss of appetite or irritability.

Causes and Risk Factors:
- Diet: A diet low in fiber and fluids can contribute to constipation in children.
- Lack of physical activity: Sedentary behavior and lack of physical activity can lead to constipation.
- Toilet training: Children who are in the process of toilet training may withhold stool, leading to constipation.
- Medical conditions: Certain medical conditions such as hypothyroidism, Hirschsprung's disease, or irritable bowel syndrome may predispose children to constipation.
- Medications: Some medications, such as certain pain medications or iron supplements, can cause constipation as a side effect.
- Family history: Children with a family history of constipation may be more likely to experience the condition.

Epidemiology:

Constipation is a common gastrointestinal problem in children, affecting up to 30% of pediatric patients. It is one of the most common reasons for pediatric gastroenterology consultations and outpatient visits.

Diagnosis:
- Clinical Evaluation: The diagnosis of constipation is based on a thorough clinical history and physical examination. The APh will assess the child's symptoms, dietary habits, and toilet habits.
- Stool Examination: Stool examination may be performed to rule out underlying conditions such as infections or malabsorption.
- Imaging Studies: Abdominal X-rays or anorectal manometry may be performed to evaluate the severity of constipation and assess for structural abnormalities.
- Blood tests: to check for underlying medical conditions that may be contributing to constipation

Treatment:
- Dietary Modifications: Increasing dietary fiber intake by incorporating fruits, vegetables, whole grains, and legumes into the child's diet can help promote regular bowel movements. Adequate fluid intake is also essential.
- Toilet Training: Establishing a regular toilet routine and encouraging the child to sit on the toilet after meals can help prevent stool withholding and promote regular bowel movements.

- **Medications:** Laxatives or stool softeners may be prescribed to help relieve constipation in children with severe symptoms or chronic constipation.
- **Behavioral Therapy:** Positive reinforcement and toilet training may be used to help children overcome stool withholding behaviors.
- **Regular Physical Activity:** can help promote bowel regularity
- **Education and Support:** Providing education and support to parents and caregivers about the importance of bowel habits, dietary habits, and toilet training techniques can help manage and prevent constipation in children.

13.11. Diarrhea

> ➢ *Diarrhea in children is characterized by loose or watery stools occurring more frequently than usual, often accompanied by abdominal pain, cramps, fever, or vomiting.*
>
> ➢ *It is commonly caused by viral or bacterial infections, food intolerance, or changes in diet.*
>
> ➢ *Management involves fluid and electrolyte replacement, continued feeding, and monitoring for signs of dehydration or complications.*

Symptoms:
- Frequent, loose, or watery stools: Diarrhea is characterized by an increase in the frequency, looseness, or watery consistency of stools.
- Abdominal pain or cramping
- Fever: especially if the diarrhea is caused by an infection
- Nausea and vomiting
- Dehydration: may manifest as decreased urination, dry mouth, sunken eyes, or lethargy
- Blood or mucus in stool

Causes and Risk Factors:
- Contaminated food or water: Consumption of contaminated food or water, especially in areas with poor sanitation, increases the risk of infectious diarrhea.
- Poor hygiene: Inadequate handwashing and poor hygiene practices can contribute to the spread of diarrheal illnesses.
- Exposure to infectious agents: Children who are exposed to bacteria, viruses, or parasites are at increased risk of developing diarrhea.

- Medical conditions: Certain medical conditions such as inflammatory bowel disease (IBD), lactose intolerance, or celiac disease may predispose children to diarrhea.
- Medications: Some medications, such as antibiotics or nonsteroidal anti-inflammatory drugs (NSAIDs), can cause diarrhea as a side effect.
- Travel: Traveling to regions with poor sanitation or inadequate access to clean water increases the risk of traveler's diarrhea.

Epidemiology:

Diarrhea is a common gastrointestinal problem in children worldwide, particularly in developing countries. It is one of the leading causes of morbidity and mortality in children under the age of five, especially in resource-limited settings.

Diagnosis:
- Clinical Evaluation: The diagnosis of diarrhea is primarily based on a thorough clinical history and physical examination. The APh will assess the child's symptoms, including the duration, frequency, and consistency of stools.
- Stool Examination: Stool culture, microscopy, or antigen testing may be performed to check for the presence of infectious agents such as bacteria, viruses, or parasites.
- Blood Tests: to assess for signs of dehydration or electrolyte imbalances
- Imaging Studies: Abdominal X-rays or ultrasound may be performed to evaluate for underlying causes of diarrhea, such as bowel obstruction or inflammation.

Treatment:
- Fluid Replacement:

    The cornerstone of diarrhea treatment in children is fluid replacement to prevent or correct dehydration. Oral rehydration solutions (ORS) containing electrolytes and glucose are recommended for mild to moderate dehydration.

- Nutritional Support:

    Children with diarrhea should continue to eat a normal diet if possible. Breastfeeding should be continued in infants, and formula-fed infants should receive their usual feeds. Avoiding certain foods or beverages that may exacerbate diarrhea, such as sugary drinks or fatty foods, may be beneficial.

- Medications:
    In some cases, antimicrobial medications may be prescribed for bacterial or parasitic causes of diarrhea. However, antibiotics are not routinely recommended for viral diarrhea. Antidiarrheal medications such as loperamide may be used in older children with persistent diarrhea, but they are not recommended for use in young children or in cases of bloody diarrhea.
- Prevention: Handwashing, safe food and water practices, and vaccination against rotavirus (where available) can help reduce the risk of diarrhea in children.

13.12. Conjunctivitis

> ➢ *Conjunctivitis, or pink eye, in children is inflammation of the conjunctiva, causing redness, itching, discharge, and sometimes blurred vision or sensitivity to light.*
> ➢ *It can be viral, bacterial, or allergic in origin, spreading easily through contact.*
> ➢ *Treatment involves symptom relief with warm compresses, eye drops, and proper hygiene practices to prevent spread and complications.*

Symptoms:
- Redness: The whites of the eyes may appear red or pink.
- Eye discharge: Children with conjunctivitis may have discharge from one or both eyes. The discharge can vary in consistency and color, ranging from clear and watery to thick and yellow or green.
- Itchiness or irritation: The affected eye(s) may feel itchy, irritated, or gritty.
- Swelling: Swelling of the eyelids or conjunctiva (the thin, transparent membrane covering the white part of the eye) may occur.
- Tearing: Excessive tearing or watering of the eyes may be present.
- Crusting: In cases of bacterial conjunctivitis, crusts or scales may form on the eyelashes, especially upon waking in the morning.
- Sensitivity to light: Children with conjunctivitis may experience sensitivity to light (photophobia).

Causes and Risk Factors:
- Viral or bacterial infection: Conjunctivitis can be caused by viral or bacterial infections, which can be easily spread in settings such as daycare centers or schools.
- Allergies: Allergic conjunctivitis may occur in children with allergies to pollen, dust mites, pet dander, or other environmental allergens.
- Contact with irritants: Exposure to irritants such as smoke, chemicals, or chlorine in swimming pools may trigger non-infectious conjunctivitis.
- Close contact: Close contact with an infected patient, such as through touching or sharing personal items like towels or pillowcases, increases the risk of acquiring infectious conjunctivitis.
- Poor hygiene: Poor hand hygiene or inadequate cleaning of contact lenses can contribute to the transmission of infectious conjunctivitis.

Epidemiology:

Conjunctivitis is a common eye condition in children, with viral and bacterial forms being the most prevalent. The condition can affect children of all ages but is particularly common in school-aged children and those attending daycare centers.

Diagnosis:
- Clinical Examination: Diagnosis of conjunctivitis is primarily based on clinical signs and symptoms observed during a physical examination of the eyes.
- Medical History: The APh may inquire about recent exposure to infectious patients, environmental allergens, or irritants.
- Eye Swab: In cases of severe or persistent conjunctivitis, a swab of the conjunctival discharge may be taken for laboratory analysis to identify the causative organism (bacterial or viral).
- Allergy Testing: may be recommended in cases of suspected allergic conjunctivitis to identify specific allergens triggering the symptoms

Treatment:
- Viral Conjunctivitis:

    Most cases of viral conjunctivitis are self-limiting and resolve on their own without specific treatment. Supportive measures such as applying warm compresses to the eyes and using artificial tears may help alleviate symptoms. Antiviral medications may be prescribed in severe or prolonged cases.

- Bacterial Conjunctivitis:

    Antibiotic eye drops or ointments are often prescribed for bacterial conjunctivitis to help shorten the duration of symptoms and reduce the risk of transmission to others. Proper hygiene practices, such as frequent handwashing and avoiding touching the eyes, are important to prevent the spread of infection.

- Allergic Conjunctivitis:

    Avoiding allergens whenever possible and using antihistamine eye drops or oral medications can help manage symptoms of allergic conjunctivitis. Cold compresses may provide relief from itchiness and swelling.

13.13. Strep Throat

> ➤ Strep throat in children is a bacterial infection of the throat and tonsils caused by group A Streptococcus bacteria, presenting with sore throat, fever, difficulty swallowing, and swollen lymph nodes.
>
> ➤ Diagnosis is confirmed through throat swab testing.
>
> ➤ Treatment involves antibiotics to prevent complications like rheumatic fever or kidney inflammation, along with pain relief measures to alleviate symptoms.

Symptoms:

- Sore throat: Children with strep throat typically experience a sore throat that can be moderate to severe and may worsen with swallowing.
- Fever and chills
- Red and swollen tonsils: The tonsils may appear red, swollen, and may have white or yellow patches or streaks of pus.
- Dysphagia: Pain or discomfort while swallowing may occur due to the inflamed throat.
- Swollen lymph nodes: may be palpable in the neck
- Headache: Children with strep throat may experience headaches, often accompanying the fever.
- Abdominal pain: Some children may complain of stomach pain or nausea, especially younger children.

- Rash: In some cases, children with strep throat may develop a rash known as scarlet fever, characterized by a red rash that feels like sandpaper and may start on the neck and chest before spreading to the rest of the body.

Causes and Risk Factors:
- Age: Strep throat can affect children of all ages, but it is more common in school-aged children between 5 and 15 years old.
- Close contact: Exposure to an infected person, particularly in crowded environments such as schools or daycare centers, increases the risk of contracting strep throat.
- Weakened immune system: Children with weakened immune systems due to underlying medical conditions or recent illness may be more susceptible to strep throat.
- Season: Strep throat tends to occur more frequently during the fall and winter months.
- Poor hygiene: Poor hand hygiene and sharing of utensils, cups, or towels with an infected patient can contribute to the spread of strep throat.

Epidemiology:

Strep throat is a common bacterial infection, particularly among school-aged children. Group A Streptococcus (GAS) bacteria are the most common cause of strep throat, accounting for approximately 15-30% of sore throats in children. The infection can occur throughout the year but tends to peak during the school year when close contact among children is more common.

Strep Infection Risk Score

The Centor Score is a clinical tool used to assess the probability of streptococcal pharyngitis in patients presenting with sore throat.
- Presence of Fever: Assigns 1 point if the patient has a documented fever.
- Tonsillar Exudates: Assigns 1 point if there are visible white or yellow patches on the tonsils.
- Tender Anterior Cervical Lymphadenopathy: Assigns one 1 if there are tender lymph nodes in the anterior cervical region.
- Absence of Cough: Assigns 1 point if the patient reports no cough.

The Centor Score ranges from 0 to 4, with higher scores indicating a higher likelihood of streptococcal infection.

Diagnosis:
- Throat Swab: A sample from the back of the throat is tested for the presence of Group A Streptococcus bacteria using rapid antigen tests or culture methods.
- Physical Examination: The APh will examine the child's throat and tonsils for signs of inflammation, redness, swelling, and the presence of pus.
- Medical History: The APh may inquire about the child's symptoms, recent exposure to strep throat, and any underlying medical conditions.

Treatment:
- Antibiotics:
  - If strep throat is confirmed by a positive throat swab, treatment typically involves a course of oral antibiotics, such as penicillin or amoxicillin, to eliminate the bacteria and prevent complications.
  - Applying Centor Score is used to help guide the decision whether to prescribe antibiotics for patients:
    - Centor Score of 0 or 1: Antibiotics are generally not recommended due to the low likelihood of streptococcal infection.
    - Centor Score of 2 or 3: Antibiotics may be considered in certain cases, especially if the patient has additional risk factors for streptococcal infection or if there's high suspicion based on clinical judgment.
    - Centor Score of 4: Antibiotics are often recommended, as the likelihood of streptococcal infection is higher.
- Symptom relief: Over-the-counter pain relievers such as ibuprofen or acetaminophen can help alleviate pain, fever, and discomfort associated with strep throat. Gargling with warm salt water or using throat lozenges may also provide relief for sore throat symptoms.
- Rest and hydration: to support the body's recovery process
- Isolation: Infected children should stay home from school or daycare until at least 24 hours after starting antibiotic treatment to prevent spreading the infection to others.

13.14. Acute Gastroenteritis

> ➢ *Acute gastroenteritis in children is a common condition characterized by diarrhea, vomiting, abdominal pain, and fever.*
>
> ➢ *It is usually caused by viral infections such as rotavirus or norovirus.*
>
> ➢ *It is typically self-limiting, managed with supportive care including oral rehydration solutions, fluid intake, and symptomatic treatment, with antibiotics reserved for specific cases such as bacterial gastroenteritis.*

Symptoms:
- Diarrhea: Watery or loose stools are the hallmark symptom of acute gastroenteritis. Diarrhea may be accompanied by abdominal cramps and urgency.
- Vomiting: Children with acute gastroenteritis may experience vomiting, which can range from mild to severe and may lead to dehydration.
- Fever: Low-grade fever is common in children with gastroenteritis, although some may develop a higher fever.
- Abdominal pain: Children may experience generalized abdominal discomfort or cramping.
- Nausea: Some children may feel nauseous or have a loss of appetite.
- Dehydration: Signs of dehydration may include dry mouth, sunken eyes, decreased urine output, lethargy, and irritability.
- Fatigue: Children may feel tired or weak due to fluid loss and electrolyte imbalances.

Causes and Risk Factors:
- Age: Infants and young children are at a higher risk of developing acute gastroenteritis due to their immature immune systems and frequent hand-to-mouth behaviors.
- Exposure: Close contact with infected patients, contaminated food or water, or exposure to contaminated surfaces increases the risk of gastroenteritis.
- Poor hygiene: Lack of proper handwashing, especially after using the toilet or changing diapers, can facilitate the spread of gastroenteritis-causing pathogens.
- Crowded environments: Settings such as daycare centers, schools, and childcare facilities where children are in close proximity increase the risk of transmission.

- Travel: Traveling to regions with poor sanitation or hygiene practices may increase the risk of acquiring gastroenteritis.

Epidemiology:

Acute gastroenteritis is a common illness in children worldwide, with millions of cases reported each year. Viral pathogens, such as rotavirus and norovirus, are among the leading causes of acute gastroenteritis in children, particularly in infants and young children. Bacterial pathogens, including Salmonella, Escherichia coli, and Campylobacter, may also cause gastroenteritis, especially in older children. The condition can occur at any time of the year but is more prevalent during the winter months.

Diagnosis:

- Clinical Assessment: The APh typically diagnoses acute gastroenteritis based on the child's clinical presentation, including symptoms such as diarrhea, vomiting, and fever, along with a history of recent illness or exposure.
- Stool Sample Analysis: In some cases, a stool sample may be collected and analyzed to identify the causative pathogen, especially if the illness is severe, persistent, or if there are concerns about bacterial or parasitic infections.

Treatment:

- Fluid Replacement:

    The primary goal of treatment for acute gastroenteritis in children is to prevent dehydration by replacing lost fluids and electrolytes. Oral rehydration solutions (ORS) containing electrolytes and glucose are recommended for mild to moderate dehydration.

- Nutritional Support:

    Children should continue to breastfeed or receive formula feeds if tolerated. For older children, a bland diet including crackers, rice, bananas, and toast (BRAT diet) may help ease symptoms.

- Medications:

    Antidiarrheal medications are generally not recommended for children with acute gastroenteritis, as they may prolong the illness or lead to complications. However, antiemetic medications may be prescribed to alleviate severe vomiting in some cases.

- Monitoring:

    Parents should monitor their child's symptoms closely, including fluid intake, urine output, and signs of dehydration or worsening symptoms. Seek medical attention if dehydration or other concerning symptoms develop.

13.15. Sinusitis

> Sinusitis in children is inflammation of the sinuses often caused by viral infections, leading to symptoms like nasal congestion, facial pain, headache, and coughing.
>
> Bacterial sinusitis may develop from viral infections, and symptoms lasting more than 10 days may require antibiotics.
>
> Treatment mainly involves symptomatic relief, saline nasal irrigation, and adequate hydration to promote recovery.

Symptoms:

- Nasal congestion: difficulty breathing through the nose due to blockage
- Nasal discharge: thick, discolored nasal discharge
- Cough: often worsens at night or upon waking
- Facial pain or pressure: Pain or pressure may be felt in the forehead, cheeks, or around the eyes.
- Headache: especially if sinus pressure is significant
- Fever: Low-grade fever may occur, particularly with bacterial sinusitis.
- Bad breath
- Fatigue: Children may feel tired or irritable, especially if symptoms disrupt sleep.

Causes and Risk Factors:

- Viral infections: Common colds and other respiratory viruses can lead to sinusitis.
- Allergies: Allergic rhinitis can increase the risk of developing sinusitis.
- Anatomic factors: Structural abnormalities of the nose or sinuses, such as nasal polyps or deviated septum, can predispose children to sinusitis.
- Immune system disorders: Conditions that weaken the immune system, such as HIV/AIDS or certain medications, can increase susceptibility to sinus infections.

Epidemiology:

Sinusitis is relatively common in children, with viral upper respiratory infections being the most common cause. Bacterial sinusitis, while less common, can occur as a complication of viral infections or as a primary bacterial infection. Sinusitis can affect children of all ages, but it's more prevalent in school-aged children.

Diagnosis:

- Clinical Assessment: The diagnosis of sinusitis is primarily based on the child's clinical presentation. The APh will take note if there is:
    - Persistence of symptoms for more than 10 days without improvement.
    - Severe symptoms (e.g., fever ≥ 102°F, purulent nasal discharge) persisting for at least 3 consecutive days.
    - Worsening symptoms following initial improvement ("double sickening").
- Physical examination: The APh will examine for findings consistent with sinusitis, such as sinus tenderness or purulent nasal discharge.
- Imaging studies: Sinus X-rays or CT scans, are not routinely recommended for diagnosing uncomplicated cases of acute sinusitis in children.

Treatment:

- Supportive care: Treatment for sinusitis in children often involves supportive measures to alleviate symptoms and promote comfort. This may include:
    - Nasal saline irrigation or sprays to help relieve nasal congestion
    - Humidification to keep the air moist, especially during dry weather
    - Pain relievers such as acetaminophen or ibuprofen to alleviate discomfort and reduce fever
- Antibiotics:

    Antibiotics may be prescribed for children with bacterial sinusitis or those at risk of complications. The choice of antibiotic depends on the child's age, severity of symptoms, and suspected bacterial pathogens. Amoxicillin is commonly used as the first-line antibiotic for uncomplicated cases.

- **Decongestants:** Oral or topical decongestants may be used to help relieve nasal congestion, but they should be used with caution in children due to the risk of side effects and rebound congestion.
- **Nasal Corticosteroids:** Intranasal corticosteroid sprays may be beneficial in children with allergic rhinitis or chronic sinusitis to reduce inflammation and symptoms.
- **Surgery:** In rare cases of chronic or recurrent sinusitis that does not respond to medical treatment, surgical intervention such as adenoidectomy or sinus surgery may be considered.

13.16. Hand, Foot, and Mouth Disease

> ➤ *Hand, Foot, and Mouth Disease (HFMD) is a common viral infection in children caused by Coxsackievirus or Enterovirus, presenting with fever, sore throat, and characteristic blisters or sores on the hands, feet, and inside the mouth.*
>
> ➤ *It spreads through respiratory droplets or contact with contaminated surfaces, typically resolves within a week without specific treatment.*
>
> ➤ *Management focuses on relieving symptoms and preventing dehydration.*

Symptoms:
- Fever: HFMD often begins with a mild fever, usually below 101°F (38.3°C).
- Sore throat: Painful sores may develop in the mouth, making swallowing uncomfortable.
- Rash: Small, red spots or tiny blisters may appear on the palms of hands, soles of feet, and sometimes on the buttocks. The rash may be accompanied by mild itching.
- Irritability: Due to discomfort caused by the sores in the mouth and throat, children may become irritable.
- Loss of appetite: Painful mouth sores can lead to decreased appetite and difficulty eating or drinking.

Causes and Risk Factors:
- Age: Children under 5 years old, particularly those under 2, are most commonly affected by HFMD.
- Exposure: HFMD spreads through close contact with infected patients, as well as contact with contaminated surfaces or objects.

Epidemiology:

HFMD is caused by various enteroviruses, most commonly Coxsackievirus A16 and Enterovirus 71. It's a highly contagious disease, with outbreaks often occurring in childcare settings, schools, and other crowded environments. While it can happen at any time of the year, it's more prevalent in late summer and early fall.

Diagnosis:

- Clinical Assessment: Diagnosis of HFMD is typically based on clinical symptoms. The APh may also conduct a physical examination to identify characteristic skin lesions and mouth sores.
- Laboratory Tests: Viral cultures or polymerase chain reaction (PCR) tests may be performed in severe cases or outbreaks to confirm the presence of the virus.

Treatment:

There is no specific treatment for HFMD, as it's a viral illness that typically resolves on its own within 7-10 days. Treatment focuses on relieving symptoms and providing comfort to the affected child:

- Pain Relief: Over-the-counter pain relievers such as acetaminophen or ibuprofen can help reduce fever and alleviate discomfort caused by mouth sores.
- Hydration: Encourage the child to drink plenty of fluids to prevent dehydration, especially if they have difficulty swallowing due to mouth sores.
- Topical Treatments: Oral rinses or sprays containing anesthetic agents can provide temporary relief from mouth pain.
- Rest: Ensure the child gets adequate rest to support their immune system in fighting off the infection.

Prevention:

- Hand hygiene: Regular handwashing with soap and water is crucial in preventing the spread of HFMD.
- Disinfection: Clean and disinfect frequently touched surfaces and toys, especially in childcare settings.
- Isolation: Keep infected children home from school or daycare until they are no longer contagious, typically until the fever resolves and mouth sores have healed.

13.17. Pediatric Obesity

> ➤ *Pediatric obesity is a chronic condition characterized by excessive body fat accumulation in children and adolescents, often resulting from a combination of genetic, environmental, and lifestyle factors.*
>
> ➤ *It increases the risk of various health problems such as type 2 diabetes, hypertension, and cardiovascular disease.*
>
> ➤ *It requires comprehensive management strategies including dietary modifications, increased physical activity, behavioral changes, and, in some cases, medical intervention to promote healthy weight management and prevent long-term complications.*

Symptoms:

- Increased body weight: Children with obesity have a body mass index (BMI) above the 95th percentile for their age and sex.
- Excess body fat: visible signs of excess body fat, such as a protruding abdomen or thickened waist circumference
- Physical symptoms: shortness of breath, joint pain, or fatigue during physical activity
- Psychosocial effects: Pediatric obesity can also impact mental health, leading to low self-esteem, depression, or social isolation.

Causes and Risk Factors:

- Unhealthy diet: Consuming high-calorie, low-nutrient foods and beverages, such as fast food, sugary drinks, and processed snacks, increases the risk of obesity.
- Sedentary lifestyle: Lack of physical activity and excessive screen time contribute to weight gain and obesity.
- Genetics: Genetic factors can influence a child's susceptibility to obesity.
- Family factors: Environmental factors within the family, such as parental obesity, socioeconomic status, and cultural norms around diet and physical activity, can contribute to pediatric obesity.
- Medical conditions: Certain medical conditions or medications may increase the risk of weight gain and obesity in children.

Epidemiology:

Pediatric obesity has become a significant public health concern worldwide. According to the World Health Organization (WHO), the prevalence of obesity among children and adolescents has increased dramatically over the past few decades. It's estimated that over 340 million children and adolescents aged 5-19 were overweight or obese globally in 2016.

Diagnosis:

Diagnosis of pediatric obesity is based on measurements of body weight and height to calculate BMI, followed by interpretation using growth charts specific to age and sex. The APh may also assess other factors such as family history, dietary habits, physical activity levels, and any underlying medical conditions.

Treatment:

- Lifestyle modifications: The cornerstone of pediatric obesity treatment involves implementing healthy lifestyle changes, including:
    - Dietary changes: encouraging a balanced diet rich in fruits, vegetables, whole grains, and lean proteins while limiting high-calorie, low-nutrient foods
    - Increased physical activity: promoting regular physical activity through activities that children enjoy, such as sports, outdoor play, or recreational activities
    - Limiting screen time: reducing sedentary behaviors, such as excessive screen time (e.g., television, video games, smartphones, computers)
- Behavioral Interventions: Behavioral therapy and counseling may help children and families adopt and maintain healthy lifestyle habits.
- Medical Management: In some cases, The APP may consider pharmacological interventions, such as medications to help with weight loss or management of comorbid conditions.
- Multidisciplinary Approach:

    Treatment of pediatric obesity often involves a multidisciplinary team of healthcare professionals, including pediatricians, dietitians, psychologists, and exercise physiologists, to provide comprehensive care and support.

- Prevention:

    Prevention efforts are crucial in addressing pediatric obesity. This includes promoting breastfeeding, encouraging healthy eating habits from an early age, promoting physical activity in schools and communities, and creating supportive environments for healthy lifestyle behaviors.

13.18. Rotavirus infection

> ➤ *Rotavirus infection in children is a highly contagious viral illness causing gastroenteritis with symptoms like vomiting, diarrhea, fever, and abdominal pain.*
>
> ➤ *It spreads through fecal-oral routes and is common in young children.*
>
> ➤ *Vaccination is a key preventive measure alongside supportive care including hydration, electrolyte replacement, and monitoring for dehydration.*

Symptoms:

- Severe diarrhea: Watery diarrhea is the hallmark symptom of rotavirus infection, often accompanied by frequent bowel movements.
- Vomiting: Children with rotavirus infection may experience vomiting, which can be severe and persistent.
- Fever: Low-grade fever is common, but high fever may occur in some cases.
- Abdominal cramps or discomfort
- Dehydration: Severe diarrhea and vomiting can lead to dehydration, characterized by decreased urine output, dry mouth, sunken eyes, and lethargy.

Causes and Risk Factors:

- Age: Rotavirus infection is most common in infants and young children under 5 years old, particularly those aged 6 months to 2 years.
- Childcare settings: Rotavirus spreads easily in environments where children gather, such as daycare centers and preschools.
- Poor hygiene: Lack of handwashing and inadequate sanitation facilities can facilitate the spread of rotavirus.
- Immunocompromised patients: Children with weakened immune systems are at increased risk of severe rotavirus infection and complications.

Epidemiology:

Rotavirus is a leading cause of severe diarrhea and dehydration in infants and young children worldwide. Before the introduction of rotavirus vaccines, rotavirus gastroenteritis was responsible for millions of cases of severe illness and hundreds of thousands of deaths annually, particularly in low-income countries. Rotavirus infection occurs throughout the year but is more common during the winter months in temperate climates.

Diagnosis:
- <u>Clinical Assessment:</u> Diagnosis of rotavirus infection is typically based on clinical symptoms, particularly the presence of severe diarrhea and vomiting in young children.
- <u>Laboratory Tests:</u> Enzyme immunoassays (EIA) or polymerase chain reaction (PCR) tests, can detect the presence of rotavirus antigens or genetic material in stool samples. These tests are often used in healthcare settings to confirm the diagnosis of rotavirus gastroenteritis.

Treatment:
- <u>Fluid Replacement:</u>

    The mainstay of treatment for rotavirus infection is oral rehydration therapy to replace fluids and electrolytes lost through diarrhea and vomiting. Oral rehydration solutions (ORS) containing a balanced combination of salts and sugars are recommended to prevent dehydration.

- <u>Symptomatic Relief:</u> Over-the-counter medications such as acetaminophen or ibuprofen may be used to reduce fever and alleviate abdominal pain.
- <u>Nutritional Support:</u> Continuing breastfeeding or formula feeding is important to maintain adequate nutrition and hydration during illness.
- <u>Prevention:</u>

    Rotavirus vaccines are highly effective in preventing severe rotavirus gastroenteritis. Two rotavirus vaccines, Rotarix (RV1) and RotaTeq (RV5), are approved for use in infants in many countries and are typically administered in a series of doses starting around 2 months of age.

References
- Heikkinen, T., & Järvinen, A. (2003). The common cold. The Lancet, 361(9351), 51-59.
- Lieberthal, A. S., Carroll, A. E., & et al. (2013). The diagnosis and management of acute otitis media. Pediatrics, 131(3), e964-e999.
- National Asthma Education and Prevention Program. (2007). Expert panel report 3 (EPR-3): Guidelines for the diagnosis and management of asthma-summary report 2007. Journal of Allergy and Clinical Immunology, 120(5), S94-S138.

- Dykewicz, M. S., & Hamilos, D. L. (2010). Rhinitis and sinusitis. Journal of Allergy and Clinical Immunology, 125(2 Suppl 2), S103-S115.

- Sidbury, R., Davis, D. M., & et al. (2014). Guidelines of care for the management of atopic dermatitis: Section 3. Management and treatment with phototherapy and systemic agents. Journal of the American Academy of Dermatology, 71(2), 327-349.

- Subcommittee on Urinary Tract Infection, Steering Committee on Quality Improvement and Management, Roberts, K. B., & et al. (2016). Urinary tract infection: Clinical practice guideline for the diagnosis and management of the initial UTI in febrile infants and children 2 to 24 months. Pediatrics, 138(6), e20163026.

- American Academy of Pediatrics, Provisional Committee on Quality Improvement, Subcommittee on Febrile Seizures. (2011). Practice parameter: The neurodiagnostic evaluation of the child with a first simple febrile seizure. Pediatrics, 127(2), 389-394.

- Geelhoed, G. C., Macdonald, W. B., & et al. (1995). Single-dose oral dexamethasone in the treatment of croup: A randomized, placebo-controlled trial. Pediatrics, 95(1), 105-108.

- Tabbers, M. M., DiLorenzo, C., & et al. (2014). Evaluation and treatment of functional constipation in infants and children: evidence-based recommendations from ESPGHAN and NASPGHAN. Journal of Pediatric Gastroenterology and Nutrition, 58(2), 258-274.

- Guarino, A., Ashkenazi, S., & et al. (2014). European Society for Pediatric Gastroenterology, Hepatology, and Nutrition/European Society for Pediatric Infectious Diseases evidence-based guidelines for the management of acute gastroenteritis in children in Europe: update 2014. Journal of Pediatric Gastroenterology and Nutrition, 59(1), 132-152.

- Rietveld, R. P., & Van Weert, H. C. (2003). Differences in outcome of acute conjunctivitis in children: a follow-up study in primary care. Family Practice, 20(6), 575-579.

- Shulman, S. T., Bisno, A. L., & et al. (2012). Clinical practice guideline for the diagnosis and management of group A streptococcal pharyngitis: 2012 update by the Infectious Diseases Society of America. Clinical Infectious Diseases, 55(10), 1279-1282.

- O'Ryan, M., Lucero, Y., & et al. (2019). Etiology of diarrhea in children <5 years of age in Bolivia. BMC Research Notes, 12(1), 1-6.

- Chow, A. W., Benninger, M. S., & et al. (2012). IDSA clinical practice guideline for acute bacterial rhinosinusitis in children and adults. Clinical Infectious Diseases, 54(8), e72-e112.

- Ho, M., Chen, E. R., & et al. (1999). An epidemic of enterovirus 71 infection in Taiwan. New England Journal of Medicine, 341(13), 929-935.

- Long, S. S., & Prober, C. G. (2012). Principles and practice of pediatric infectious diseases (Vol. 1037). Elsevier Health Sciences.

- Barlow, S. E., & Expert Committee. (2007). Expert committee recommendations regarding the prevention, assessment, and treatment of child and adolescent overweight and obesity: summary report. Pediatrics, 120(Supplement 4), S164-S192.
- Ruuska, T., & Vesikari, T. (1990). Rotavirus disease in Finnish children: use of numerical scores for clinical severity of diarrhoeal episodes. Scandinavian Journal of Infectious Diseases, 22(3), 259-267.

Chapter 14: Ophthalmologic Disorders

Reviewed by
Linda Vu, MD, FACS

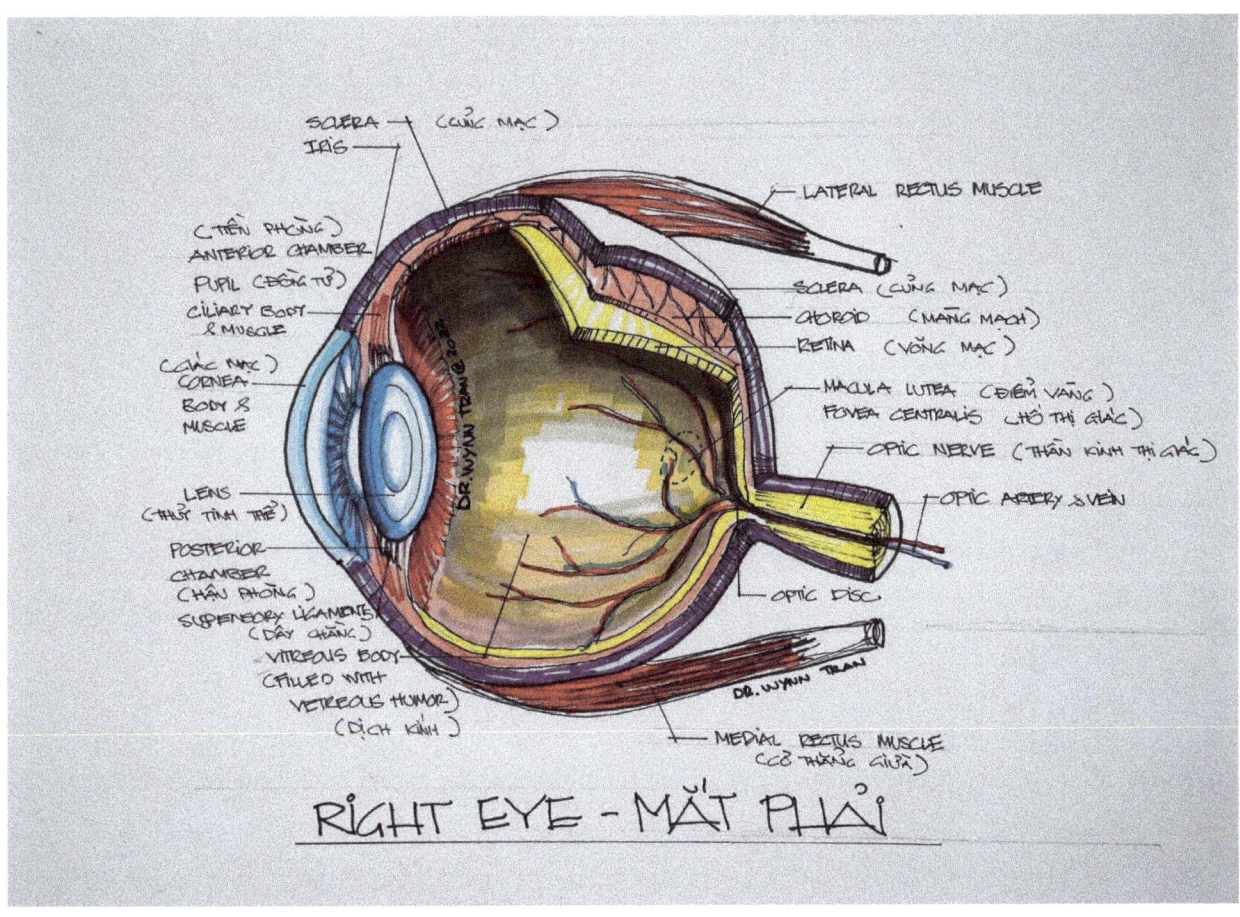

The APh should be familiar with the presentation, diagnosis, and management of these common eye disorders to provide appropriate care and referral to the optometrist or ophthalmologist when necessary.

14.1. Refractive Errors

> ➢ *Refractive errors are common vision problems resulting from irregularities in the shape of the eye, leading to blurred vision.*
> ➢ *Types include myopia (nearsightedness), hyperopia (farsightedness), astigmatism, and presbyopia.*
> ➢ *Treatment options include corrective lenses, such as glasses or contact lenses, and refractive surgery to improve vision clarity.*

Symptoms:

- Blurred vision
- Eyestrain: eye discomfort or fatigue, especially after prolonged reading or other close-up tasks
- Headaches: particularly after extended periods of visual concentration
- Squinting
- Difficulty seeing at night

Causes and Risk Factors:

- Genetics: Family history of refractive errors can increase the risk of developing similar vision problems.
- Age: Certain refractive errors, such as presbyopia, commonly occur with aging.
- Environmental factors: Prolonged close-up work, such as reading or using digital devices, may contribute to the development of myopia.
- Medical conditions: Certain medical conditions, such as diabetes or eye diseases like cataracts, can increase the risk of refractive errors.

Epidemiology:

Refractive errors are a common vision problem worldwide, affecting patients of all ages. The prevalence of refractive errors varies depending on factors such as geographic location, ethnicity, and age group. Myopia, in particular, has been increasing in prevalence, especially in urban areas with high levels of education and screen use.

Diagnosis:

Diagnosis of refractive errors is typically performed by an eye care professional, such as an optometrist or ophthalmologist, through a comprehensive eye examination.

- Visual Acuity Testing: assessing how well a person can see at various distances using an eye chart
- Refraction: determining the appropriate lens prescription by asking the person to look through a series of lenses to find the one that provides the clearest vision
- Eye Health Evaluation: examining the structures of the eye to detect any abnormalities or underlying eye conditions

Treatment:
- Eyeglasses:

    Prescription eyeglasses are a common and effective treatment for correcting refractive errors. Eyeglasses use lenses with specific optical powers to correct nearsightedness, farsightedness, astigmatism, or presbyopia.

- Contact Lenses:

    Contact lenses provide an alternative to eyeglasses for correcting refractive errors. They are available in various types, including soft lenses, rigid gas-permeable lenses, and specialty lenses for astigmatism or presbyopia.

- Refractive Surgery:

    LASIK (laser-assisted in situ keratomileusis) or PRK (photorefractive keratectomy) can permanently reshape the cornea to correct refractive errors. These procedures are typically performed by an ophthalmologist and are suitable for certain candidates based on factors such as age, eye health, and refractive stability.

- Orthokeratology (Ortho-K): Specialized rigid contact lenses worn overnight to temporarily reshape the cornea and correct refractive errors during the day.
- Low-Vision Aids:

    For patients with severe refractive errors or other vision impairments that cannot be fully corrected with conventional methods, low-vision aids such as magnifiers or telescopic lenses may be helpful for improving visual function.

14.2. Cataracts

> ➢ *Cataracts are a common age-related condition characterized by clouding of the eye's natural lens, leading to blurry vision, glare, and difficulty seeing at night.*
>
> ➢ *They can also occur in younger individuals due to factors like trauma, diabetes, or medication use.*
>
> ➢ *Treatment involves surgical removal of the cataract and replacement with an artificial lens to restore vision clarity.*

Symptoms:

- Blurry or cloudy vision: the most common symptom, usually worsens over time.
- Difficulty seeing at night
- Sensitivity to bright lights cause visual discomfort and glare, with increased difficulty seeing.
- Frequent changes in glasses prescription: Cataracts can cause changes in the refractive index of the lens material, causing changes in refraction.
- Colors appear faded or yellowed: due to changes in the lens
- Seeing halos or rings around lights, especially at night.

Causes and Risk Factors:

- Aging is the primary risk factor for cataracts, with the condition becoming more common as patients get older.
- Prolonged exposure to ultraviolet (UV) radiation from sunlight or artificial sources can increase the risk of cataracts.
- Smoking cigarettes or exposure to secondhand smoke is associated with an increased risk of cataracts.
- Diabetes: patients with diabetes are at higher risk of developing cataracts, particularly at a younger age.
- Family history may increase the likelihood of developing the condition
- Certain medications: Long-term use of corticosteroids or other medications, such as statins, may increase the risk of cataracts.
- Previous eye injuries or trauma can increase the risk of developing cataracts later in life.
- Medical conditions: Obesity or hypertension may also be associated with an increased risk of cataracts.

Epidemiology:

Cataracts are a leading cause of vision impairment and blindness worldwide, particularly among older adults. The prevalence of cataracts increases with age, and it's estimated that more than half of all Americans aged 80 and older have cataracts or have undergone cataract surgery.

Diagnosis:

Cataracts are diagnosed through a comprehensive eye examination by an optometrist or ophthalmologist.

- <u>Visual Acuity Testing:</u> assessing how well a person can see at various distances using an eye chart
- <u>Slit-Lamp Examination:</u> using a special microscope to examine the structures of the eye, including the lens, for signs of cataracts
- <u>Dilated Eye Exam:</u> widening the pupil with eye drops to allow for a more thorough examination of the lens and other structures inside the eye
- <u>Measurement of Intraocular Pressure:</u> checking for elevated intraocular pressure, which may indicate other eye conditions such as glaucoma

Treatment:

- <u>Regular Monitoring:</u> may be recommended for patients with mild cataracts or those who are not yet experiencing significant vision problems to track changes in vision over time
- <u>Glasses or Contact Lenses:</u> may help improve vision temporarily, particularly in the early stages of cataracts
- <u>Cataract surgery:</u> Once the vision is not improved adequately with changes in prescription, the most common treatment for cataracts is surgical removal of the cloudy lens and replacement with an artificial intraocular lens (IOL). Cataract surgery is a safe and effective procedure that is typically performed on an outpatient basis.

14.3. Glaucoma

> ➤ Glaucoma is a group of eye conditions characterized by damage to the optic nerve, often caused by elevated intraocular pressure, leading to progressive vision loss.
>
> ➤ It is a leading cause of blindness worldwide and can develop slowly over time without noticeable symptoms, making regular eye exams crucial for early detection.
>
> ➤ Management includes medications, laser therapy, or surgery to lower intraocular pressure and preserve vision.

Symptoms:

- Open-angle glaucoma: Most cases develop gradually and are often asymptomatic until later stages.
    - Gradual loss of peripheral vision (tunnel vision)
    - Patchy blind spots in the visual field
    - Difficulty adjusting to low light conditions
- Closed-angle glaucoma: characterized by impaired drainage of aqueous humor from the eye due to a narrow or closed angle between the iris and cornea
    - Severe eye pain or headache
    - Blurred or hazy vision
    - Halos around lights
    - Redness in the eye
    - Nausea and vomiting

Causes and Risk Factors:

- Age increases the risk of glaucoma, particularly after age 40.
- Family history: Having a close relative with glaucoma increases the risk of developing the condition.
- Ethnicity: Certain ethnic groups, such as African Americans and Hispanics, have a higher risk of developing glaucoma.
- High intraocular pressure: Elevated pressure inside the eye is a significant risk factor for glaucoma.
- Thin central cornea: Patients with thinner corneas may have an increased risk of glaucoma.
- Medical conditions: Diabetes, hypertension, and cardiovascular disease, may increase the risk of glaucoma.

- Eye conditions: Previous eye injuries, inflammation, or surgeries may increase the risk of glaucoma.
- Long-term corticosteroid use: Prolonged use of corticosteroid medications, whether in the form of eye drops, oral pills, or injections, may increase the risk of glaucoma.

Epidemiology:

Glaucoma is a leading cause of irreversible blindness worldwide. It affects millions of patients, with the prevalence increasing with age. The exact prevalence of glaucoma varies by geographic region and population demographics.

Diagnosis:

Diagnosis of glaucoma involves a comprehensive eye examination by an eye care professional, such as an optometrist or ophthalmologist. The examination may include:

- <u>Measurement of Intraocular Pressure:</u> Tonometry is used to measure the pressure inside the eye.
- <u>Evaluation of the Optic Nerve:</u> Dilated fundus examination allows for visualization of the optic nerve to assess for signs of damage or abnormalities.
- <u>Visual Field Testing:</u> Perimetry is used to assess the visual field and detect any areas of vision loss or blind spots.
- <u>Gonioscopy:</u> This test evaluates the drainage angle of the eye to determine if there is any obstruction to fluid outflow.
- <u>Measurement of Central Corneal Thickness:</u> Pachymetry measures the thickness of the cornea, which can affect intraocular pressure readings.

Treatment:

Acute closed-angle glaucoma is a medical emergency and requires immediate treatment to lower intraocular pressure and prevent permanent vision loss.

- <u>Regular Monitoring:</u> Patients with glaucoma require ongoing monitoring by an eye care professional to assess the progression of the disease and adjust treatment as needed.
- <u>Eye Drops:</u> Medications in the form of eye drops are often used as the first-line treatment to lower intraocular pressure. These medications may include prostaglandin analogs, beta-blockers, alpha-adrenergic agonists, carbonic anhydrase inhibitors, and Rho kinase inhibitors.
- <u>Oral Medications:</u> to help lower intraocular pressure

- Laser Therapy: Trabeculoplasty or iridotomy can help improve the drainage of fluid from the eye and reduce intraocular pressure.
- Surgery: Trabeculectomy or implantation of drainage devices may be recommended for patients with advanced or uncontrolled glaucoma.

14.4. Age-Related Macular Degeneration

> ➤ *Age-related macular degeneration (AMD) is a progressive eye disease affecting the macula, causing central vision loss.*
>
> ➤ *It is the leading cause of vision impairment and blindness in older adults.*
>
> ➤ *Treatment may include oral antioxidants supplements, anti-VEGF injections, laser therapy, or photodynamic therapy to slow progression and preserve remaining vision.*

Symptoms:
- Blurred or distorted central vision: One of the most common symptoms of AMD is a gradual loss of central vision, which may cause objects to appear blurry or distorted.
- Dark or empty areas in central vision: AMD can cause blind spots or areas of reduced vision in the center of the visual field.
- Difficulty reading or recognizing faces: As AMD progresses, patients may have difficulty reading fine print, recognizing faces, or performing tasks that require detailed vision.
- Changes in color perception: Some patients with AMD may experience changes in color perception, such as seeing less vibrant colors or difficulty distinguishing between different shades.
- Straight lines appear wavy: A common early sign of AMD is the appearance of straight lines as wavy or distorted.

Causes and Risk Factors:
- Advanced age is the primary risk factor for AMD, with the condition becoming more common in patients over the age of 50.
- Family history
- Smoking: significant modifiable risk factor for AMD
- Race and ethnicity: AMD is more common among Caucasians than other racial or ethnic groups.
- Obesity: Being overweight or obese is associated with an increased risk of developing AMD.

- Cardiovascular disease: Hypertension, high cholesterol, and atherosclerosis, may increase the risk of AMD.
- Sunlight exposure: Prolonged exposure to ultraviolet (UV) radiation from sunlight may increase the risk of AMD.
- Gender: Women may be at slightly higher risk than men.

Epidemiology:

AMD is a leading cause of vision loss and blindness among older adults worldwide. The prevalence of AMD increases with age, and it's estimated that millions of patients are affected by the condition globally. As the population ages, the prevalence of AMD is expected to rise, making it a significant public health concern.

Diagnosis:

Diagnosis of AMD is typically made through a comprehensive eye examination by an eye care professional, such as an optometrist or ophthalmologist. The examination may include:

- Visual Acuity Testing: assessing how well a person can see at various distances using an eye chart
- Dilated Fundus Examination: using special instruments to examine the retina and macula for signs of AMD, such as drusen (yellow deposits) or pigment changes
- Fluorescein Angiography: injecting a dye into the bloodstream and taking photographs of the retina to evaluate blood flow and identify abnormal blood vessels
- Optical Coherence Tomography (OCT): This non-invasive imaging technique allows for detailed cross-sectional imaging of the retina, including the macula, to assess structural changes associated with AMD.

Treatment:

- Regular Monitoring: Patients with AMD require ongoing monitoring by an eye care professional to assess the progression of the disease and adjust treatment as needed.
- Oral Antioxidant Supplements:
    Commercially available formulations of high amounts of vitamins and minerals can slow progression of AMD from early to intermediate disease. The supplements will not reverse any damage already present.

- Anti-VEGF Injections:

    Intravitreal injections of anti-vascular endothelial growth factor (anti-VEGF) medications, such as ranibizumab, aflibercept, or bevacizumab, may be used to treat neovascular AMD by blocking abnormal blood vessel growth and reducing fluid leakage in the macula.

- Photodynamic Therapy: PDT involves injecting a light-sensitive drug into the bloodstream and then applying laser therapy to activate the drug and destroy abnormal blood vessels in the macula.

- Laser Therapy: to seal leaking blood vessels or destroy abnormal blood vessels in the retina

- Low-Vision Aids: For patients with advanced AMD and significant vision loss, magnifiers, telescopic lenses, or electronic devices may help improve visual function and quality of life.

14.5. Diabetic Retinopathy

> ➤ *Diabetic retinopathy is a complication of diabetes that affects the blood vessels in the retina, leading to vision impairment and blindness.*
>
> ➤ *It can cause symptoms such as blurred vision, floaters, and difficulty seeing at night.*
>
> ➤ *Treatment involves managing diabetes through blood sugar control, along with laser therapy, injections, or surgery to prevent or delay vision loss.*

Symptoms:

- Blurred vision or difficulty focusing on objects may occur as diabetic retinopathy progresses or worsens.

- Floaters: Dark spots or floaters may appear in the field of vision.

- Impaired color vision: Changes in color perception or difficulty distinguishing between colors may occur.

- Fluctuating vision: particularly in patients with unstable blood sugar levels

- Vision loss: In advanced stages of diabetic retinopathy, vision loss may occur, sometimes leading to blindness if left untreated.

Causes and Risk Factors:

- Duration of diabetes: The longer a person has diabetes, the higher the risk of developing diabetic retinopathy.

- Poorly controlled blood sugar: Chronic hyperglycemia is a major risk factor for diabetic retinopathy.
- Hypertension increases the risk of developing diabetic retinopathy and can worsen its progression.
- High cholesterol: Elevated levels of cholesterol and triglycerides may increase the risk of diabetic retinopathy.
- Pregnancy: Pregnant women with diabetes are at increased risk.
- Ethnicity: Certain ethnic groups, including African Americans, Hispanics, and Native Americans, have a higher prevalence of diabetic retinopathy.
- Smoking increases the risk of developing diabetic retinopathy and can worsen its progression.
- Diabetic nephropathy is often associated with diabetic retinopathy and may increase the risk of vision loss.

Epidemiology:

Diabetic retinopathy is a leading cause of vision loss and blindness among working-age adults worldwide. The prevalence of diabetic retinopathy is closely linked to the prevalence of diabetes, with an estimated one-third of patients with diabetes affected by some form of diabetic retinopathy. As the global burden of diabetes continues to rise, the incidence and prevalence of diabetic retinopathy are expected to increase as well.

Diagnosis:

- Visual Acuity testing: assessing how well a person can see at various distances using an eye chart
- Dilated Fundus Examination: examining the retina and blood vessels at the back of the eye for signs of diabetic retinopathy, such as microaneurysms, hemorrhages, or neovascularization
- Fluorescein Angiography: injecting a dye into the bloodstream and taking photographs of the retina to evaluate blood flow and identify abnormal blood vessels
- Optical Coherence Tomography (OCT): This non-invasive imaging technique allows for detailed cross-sectional imaging of the retina, including the macula, to assess for structural changes associated with diabetic retinopathy, such as macular edema or retinal thinning.

Treatment:

- Optimal Diabetes Management: Tight control of blood sugar levels, blood pressure, and cholesterol is essential for preventing or delaying the progression of diabetic retinopathy.

- Regular Eye Examinations: Patients with diabetes should undergo regular eye examinations to detect diabetic retinopathy early and monitor for changes in the condition over time.
- Intravitreal Injections:

    Anti-vascular endothelial growth factor (anti-VEGF) medications or corticosteroids may be injected into the eye to reduce swelling (macular edema) and inhibit abnormal blood vessel growth (neovascularization).
- Laser Therapy: Laser photocoagulation or panretinal photocoagulation may be used to seal leaking blood vessels or destroy abnormal blood vessels in the retina.
- Vitrectomy:

    In advanced cases of diabetic retinopathy with vitreous hemorrhage or tractional retinal detachment, vitrectomy surgery may be performed to remove blood and scar tissue from the eye and repair retinal detachment.

14.6. Dry Eye Syndrome

> ➤ *Dry eye syndrome is a common condition characterized by insufficient tear production or poor tear quality, leading to discomfort, redness, and blurred vision.*
>
> ➤ *It may result from aging, certain medications, environmental factors, or underlying health conditions.*
>
> ➤ *Treatment involves lubricating eye drops, lifestyle changes, and sometimes prescription medications or procedures to manage symptoms and improve tear production.*

Symptoms:

- Dryness: dry, gritty, or scratchy sensation in the eyes, often described as feeling like sand is in the eye
- Redness of the eyes, especially along the edges of the eyelids
- Burning or stinging sensation in the eyes, particularly after periods of prolonged focus, such as reading or using digital devices
- Watery eyes: Paradoxically, dry eye syndrome can sometimes lead to excessive tearing as the eyes attempt to compensate.
- Blurred or fluctuating vision, particularly when performing tasks that require visual concentration

- Increased sensitivity to light
- Eye fatigue or discomfort, particularly after extended periods of reading, driving, or screen time
- Mucus discharge: stringy or mucus-like discharge from the eyes, especially upon waking in the morning

Causes and Risk Factors:
- Age increases the risk of dry eye syndrome, particularly in patients over 50.
- Gender: Women are more likely to develop dry eye syndrome compared to men, particularly during hormonal changes such as pregnancy, menopause, or while taking certain medications such as oral contraceptives.
- Environmental factors: Prolonged exposure to dry or windy environments, air conditioning, heating, or smoke can increase the risk of dry eye syndrome.
- Contact lens use: particularly if lenses are worn for extended periods or not properly cleaned and maintained
- Medical conditions: Autoimmune diseases (e.g., Sjögren's syndrome, rheumatoid arthritis), diabetes, thyroid disorders, or allergic conjunctivitis, may increase the risk of dry eye syndrome.
- Medications: Antihistamines, decongestants, antidepressants, hormone replacement therapy, and certain acne medications, can cause or worsen dry eye symptoms.
- Screen use: Prolonged use of digital devices, computers, or smartphones can lead to decreased blinking and increased evaporation of tears, contributing to dry eye syndrome.

Epidemiology:

Dry eye syndrome is a common eye condition that affects millions of patients worldwide. The prevalence of dry eye syndrome varies by geographic region and population demographics, with estimates ranging from 5% to 50% of the population affected. Dry eye syndrome is more common in older adults, women, and patients with certain medical conditions or environmental exposures.

Diagnosis:
- <u>Symptom Assessment:</u> evaluation of symptoms such as dryness, burning, irritation, or visual disturbances
- <u>Tear Film Evaluation:</u> measurement of tear production and quality using tests such as the Schirmer's test, tear breakup time (TBUT) test, or tear osmolarity test

- Corneal and Conjunctival Evaluation: examination of the cornea and conjunctiva for signs of dryness, inflammation, or damage
- Evaluation of Eyelids and Meibomian Glands: These contribute to the oil layer of the tear film which plays a crucial role in tear production and distribution.
- Fluorescein or Lissamine Green Staining: application of special dyes to the surface of the eye to detect abnormalities or damage to the cornea and conjunctiva

Treatment:
- Artificial Tears: Over-the-counter artificial tear eye drops are often used to provide lubrication and relieve symptoms of dryness and irritation.
- Prescription Eye Drops: Medications with cyclosporine (Restasis), lifitegrast (Xiidra), or corticosteroids may be prescribed to reduce inflammation and improve tear production.
- Lid Hygiene: Warm compresses, eyelid massages, and lid scrubs may help improve meibomian gland function and reduce blockage of the glands.
- Moisture Chamber Glasses: can help protect the eyes from environmental factors and reduce tear evaporation
- Punctal Plugs: Tiny plugs inserted into the tear ducts (puncta) can help block tear drainage and keep tears in the eyes longer.
- Nutritional Supplements: Omega-3 fatty acids, flaxseed oil, or fish oil supplements may help improve tear quality and reduce inflammation.
- Novel Treatments: Varenicline solution is a nasal spray used to induce natural tears, improving tear production. Perfluorohexyloctane ophthalmic solution is a supplement to the lipid layer of the tear film.

14.7. Conjunctivitis

> ➤ *Conjunctivitis, or pink eye, in adults is inflammation of the conjunctiva, presenting with redness, itching, discharge, and sometimes blurred vision.*
> ➤ *It can be viral, bacterial, or allergic in origin, spreading easily through contact.*
> ➤ *Treatment involves symptom relief with warm compresses, lubricating eye drops, and proper hygiene practices to prevent spread and complications.*

Symptoms:
- Redness in the white of the eye or inner eyelid
- Watery or mucous discharge from the eye
- Itching or burning sensation in the eye
- Gritty feeling in the eye
- Swelling of the eyelids
- Sensitivity to light
- Crusting of eyelids or lashes, particularly upon waking in the morning

Causes and Risk Factors:
- Viral or bacterial infections: Viral and bacterial conjunctivitis are the most common forms of pink eye and can be highly contagious.
- Allergies: Allergic conjunctivitis can occur due to exposure to allergens such as pollen, dust, pet dander, or certain irritants.
- Contact lens use: Improper cleaning or wearing contact lenses for extended periods can increase the risk of developing bacterial or allergic conjunctivitis.
- Environmental factors: Exposure to smoke, pollutants, or other irritants can irritate the eyes and contribute to the development of conjunctivitis.
- Poor hygiene: Touching the eyes with unwashed hands or sharing personal items such as towels or cosmetics can spread infectious conjunctivitis.
- Pre-existing eye conditions: Patients with dry eye syndrome or blepharitis may be more prone to developing conjunctivitis.

Epidemiology:
- Conjunctivitis is a common eye condition that can affect patients of all ages, including adults.
- Viral conjunctivitis is the most common form of pink eye and is highly contagious, particularly in crowded environments such as schools, daycare centers, or workplaces.
- Bacterial conjunctivitis is also common and can occur sporadically or in outbreaks, particularly in healthcare settings or among patients with compromised immune systems.

Diagnosis:
Conjunctivitis is usually diagnosed based on a medical history and physical examination of the eye. Cultures or tests of eye discharges are rarely needed but may be performed if the infection does not respond to initial

treatment, to identify specific bacteria or viruses, or in cases of severe infections.

Treatment:

Most cases of viral pink eye are self-limiting and do not require specific treatment.

- Symptomatic Relief: Cool compresses, artificial tears, and over-the-counter (OTC) antihistamine or decongestant eye drops can alleviate itching and redness.
- Viral Conjunctivitis: In severe cases, a healthcare provider may prescribe antiviral eye drops or ointments.
- Bacterial Conjunctivitis:
    - Antibiotic eye drops or ointments are typically prescribed to treat bacterial pink eye. Topical antibiotics such as erythromycin, bacitracin, or polymyxin B are commonly used. Improvement is usually seen within a few days of starting treatment, and it's essential to complete the full course of antibiotics as prescribed.
- Allergic Conjunctivitis:

    Avoiding exposure to allergens is the primary strategy for managing allergic pink eye. Over-the-counter or prescription antihistamine eye drops, mast cell stabilizers, or nonsteroidal anti-inflammatory drugs (NSAIDs) may provide relief from symptoms. Cold compresses and artificial tears can also help soothe irritated eyes.
- Home Care:

    Practicing good hygiene, such as washing hands frequently, avoiding rubbing or touching the eyes, and using clean towels and pillowcases, can help prevent the spread of infectious conjunctivitis. Patients with pink eyes should avoid wearing contact lenses and eye makeup until symptoms resolve.

14.8. Blepharitis

> ➢ *Blepharitis is a common eyelid inflammation characterized by redness, itching, irritation, and crusty eyelids, often caused by bacteria or dysfunction of the oil glands.*
>
> ➢ *It can lead to discomfort, blurry vision, and recurrent eye infections.*
>
> ➢ *Treatment involves warm compresses, eyelid hygiene, antibiotic ointments, and sometimes steroid drops to alleviate symptoms and prevent complications.*

Symptoms:

- Redness and swelling of the eyelids
- Itching or burning sensation in the eyes
- Irritation or gritty feeling in the eyes
- Excessive tearing or watery eyes
- Crusting or scales along the eyelid margins, particularly upon waking in the morning
- Sensitivity to light
- Blurred vision
- Foreign body sensation or discomfort in the eyes
- Thickened or misdirected eyelashes

Causes and Risk Factors:

- Poor eyelid hygiene: Inadequate cleansing of the eyelids can lead to the accumulation of debris, oil, and bacteria along the eyelid margins, increasing the risk of blepharitis.
- Skin conditions: Patients with seborrheic dermatitis, rosacea, or eczema are at higher risk of developing blepharitis.
- Demodex infestation: Overgrowth of Demodex mites on the eyelids has been associated with blepharitis.
- Meibomian gland dysfunction: Dysfunction of the meibomian glands, which produce the oily component of tears, can contribute to the development of blepharitis.
- Contact lens wear: Improper use, hygiene, or extended wear of contact lenses can increase the risk of blepharitis, particularly anterior blepharitis.
- Allergies: Allergic reactions to cosmetics, eye makeup, or environmental allergens may contribute to blepharitis.

- Systemic conditions: Certain systemic conditions such as autoimmune disorders or hormonal imbalances may be associated with an increased risk of blepharitis.
- Age: Blepharitis can occur at any age but is more common in older adults.

Epidemiology:
- Blepharitis is a common eyelid condition that can affect patients of all ages, including children and adults.
- It is estimated to affect up to 50% of the population to some degree.
- Blepharitis is more prevalent in older adults and tends to be more chronic in nature.

Diagnosis:
- Physical Examination: The physical exam should include:
    - inspection of the eyelid margins, base of the eyelashes, and meibomian glands under magnification
    - evaluation for signs of skin conditions that can contribute to blepharitis, such as seborrheic dermatitis or rosacea
- Eye Swab: swabbing the eyelid margin for laboratory analysis to detect bacteria, fungi, or Demodex mites, if standard treatments fail

Treatment:
- Lid Hygiene:
    - The cornerstone of blepharitis treatment is daily eyelid hygiene to remove debris, oil, and bacteria from the eyelid margins. This may include warm compresses and gentle scrubbing of the eyelids with a clean washcloth or commercially available eyelid scrub solution.
    - In cases of Demodex infestation, treatment with tea tree oil-based eyelid cleansers or other Demodex-targeted therapies may be recommended.
- Topical Antibiotics: In cases of bacterial blepharitis, topical antibiotics such as erythromycin ointment or azithromycin ophthalmic solution may be prescribed to reduce bacterial colonization and inflammation.
- Artificial Tears: Lubricating eye drops or ointments can help alleviate dryness and discomfort associated with blepharitis.
- Topical Corticosteroids:

    Short-term use of topical corticosteroid ointments or drops may be prescribed to reduce inflammation and alleviate symptoms, particularly in cases of severe or chronic blepharitis.

- **Management of Underlying Conditions:** Treating underlying skin conditions such as rosacea or seborrheic dermatitis may help improve blepharitis symptoms.
- **Meibomian Gland Expression:**
    Mechanical expression or massage of the meibomian glands may help improve meibomian gland function and reduce inflammation in cases of meibomian gland dysfunction-associated blepharitis.

14.9. Keratitis

> ➢ *Keratitis is inflammation of the cornea, the clear outer layer of the eye, typically caused by infection, injury, or underlying conditions such as dry eye or autoimmune diseases.*
> ➢ *Symptoms include eye pain, redness, blurred vision, and sensitivity to light.*
> ➢ *Treatment involves antibiotics, antiviral medications, corticosteroids, or other medications depending on the cause, along with supportive measures to promote healing and prevent vision loss.*

Symptoms:
- Eye pain or discomfort
- Redness of the eye
- Sensitivity to light
- Blurred or decreased vision
- Excessive tearing or discharge from the eye
- Foreign body sensation or gritty feeling in the eye
- Watery or mucous discharge
- Swelling or inflammation of the eyelids
- Eye irritation or itching

Causes and Risk Factors:
- Infections: Bacterial, viral, fungal, or parasitic infections can cause keratitis.
- Trauma: Injury to the cornea, such as scratches (corneal abrasions), foreign bodies, or chemical exposure, can lead to keratitis.

- Contact lens wear: Prolonged contact lens use, improper lens care, or sleeping in contact lenses can increase the risk of developing infectious keratitis.
- Reduced immune function: Conditions or medications that suppress the immune system, such as HIV/AIDS, corticosteroids, or chemotherapy, can increase susceptibility to infectious keratitis.
- Dry eye syndrome: Insufficient tear production or poor tear quality can lead to dryness and damage to the cornea, increasing the risk of developing keratitis.
- Eye conditions: Pre-existing blepharitis, conjunctivitis, or corneal dystrophies may predispose patients to keratitis.
- Environmental factors: Exposure to ultraviolet (UV) radiation, dusty or windy environments, or contact with contaminated water sources can increase the risk of developing keratitis.

Epidemiology:
- The incidence and prevalence of keratitis vary depending on the underlying cause and geographic region.
- Infectious keratitis is more common in tropical and subtropical regions, where environmental factors and poor hygiene practices may contribute to its development.
- Contact lens-related keratitis is more prevalent in developed countries, particularly among patients who wear contact lenses for extended periods or do not adhere to proper lens care guidelines.

Diagnosis:
- <u>Clinical Examination:</u> Diagnosis is often based on clinical symptoms and an examination of the eye.
- <u>Slit Lamp Examination:</u> to observe the extent and depth of corneal involvement
- <u>Corneal Staining:</u> application of special dyes (e.g., fluorescein) that highlight areas of damage on the cornea
- <u>Microbiological Testing:</u> Samples from the corneal surface may be taken for culture or PCR testing to identify specific infectious agents.

Treatment:
- <u>Infectious Keratitis:</u>
  - Bacterial keratitis: Topical or oral antibiotics are typically prescribed to treat bacterial infections. The choice of antibiotic depends on the suspected or identified bacterial pathogen.

- - Viral keratitis: Antiviral medications may be used to treat viral infections such as herpes simplex keratitis. Topical corticosteroids may also be prescribed to reduce inflammation.
  - Fungal keratitis: Antifungal medications, such as voriconazole or natamycin, are used to treat fungal infections. In severe cases, surgical debridement of the infected tissue may be necessary.
- Non-Infectious Keratitis:
  - Treatment of non-infectious keratitis may include topical corticosteroids, lubricating eye drops, or other anti-inflammatory medications to reduce inflammation and promote healing.
  - Management of underlying conditions such as dry eye syndrome or autoimmune disorders may also be necessary to prevent recurrence.
- Symptomatic relief: Cool compresses, artificial tears, and pain-relieving medications may be used to alleviate symptoms such as pain, redness, and discomfort.
- Corneal Transplantation: In severe cases of keratitis that do not respond to conservative treatment measures, corneal transplantation (keratoplasty) may be considered to replace the damaged corneal tissue with healthy donor tissue.

14.10. Chalazion

> - *A chalazion is a painless, slow-growing lump or cyst in the eyelid caused by the blockage of an oil gland.*
> - *It typically appears as a small, firm bump under the skin.*
> - *It often resolves on its own but may require warm compresses, antibiotic ointments, or steroid injections for treatment, and in rare cases, surgical removal.*

Symptoms:
- Swelling: A chalazion typically appears as a firm, painless lump or nodule on the eyelid, usually on the upper eyelid.
- Redness: The area surrounding the chalazion may become red or inflamed.
- Tenderness: In some cases, the eyelid may feel tender or sensitive to touch, particularly if the chalazion is large or inflamed.

- Blurred vision: Rarely, if a chalazion grows large enough to press against the eyeball, it may cause blurred or distorted vision.

Causes and Risk Factors:
- Blepharitis: Chronic inflammation of the eyelid margins, known as blepharitis, is a common risk factor for developing chalazia. Blepharitis can lead to blockage of the meibomian glands, predisposing patients to chalazion formation.
- Meibomian gland dysfunction: Dysfunction or blockage of the meibomian glands, which produce the oily component of tears, can increase the risk of developing chalazia.
- Skin conditions: Rosacea or seborrheic dermatitis may be associated with an increased risk of chalazion formation.
- Contact lens wear: Long-term use of contact lenses or improper lens hygiene may increase the risk of developing chalazia.
- Poor eyelid hygiene: Inadequate eyelid hygiene, such as failure to remove eye makeup or clean the eyelids properly, may contribute to the development of chalazion.

Epidemiology:
- Chalazia are common eyelid conditions that can occur at any age but are most commonly seen in adults.
- They are slightly more common in women than men.
- Patients with a history of blepharitis or meibomian gland dysfunction are at higher risk of developing chalazia.

Diagnosis:
- <u>Clinical Examination:</u> Inspection and palpation of the eyelid by an ophthalmologist is usually sufficient for diagnosis.
- <u>Slit Lamp Examination:</u> An ophthalmologist may use a slit lamp microscope to examine the eye and eyelid structures in detail.
- <u>Biopsy:</u> rarely required but may be performed if a chalazion is atypical, recurrent, or resistant to treatment to rule out more serious conditions like eyelid cancer

A stye (hordeolum) vs. a chalazion:
- Location and Pain: Styes are typically painful and appear at the base of an eyelash, representing an acute bacterial infection of the eyelash follicle. Chalazia are usually painless and develop further up on the eyelid as a result of a blocked oil gland.

- Appearance: Styes often present as red, swollen bumps that resemble pimples, while chalazia tend to be larger, less defined, and may not appear as red or tender.
- Duration: Styes generally resolve more quickly, often within a few days to a week. Chalazia grows more slowly and can persist for weeks to months if untreated.

Treatment:
- <u>Warm Compresses:</u> Applying warm compresses to the affected eyelid for 10-15 minutes several times a day can help soften the contents of the chalazion, promote drainage, and reduce inflammation.
- <u>Lid Hygiene:</u> Gentle cleansing of the eyelids with warm water and mild soap or baby shampoo can help prevent further blockage of the meibomian glands and reduce the risk of recurrence.
- <u>Massage:</u> Massaging the eyelid gently with clean fingers or a clean cotton swab after applying warm compresses may help facilitate drainage of the chalazion.
- <u>Topical Antibiotics:</u> Antibiotic ointment or drops can help prevent infection or reduce inflammation.
- <u>Steroid Injections:</u> For larger or persistent chalazion, corticosteroid medication may be injected directly into the chalazion to help reduce inflammation and promote resolution.
- <u>Surgical drainage:</u>

    If conservative measures are unsuccessful or the chalazion does not improve on its own, an ophthalmologist may perform a minor surgical procedure to drain the chalazion and remove its contents. This procedure, known as incision and curettage, is typically performed under local anesthesia in an office setting.

14.11. Ptosis

> ➢ *Ptosis is drooping of the upper eyelid, often due to weakened or stretched eyelid muscles, nerve damage, or aging.*
> ➢ *It can affect one or both eyes, leading to vision obstruction, eyestrain, or a tired appearance.*
> ➢ *Treatment involves surgery to repair the muscle or tissues supporting the eyelid, depending on the underlying cause and severity.*

Symptoms:
- Drooping of the upper eyelid, which may affect one or both eyes
- Difficulty keeping the eye open, leading to partial or complete obstruction of the visual field
- Eyestrain or fatigue due to efforts to elevate the eyelid
- Impaired vision in severe cases, particularly if the ptosis obstructs the pupil and affects visual acuity
- Head tilting or chin elevation to compensate for the drooping eyelid

Causes and Risk Factors:
- Aging: Ptosis is more common in older adults due to age-related weakening of the muscles and ligaments that support the eyelid.
- Congenital factors: Some patients may be born with ptosis due to congenital abnormalities or developmental issues affecting the eyelid muscles or nerves.
- Eye trauma: Injury or trauma to the eye or eyelid muscles can lead to ptosis.
- Neurological conditions: Certain neurological disorders, such as myasthenia gravis, Horner syndrome, or third nerve palsy, may cause ptosis as a result of muscle weakness or nerve damage.
- Medical conditions: Diabetes, thyroid disorders, or muscular dystrophy may be associated with ptosis.
- Medications: Muscle relaxants or antihypertensive drugs may cause ptosis as a side effect.

Epidemiology:
- Ptosis can occur at any age but is more common in older adults.
- Congenital ptosis is relatively rare, occurring in approximately 1 in 1000 births.
- Acquired ptosis is more prevalent in older adults, with increasing incidence with advancing age.

Diagnosis:
- <u>Clinical Assessment:</u> Diagnosis of ptosis is based on a clinical examination of the eyelids and eye movements.
    - Measurement of visual acuity is important to evaluate the impact of ptosis on vision.
    - Evaluation of eyelid position: The degree of eyelid drooping is assessed by measuring the margin reflex distance (MRD) or the distance between the upper eyelid margin and the pupil.

- o Assessment of eyelid function: Examination of eyelid muscle strength, levator function, and presence of associated neurological signs may help identify underlying causes of ptosis.
- Evaluation of Systemic Health: Assessment of medical history, systemic symptoms, and risk factors for underlying medical conditions associated with ptosis may be necessary.

Treatment:
- Observation: Mild cases of ptosis without significant impact on vision may be monitored without intervention.
- Eyelid Crutches: Temporary measures such as eyelid crutches or tape may be used to temporarily elevate the eyelid and improve vision.
- Eyelid Exercises: Strengthening exercises for the eyelid muscles may be recommended in mild cases of ptosis.
- Surgical Correction: most common treatment approach, involving tightening or repositioning of the levator to elevate the eyelid and improve symmetry
- Blepharoplasty: may be performed to remove excess tissue and improve eyelid appearance in cases of age-related ptosis associated with excess skin or fat deposits
- Treatment of Underlying Conditions: Management of neurological disorders or systemic diseases may be necessary to address the underlying cause.

14.12. Retinal Detachment

> ➤ *Retinal detachment is a serious eye condition where the retina detaches from its normal position, leading to vision loss if not promptly treated.*
> ➤ *Symptoms include sudden flashes of light, floaters, and a curtain-like shadow across the field of vision.*
> ➤ *Urgent medical attention and surgical repair to prevent permanent vision loss is required.*

Symptoms:
- Sudden onset of floaters
- Flashes of light in the affected eye, often described as seeing "lightning bolts" or "streaks"

- Blurred or distorted vision, which may progress rapidly
- Shadow or curtain-like obstruction in the peripheral or central visual field
- Decreased or loss of vision, particularly if the macula becomes detached

Causes and Risk Factors:
- Age increases risk of retinal detachment, particularly after age 40.
- Previous eye surgery or injury: Patients who have undergone cataract surgery, LASIK, or other eye procedures are at higher risk.
- Severe myopia: Patients with severe nearsightedness have a greater risk of retinal detachment due to elongation of the eyeball.
- Family history
- Medical history: Patients who have experienced retinal detachment in one eye are at higher risk of it occurring in the other eye.
- Eye diseases: Conditions such as lattice degeneration, retinoschisis, or diabetic retinopathy increase the risk of retinal detachment.
- Trauma: Blunt trauma to the eye can cause retinal tears or detachments.
- Posterior vitreous detachment (PVD): The separation of the vitreous gel from the retina can lead to traction on the retina and increase the risk of tears and detachments.

Epidemiology:
- The overall incidence of retinal detachment is relatively low, estimated at around 6.3 to 17.9 per 100,000 people.
- Retinal detachment is more common in older adults, with peak incidence in the sixth and seventh decades of life.
- Men have a slightly higher risk of retinal detachment compared to women.
- Myopia is a significant risk factor, with patients with high myopia (greater than -6 diopters) having a much higher risk compared to those with low myopia.

Diagnosis:
- <u>Dilated Eye Examination:</u> A comprehensive eye examination with pupil dilation allows the ophthalmologist to examine the retina and detect any tears, holes, or detachments.

- Retinal Imaging: Techniques such as fundus photography, optical coherence tomography (OCT), or ultrasound may be used to visualize the retina and assess the extent of detachment.
- Visual Field Testing: Testing peripheral vision can help detect any visual field defects caused by retinal detachment.
- Measurement of Intraocular Pressure: Elevated intraocular pressure may indicate secondary complications such as glaucoma.

Treatment:
- Surgical Repair: The primary treatment for retinal detachment is surgical repair, which aims to reattach the retina and prevent vision loss. Surgical techniques may include:
    - Scleral buckle: placing a silicone band around the outside of the eye to provide support and indent the eye inward, bringing the detached retina into contact with the underlying tissue
    - Vitrectomy: removing the vitreous gel and any scar tissue from the eye and replacing it with a gas bubble or silicone oil to help reattach the retina
    - Pneumatic retinopexy: injecting a gas bubble into the vitreous cavity and positioning the patient's head in a specific position to help reposition the detached retina
- Laser or Cryotherapy: to create scars or adhesions around retinal tears or holes to prevent further detachment
- Observation: In cases of small, asymptomatic retinal breaks without detachment, close monitoring may be recommended to detect any progression.

14.13. Uveitis

> *Uveitis is inflammation of the uvea, the middle layer of the eye, often caused by autoimmune disorders, infections, or underlying conditions.*
> *Symptoms include eye pain, redness, blurred vision, and sensitivity to light.*
> *Treatment involves corticosteroid eye drops, oral medications, or immunosuppressive therapy to reduce inflammation and prevent complications such as vision loss or glaucoma.*

Symptoms:
- Eye redness

- Eye pain
- Blurred vision
- Sensitivity to light
- Floaters
- Decreased vision
- Eye discharge
- Eye discomfort

Causes and Risk Factors:
- Autoimmune diseases
- Inflammatory disorders
- Infections
- Trauma or injury to the eye
- Genetics
- Exposure to certain toxins or chemicals
- Systemic inflammatory conditions
- Previous eye surgery

Epidemiology:

Uveitis is relatively uncommon, but it can affect patients of any age. The exact prevalence varies depending on the population studied and the definition of uveitis used. However, it is estimated to affect approximately 38 to 714 per 100,000 people. Uveitis may occur as an isolated incident or be associated with systemic diseases.

Diagnosis:
- Medical History and Physical Examination: Assessment of symptoms, risk factors, and any systemic conditions associated with the eyes.
- Eye Examination: including visual acuity testing, intraocular pressure measurement, slit-lamp examination, and dilated fundus examination
- Laboratory Tests: to assess for autoimmune diseases, infectious causes, and systemic inflammation (e.g., complete blood count, erythrocyte sedimentation rate, C-reactive protein)
- Imaging Studies: optical coherence tomography (OCT), fluorescein angiography, or ultrasound to evaluate the extent and severity of inflammation
- Uveitis Classification: based on the location of inflammation within the eye (anterior, intermediate, posterior, or panuveitis)

Treatment:
- Topical Corticosteroids: eye drops to reduce inflammation and manage symptoms
- Systemic Corticosteroids: oral or intravenous corticosteroids for severe or refractory cases
- Immunosuppressive Therapy: methotrexate, azathioprine, or mycophenolate mofetil to control inflammation and reduce the need for corticosteroids
- Biologic Agents: In cases of severe or refractory uveitis, biologic agents such as tumor necrosis factor (TNF) inhibitors or interleukin inhibitors may be used.
- Management of associated systemic diseases or infections contributing to uveitis
- Treatment of complications such as glaucoma, cataracts, or macular edema.

14.14. Floaters

> ➤ *Floaters are tiny specks, spots, or cobweb-like shapes that drift across your field of vision.*
> ➤ *They are often caused by age-related changes in the vitreous humor, the gel-like substance in the eye.*
> ➤ *While usually harmless, sudden onset or increased floaters may indicate retinal tear or detachment, requiring prompt evaluation by an eye specialist to rule out serious conditions.*

Symptoms:
- Appearance of floaters: small shapes in your vision that appear as specks, strings, or cobwebs
- Moving with eye movements: floaters move as the eyes move, often drifting when the eyes stop
- Darting away when trying to look at them directly
- More noticeable against plain, bright backgrounds

Causes and Risk Factors:
- Age: People over the age of 50 are at a higher risk.
- Myopia: increases the likelihood of floaters
- Eye trauma

- Eye surgery: Procedures like cataract surgery can cause floaters.
- Diabetic retinopathy: Diabetes can affect the eyes and lead to floaters.
- Inflammation inside the eye

Epidemiology:

The prevalence of eye floaters increases with age. Most people start to notice them by the age of 50, although they can occur at any age. They are more common in people who are nearsighted or have had cataract operations.

Diagnosis:

- <u>Dilated Eye Exam</u>:

    This is the primary method for diagnosing floaters. An eye doctor (ophthalmologist or optometrist) uses eye drops to dilate the pupils and examines the health of the eye and the vitreous humor.

- <u>Ultrasound of the Eye:</u> In some cases, especially if it's difficult to see into the back of the eye, an ultrasound might be used.

Treatment:

Most floaters do not need treatment. They are more of an annoyance than a problem and can become less noticeable over time.

- <u>Laser Vitreolysis:</u>

    A laser can sometimes be used to break up floaters, making them less noticeable. This procedure is not universally recommended due to potential risks.

- <u>Vitrectomy:</u>

    In severe cases, the vitreous humor may be removed and replaced with a saline solution. This procedure carries risks, such as retinal detachment and cataracts, and is usually reserved for extreme cases where floaters significantly impair vision.

14.15. Presbyopia

> ➤ *Presbyopia is a common age-related condition characterized by the gradual loss of near vision due to the stiffening of the eye's lens, making it difficult to focus on close objects.*
>
> ➤ *Symptoms typically start around age 40 and worsen over time.*
>
> ➤ *Reading glasses, bifocals, or multifocal lenses to correct near vision while maintaining distance vision may be required.*

Symptoms:
- Difficulty focusing on close objects, particularly when reading or performing close-up tasks
- Blurred vision when viewing near objects
- Eye strain or fatigue, especially after prolonged periods of reading or close work
- Headaches or discomfort, particularly when trying to focus on close objects for extended periods
- Difficulty seeing clearly in low-light conditions
- Needing to hold reading material at arm's length to see it clearly

Causes and Risk Factors:
- Age: Presbyopia is a normal age-related change in vision that typically becomes noticeable around age 40, although the onset and severity may vary among patients.
- Family history: Having a family history of presbyopia may increase the likelihood of developing the condition at a younger age.
- Underlying eye conditions: Certain eye conditions or diseases, such as hyperopia, cataracts, or diabetic retinopathy, may exacerbate presbyopia or contribute to difficulties with near vision.
- Environmental factors: Prolonged exposure to activities that require close-up focusing, such as reading, computer work, or fine detail work, may contribute to the development or worsening of presbyopia.
- Systemic health conditions: Diabetes or cardiovascular disease may affect blood flow to the eyes and increase the risk of vision changes, including presbyopia.

Epidemiology:

Presbyopia is a common age-related vision problem that affects nearly everyone to some degree as they get older. It is estimated that over 1.8

billion patients worldwide are affected by presbyopia. The prevalence of presbyopia increases with age, with the majority of patients experiencing symptoms by their mid-40s to early 50s.

Diagnosis:

- Comprehensive Eye Examination:

    An ophthalmologist or optometrist will perform a thorough evaluation of the eyes, including visual acuity testing, refraction assessment, and examination of the internal structures of the eye.

- Near Vision Testing:

    The eye doctor may use a handheld or wall-mounted near vision chart to assess your ability to see clearly at close distances and determine the extent of your near vision impairment.

- Refraction Test:

    A refraction test may be performed to determine the extent of any underlying refractive errors (e.g., hyperopia, astigmatism) contributing to near vision difficulties.

Treatment:

- Reading Glasses:

    Prescription reading glasses with lenses that provide additional magnification for close-up tasks may be prescribed to compensate for the loss of near vision associated with presbyopia.

- Bifocals or Progressive Lenses:

    Bifocal or progressive lenses, which incorporate both distance and near vision correction into a single lens, may be recommended for patients with presbyopia who also have other refractive errors (e.g., myopia, astigmatism).

- Contact Lenses: Multifocal or monovision contact lenses may be used to correct presbyopia and provide clear vision at different distances.

- Refractive Surgery:

    LASIK, PRK, or lens replacement surgery may be considered to correct presbyopia by reshaping the cornea or replacing the natural lens with a multifocal or accommodating intraocular lens (IOL).

- **Over-The-Counter Reading Glasses:** Non-prescription reading glasses available at pharmacies or retail stores may provide temporary relief for patients with mild presbyopia.

14.16. Corneal Abrasion

> ➢ *A corneal abrasion is a scratch or injury to the cornea, the clear front surface of the eye, often caused by foreign objects, contact lenses, or trauma.*
> ➢ *Symptoms include eye pain, redness, tearing, and sensitivity to light.*
> ➢ *Treatment involves antibiotic eye drops, pain relief, and sometimes a protective eye patch to promote healing and prevent infection.*

Symptoms:
- Eye pain or discomfort, often described as a gritty or foreign body sensation
- Redness and inflammation of the affected eye
- Sensitivity to light
- Excessive tearing or watery eyes
- Blurred or reduced vision
- Feeling like there is something in the eye
- Eye irritation or itching
- Difficulty keeping the affected eye open
- Increased blinking or rubbing of the eye

Causes and Risk Factors:
- Trauma or injury to the eye: Corneal abrasions commonly occur as a result of foreign objects, contact lenses, fingernails, or other objects scratching or scraping the surface of the cornea.
- Contact lens wear: Improper use or hygiene of contact lenses, such as wearing them for extended periods, sleeping in contact lenses, or using expired or contaminated contact lens solution, increases the risk of corneal abrasions.
- Dry eye syndrome: Insufficient tear production or poor tear quality can lead to dry, irritated eyes, increasing the risk of corneal abrasions.

- Occupational or recreational hazards that involve exposure to airborne particles, chemicals, or environmental hazards may increase the risk of corneal abrasions.
- History of eye surgery, particularly procedures involving the cornea, may increase the risk of corneal abrasions during the healing process.
- Eye conditions: Corneal dystrophies, recurrent corneal erosions, or neurotrophic keratitis may predispose patients to corneal abrasions.
- Ocular surface abnormalities: Abnormalities of the eyelids, conjunctiva, or tear film, such as blepharitis, conjunctivitis, or meibomian gland dysfunction, can increase the risk of corneal abrasions.

Epidemiology:

Corneal abrasions are a common eye injury, accounting for a significant proportion of emergency department visits and eye-related healthcare encounters. While the exact prevalence of corneal abrasions varies by population and geographic region, they are more commonly seen in patients engaged in high-risk activities or occupations, such as contact lens wearers, outdoor workers, or athletes.

Diagnosis:

- Ocular Examination:

    An ophthalmologist or optometrist will perform a thorough evaluation of the affected eye, including visual acuity testing, assessment of eye movements, and examination of the eyelids, conjunctiva, cornea, and anterior chamber.

- Fluorescein Staining:

    The eye specialist may instill a fluorescein dye into the eye to highlight any areas of corneal abrasion or epithelial defect. The dye will fluoresce under blue light, making it easier to visualize and assess the extent of the injury.

- Slit-lamp Biomicroscopy:

    The eye specialist may use a slit lamp to examine the cornea and anterior segment of the eye in more detail, allowing for precise localization and characterization of the corneal abrasion.

Treatment:

- Lubrication: Topical lubricating eye drops or ointments may be prescribed to keep the eye moist and prevent further irritation or abrasion of the cornea.

- **Antibiotics:** Topical or oral antibiotics may be prescribed to prevent or treat bacterial infection, particularly if the corneal abrasion is associated with a contaminated foreign body or contact lens wear.
- **Pain Management:** acetaminophen or ibuprofen to alleviate eye pain or discomfort associated with corneal abrasions
- **Patching:**
  - Patching of the affected eye was previously a common practice to promote corneal healing and relieve symptoms; however, it is now generally reserved for cases with significant pain or photophobia.
- **Bandage Contact Lens:** In some cases, a therapeutic bandage contact lens may be placed on the cornea to protect the injured surface and promote healing.
- **Avoidance of Contact Lenses:** Contact lens wear should be discontinued until the corneal abrasion has healed completely to prevent further injury or infection.
- **Follow-Up Care:** may be necessary to monitor the healing progress of the corneal abrasion and adjust treatment as needed

14.17. Subconjunctival Hemorrhage

> ➢ A subconjunctival hemorrhage is a painless, bright red patch on the white part of the eye caused by broken blood vessels.
> ➢ It typically occurs spontaneously or due to minor trauma, sneezing, coughing, or straining, with no associated pain or vision loss.
> ➢ Treatment involves observation as it usually resolves on its own within a few weeks, with reassurance and avoidance of further irritation.

Symptoms:
- Sudden appearance of bright red or dark red patches on the white part of the sclera
- Blood visible beneath the clear conjunctival tissue covering the sclera
- No associated pain or discomfort in most cases
- No changes in vision or other visual symptoms
- Possible mild irritation or foreign body sensation

Causes and Risk Factors:

- Trauma or injury to the eye: Accidental trauma or eye rubbing can cause small blood vessels in the conjunctiva to rupture, leading to a subconjunctival hemorrhage.
- Systemic conditions: Hypertension, diabetes, bleeding disorders, or blood thinning medications (e.g., aspirin, anticoagulants) may increase the risk of spontaneous subconjunctival hemorrhage.
- Age: Older adults may be more susceptible to subconjunctival hemorrhage due to the natural aging process and weakening of blood vessels.
- Valsalva maneuver: Activities that increase pressure within the blood vessels, such as heavy lifting, straining during bowel movements, vomiting, or vigorous sneezing or coughing, may predispose patients to subconjunctival hemorrhage.
- Contact lens wear: Improper use, handling, or hygiene of contact lenses may increase the risk of eye trauma or irritation, leading to subconjunctival hemorrhage.

Epidemiology:

Subconjunctival hemorrhage is a common benign condition that can occur in patients of all ages, from infants to the elderly. While the exact prevalence of subconjunctival hemorrhage is difficult to determine due to its often asymptomatic nature and self-limiting course, it is estimated to affect a significant proportion of the population at some point in their lifetime. Subconjunctival hemorrhage may occur spontaneously or as a result of trauma or systemic conditions.

Diagnosis:

- Clinical Examination:

    An ophthalmologist or optometrist will perform a thorough evaluation of the affected eye, including visual acuity testing, assessment of eye movements, and examination of the external and internal structures of the eye.

- Inspection of the Eye:

    The eye doctor will visually inspect the sclera and conjunctiva for the presence of bright red or dark red patches indicative of subconjunctival hemorrhage.

- Assessment of Medical History:

    The eye doctor may inquire about any recent trauma, activities, or systemic conditions that may have contributed to the development of subconjunctival hemorrhage.

Treatment:
- Observation: In most cases, subconjunctival hemorrhage is a self-limiting condition that resolves spontaneously over time without any specific treatment.
- Lubricating Eye Drops: Artificial tears or lubricating eye drops may be recommended to soothe any mild irritation or foreign body sensation associated with subconjunctival hemorrhage.
- Avoidance of Eye Rubbing: Patients should be advised to avoid rubbing or touching the affected eye to prevent further irritation or trauma to the conjunctiva.
- Monitoring: Regular follow-up visits with an eye care professional may be recommended to monitor the resolution of subconjunctival hemorrhage and ensure no underlying eye conditions are present.

14.18. Amblyopia

> - *Amblyopia, commonly known as lazy eye, is a vision development disorder in which one eye fails to achieve normal visual acuity despite proper optical correction.*
> - *It often results from early childhood factors like strabismus, refractive errors, or visual deprivation and requires early detection.*
> - *Treatment includes patching the stronger eye or using atropine drops to encourage vision development in the weaker eye.*

Symptoms:
- Reduced vision in one eye, which may not be apparent to the affected patient
- Poor depth perception or difficulty judging distances
- Squinting or closing one eye to see more clearly
- Eyes that do not appear to work together
- Tilting or turning of the head to use the non-amblyopic eye
- Difficulty with activities requiring binocular vision, such as catching or throwing objects, or participating in sports
- Decreased visual acuity or sharpness in the amblyopic eye compared to the non-amblyopic eye
- Blurred or fuzzy vision in the amblyopic eye

Causes and Risk Factors:
- Strabismus: Amblyopia often occurs in patients with strabismus, as the brain may suppress the visual input from the misaligned eye to avoid double vision.
- Anisometropia: Significant differences in refractive error (e.g., nearsightedness, farsightedness, or astigmatism) between the two eyes can lead to amblyopia in the eye with the greater refractive error.
- Deprivation: Conditions that obstruct or deprive the visual input to one eye during critical periods of visual development, such as congenital cataracts, ptosis, or corneal opacity, can result in amblyopia.
- Family history: Having a family history of amblyopia or refractive errors may increase the risk of developing amblyopia.
- Premature infants or infants with low birth weight may be at increased risk of developing amblyopia due to incomplete visual development or other associated complications.
- Failure to detect and treat underlying eye conditions (e.g., strabismus, refractive errors) during early childhood can increase the risk of amblyopia.
- Insufficient visual stimulation or environmental factors that limit visual experiences during critical periods of visual development may contribute to amblyopia.

Epidemiology:

Amblyopia is one of the most common causes of vision impairment in children, affecting approximately 2-4% of the population. The prevalence of amblyopia varies by age, with the highest incidence occurring during early childhood when visual development is most critical. Amblyopia may persist into adulthood if left untreated, although the severity of vision loss may vary among patients.

Diagnosis:
- <u>Comprehensive Eye Examination:</u>

    An ophthalmologist will perform a thorough evaluation of the child's eyes, including visual acuity testing, assessment of eye alignment and movement, and examination of the ocular structures.

- <u>Refractive Error Assessment:</u>

    Measurement of refractive error (e.g., nearsightedness, farsightedness, astigmatism) using an autorefractor,

retinoscope, or phoropter to detect any significant differences between the two eyes.
- Evaluation of Eye Alignment: assessment of eye alignment and coordination to detect any signs of strabismus or poor eye teaming
- Visual Function Testing: Cover-uncover testing, occlusion testing, or stereopsis testing may be performed to evaluate visual function and detect amblyopia.

Treatment:
- Correction of Refractive Errors: prescribing glasses or contact lenses to correct significant refractive errors in both eyes and ensure clear and equal visual input
- Occlusion Therapy: occluding or patching the non-amblyopic eye to encourage the use of the amblyopic eye and stimulate visual development
  - Patching may be prescribed for a specified duration each day, typically several hours, depending on the severity of amblyopia.
- Atropine Penalization: Application of atropine eye drops to blur the vision in the non-amblyopic eye, similar to occlusion therapy, to encourage the use of the amblyopic eye.
- Vision Therapy: In some cases, vision therapy or orthoptics may be recommended to improve eye coordination, focusing abilities, and depth perception.
- Treatment of Underlying Eye Conditions: Prompt treatment of conditions such as strabismus or congenital cataracts may be necessary to optimize visual outcomes.

14.19. Pterygium

> *Pterygium is a noncancerous growth of tissue on the conjunctiva, often caused by excessive sun exposure, leading to a fleshy, triangular-shaped growth on the white part of the eye.*
> *It may cause redness, irritation, and blurred vision.*
> *Treatment involves lubricating eye drops, steroid eye drops, or surgical removal if it affects vision or causes significant discomfort.*

Symptoms:
- Visible growth of tissue on the conjunctiva that extends onto the cornea

- Redness or inflammation of the affected eye
- Irritation or discomfort, often described as a gritty or foreign body sensation
- Dryness or itching of the affected eye
- Blurred or distorted vision, particularly if the pterygium grows large enough to encroach upon the central visual axis
- Sensitivity to light
- Astigmatism, causing irregular or distorted corneal shape and visual disturbances

Causes and Risk Factors:

- Ultraviolet (UV) exposure: Chronic exposure to UV radiation from sunlight, particularly in sunny or tropical climates, is the primary risk factor for the development of pterygium.
- Outdoor occupation or activities: Patients who spend significant time outdoors, such as farmers, fishermen, or outdoor athletes, are at increased risk of pterygium due to prolonged UV exposure.
- Age: Pterygium is more common in patients aged 20-40 years, although it can occur at any age.
- Gender: Pterygium is more prevalent in males compared to females, possibly due to higher occupational or recreational exposure to UV radiation.
- Dry, windy environments: Exposure to dry, dusty, or windy conditions may exacerbate irritation and inflammation of the conjunctiva, contributing to the development or progression of pterygium.
- Genetic predisposition: Pterygium tends to cluster within families. There is a higher risk in Hispanics and Asians.
- Chronic eye irritation: Conditions that cause chronic eye irritation or inflammation, such as dry eye syndrome, allergies, or exposure to environmental pollutants, may increase the risk of pterygium.

Epidemiology:

Pterygium is a common ocular surface condition, particularly in regions with high levels of UV radiation exposure. The prevalence of pterygium varies geographically, with higher rates reported in sunny or tropical climates. Pterygium is more prevalent in certain occupational groups, such as outdoor workers or patients engaged in activities with prolonged UV exposure. While pterygium can affect patients of all ages, it is more commonly diagnosed in adults between the ages of 20 and 40.

Diagnosis:
- Clinical Examination: An ophthalmologist will perform visual acuity testing, slit-lamp biomicroscopy, and assessment of the ocular surface.
- Visualization of the Pterygium: Slit lamp or magnification can visualize the characteristic appearance of the pterygium as a fleshy, triangular-shaped growth on the conjunctiva extending onto the cornea.
- Measurement of pterygium size: using a ruler or calipers to measure the distance from the corneal limbus (the border between the cornea and the sclera) to the apex of the pterygium
- Documentation of associated findings: The eye doctor may document any associated signs of inflammation, redness, vascularization, or corneal involvement.

Treatment:
- Lubricating Eye Drops: Topical lubricants or artificial tears may be prescribed to relieve symptoms of dryness, irritation, and discomfort associated with pterygium.
- Steroid Eye Drops: Topical corticosteroids may be prescribed to reduce inflammation and swelling of the pterygium, particularly in cases of active inflammation or exacerbation.
- Surgical Excision:

    Removal of the pterygium may be recommended for symptomatic or visually significant lesions that cause persistent irritation, affect vision, or threaten to encroach upon the central visual axis.

- Adjuvant Therapies:

    Conjunctival autografting, amniotic membrane transplantation, mitomycin C application, or beta radiation therapy may be performed with surgical removal to reduce the risk of pterygium recurrence and promote optimal wound healing.

- UV Protection:

    Patients with pterygium should be advised to use protective eyewear, sunglasses with UV-blocking lenses, and wide-brimmed hats to minimize UV exposure and reduce the risk of pterygium progression or recurrence.

References

- Fotedar, R., Wang, J. J., & et al. (2010). Distribution of axial length and ocular biometry measured using partial coherence laser interferometry (IOL Master) in an older white population. Ophthalmology, 117(3), 417-423.
- Asbell, P. A., Dualan, I., & et al. (2005). Age-related cataract. The Lancet, 365(9459), 599-609.
- Weinreb, R. N., Aung, T., & et al. (2014). Primary open-angle glaucoma. Nature Reviews Disease Primers, 4(1), 1-19.
- Lim, L. S., Mitchell, P., & et al. (2012). Age-related macular degeneration. The Lancet, 379(9827), 1728-1738.
- Antonetti, D. A., Klein, R., & et al. (2012). Diabetic retinopathy. New England Journal of Medicine, 366(13), 1227-1239.
- Craig, J. P., Nichols, K. K., & et al. (2017). TFOS DEWS II definition and classification report. Ocular Surface, 15(3), 276-283.
- Azari, A. A., & Barney, N. P. (2013). Conjunctivitis: a systematic review of diagnosis and treatment. JAMA, 310(16), 1721-1729.
- Lindsley, K., Matsumura, S., & et al. (2012). Interventions for chronic blepharitis. Cochrane Database of Systematic Reviews, (5), CD005556.
- Jeng, B. H., Gritz, D. C., & et al. (2019). Corneal ulcer. Annals of Internal Medicine, 171(11), ITC81-ITC96.
- Satchi, K., McNab, A. A., & et al. (2006). Chalazion. Clinical & Experimental Ophthalmology, 34(9), 810-813.
- Patel, R. M., & Aakalu, V. K. (2019). Current trends in the management of congenital ptosis. Clinical Ophthalmology, 13, 503.
- Mitry, D., Charteris, D. G., & et al. (2010). The epidemiology and socioeconomic associations of retinal detachment in Scotland: a two-year prospective population-based study. Investigative Ophthalmology & Visual Science, 51(10), 4963-4968.
- Rathinam, S. R., & Cunningham Jr, E. T. (2011). Infectious causes of uveitis in the developing world. International Ophthalmology Clinics, 51(3), 1-17.
- Chan, R. V., Trope, G. E., & et al. (2013). Prevalence of posterior vitreous detachment in retinal detachment. Canadian Journal of Ophthalmology, 48(2), 165-168.
- Frick, K. D., Joy, S. M., & et al. (2013). Vision impairment and related use of medical care among elderly persons with age-related eye diseases. JAMA Ophthalmology, 131(6), 709-715.
- Basak, S. K., Basak, S., & Mohanta, A. (2005). Epidemiological and microbiological diagnosis of suppurative keratitis in Gangetic West Bengal, eastern India. Indian Journal of Ophthalmology, 53(1), 17.

- Jeng, B. H., & McCoy, A. N. (2017). Evaluation and management of red eyes in primary care. Medical Clinics, 101(3), 431-437.
- Holmes, J. M., Beck, R. W., & et al. (2003). Risk of amblyopia recurrence after cessation of treatment. J AAPOS, 7(2), 87-94.
- Clearfield, E., Hawkins, B. S., & et al. (2016). A systematic review of combination therapy and outcomes in patients with advanced pterygium. Ophthalmology and Therapy, 5(2), 287-303.

Chapter 15. Oncologic/Hematologic Disorders

Reviewed by
Quy Pham Nguyen, MD, PhD

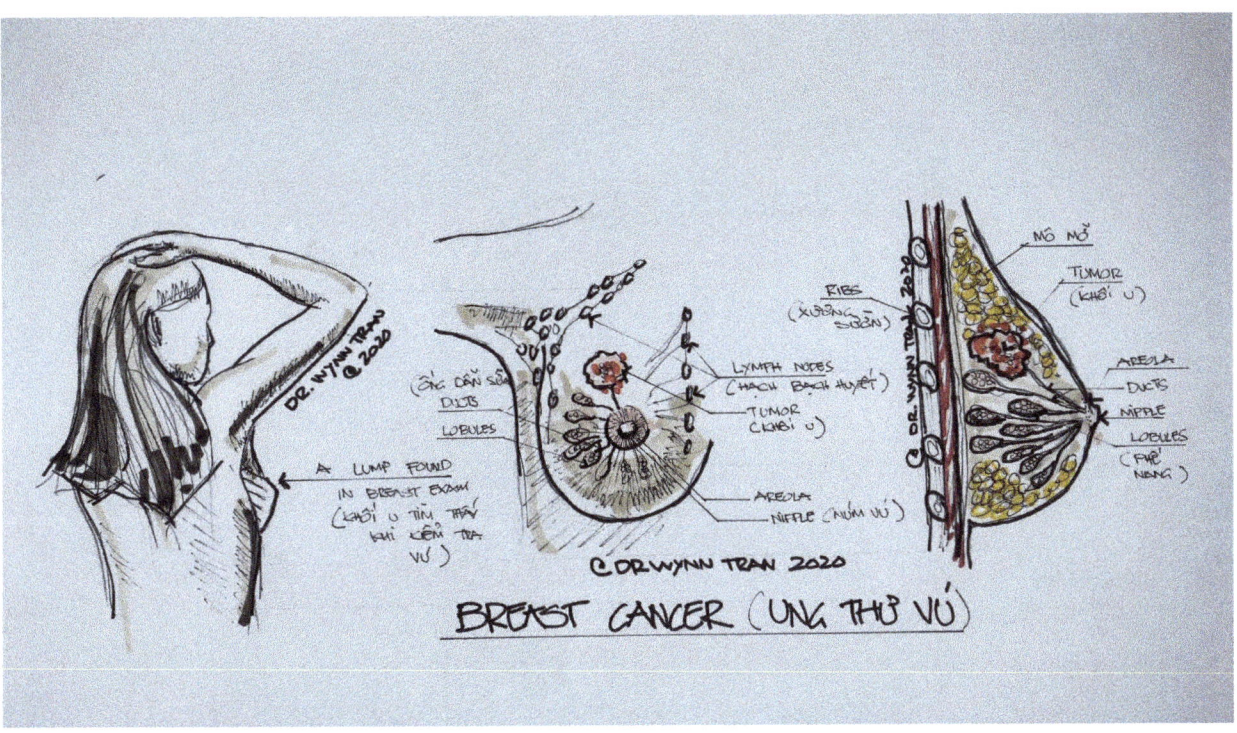

The APh should be familiar with the presentation, diagnosis, and management of these common oncologic and hematologic disorders to provide appropriate care and referral to the oncologist/hematologist when necessary.

15.1. Breast Cancer

> ➤ *Breast cancer is a malignancy originating in breast tissue, often characterized by a lump or mass, changes in breast size or shape, nipple discharge, or skin changes such as dimpling or redness.*
>
> ➤ *It is the most common cancer in women worldwide, with risk factors including age, genetics, hormonal factors, and lifestyle choices. Early detection through screening mammograms and self-exams is crucial for improving outcomes.*
>
> ➤ *Treatment involves a combination of surgery, chemotherapy, radiation therapy, hormone therapy, and targeted therapy depending on the stage and subtype of cancer.*

Symptoms:

- A lump or mass in the breast or underarm
- Changes in the size, shape, or appearance of the breast
- Nipple changes, such as inversion, discharge, or redness
- Skin changes on the breast, like dimpling or puckering
- Breast pain or tenderness that does not go away
- Swelling or lump in the lymph nodes under the arm or around the collarbone

Causes and Risk Factors:

- Gender: Breast cancer is more common in women, but men can also develop it.
- Age: Risk increases with age, with the majority of cases diagnosed in women over 50.
- Family history of breast cancer or inherited gene mutations (BRCA1, BRCA2)
- Personal history of breast cancer or certain non-cancerous breast diseases
- Hormone replacement therapy (HRT), especially long-term use
- Radiation exposure, especially to the chest area
- Obesity, especially after menopause
- Alcohol consumption and smoking
- Early menstruation (before age 12) or late menopause (after age 55)
- Not having children or having the first child after age 30

Epidemiology:

Breast cancer is the most common cancer in women worldwide, with about 2.3 million new cases diagnosed each year. It's also the second leading cause of cancer death in women, with around 685,000 deaths per year. The incidence varies globally, with higher rates in developed countries.

Diagnosis:
- Physical examination and medical history review
- Mammography: X-ray imaging of the breast to detect abnormalities
- Imaging: breast ultrasound or MRI for further evaluation
- Biopsy: removal of a small sample of tissue for examination under a microscope to confirm the presence of cancer

Treatment:
- Surgery: lumpectomy (removing the tumor and a small margin of surrounding tissue) or mastectomy (removing one or both breasts entirely). After a mastectomy, patients may choose to have breast reconstruction surgery, breast prosthesis or a flat closure.
- Radiation Therapy: using focus high-energy rays to target and kill breast cancer cells, often following surgery to eliminate any remaining cancer cells, but can also be performed in palliative setting.
- Chemotherapy:
    - Anti-cancer drugs are usually administered orally or intravenously to target and kill cancer cells. The specific drugs and regimen depend on the cancer's subtype, stage, and individual patient factors.
    - It's often used before surgery (neoadjuvant chemotherapy) to shrink tumors or after surgery (adjuvant chemotherapy) to eliminate any remaining cancer cells, reducing the risk of recurrence.
    - Chemotherapy can also be used to treat advanced or metastatic breast cancer (palliative setting), aiming to control disease progression and alleviate symptoms.
- Hormonal Therapy: For hormone receptor-positive cancers, drugs like tamoxifen or aromatase inhibitors are used to block estrogen and progesterone from supporting cancer growth.
- Targeted therapy:
    Utilizes drugs designed to specifically identify and attack cancer cells with particular genetic markers, sparing normal cells. This

approach includes treatments like HER2 inhibitors for HER2-positive breast cancers and olaparib for breast cancer with germline BRCA1/2 mutations.

- Immunotherapy:

    Involves treatments that stimulate the body's immune system to recognize and destroy cancer cells. It's particularly useful in treating triple-negative breast cancer. Current options include immune checkpoint inhibitors and monoclonal antibodies.

15.2. Lung Cancer

> ➤ Lung cancer is a malignant tumor arising from lung tissue, often associated with smoking, exposure to carcinogens, or genetic factors.
>
> ➤ Symptoms may include coughing, chest pain, shortness of breath, weight loss, and coughing up blood. Early detection through imaging tests and cessation of smoking are critical for improving survival rates.
>
> ➤ Treatment options include surgery, chemotherapy, radiation therapy, immunotherapy, and targeted therapy, depending on the stage and subtype of cancer.

Symptoms:
- Persistent cough that worsens over time
- Coughing up blood or rust-colored sputum
- Chest pain that worsens with deep breathing, coughing, or laughing
- Shortness of breath, wheezing, or hoarseness
- Recurrent respiratory infections, such as pneumonia or bronchitis
- Fatigue, weakness, or unexplained weight loss
- Bone pain, headache, or neurological symptoms

Causes and Risk Factors:
- Smoking: the primary cause of lung cancer, responsible for about 85% of cases
- Secondhand smoke exposure
- Radon exposure: Radon is a naturally occurring radioactive gas that can seep into homes.
- Occupational exposure to carcinogens such as asbestos, arsenic, chromium, and nickel
- Family history of lung cancer or genetic predisposition

- Air pollution, including indoor and outdoor pollutants
- Previous radiation therapy to the chest for other cancers

Epidemiology:

Lung cancer is the leading cause of cancer-related deaths worldwide, accounting for approximately 1.8 million deaths annually. It is more common in older adults, with the majority of cases diagnosed in patients over 65. Men are at higher risk than women, although the gap is narrowing as smoking rate among women increases.

Types:
- Non-Small Cell Lung Cancer (NSCLC): The most common type, accounting for about 85% of cases. Subtypes include adenocarcinoma, squamous cell carcinoma, and large cell carcinoma.
- Small Cell Lung Cancer (SCLC): A less common but more aggressive type, often associated with smoking. It tends to grow and spread quickly.

Diagnosis:
- Imaging Tests: chest X-ray, CT scan, MRI, or PET scan to visualize abnormalities in the lungs
- Biopsy: removal of a tissue sample for examination under a microscope to confirm cancer diagnosis and determine its type
- Sputum Cytology: examination of coughed-up sputum under a microscope to detect cancer cells
- Bronchoscopy: insertion of a thin, flexible tube with a camera into the airways to view the lungs and collect tissue samples
- Molecular Testing: Analysis of tumor tissue for specific genetic mutations or biomarkers that may guide treatment decisions

Treatment:
- Surgery: removal of the tumor and surrounding tissue, varying from wedge resection, segmentectomy to lobectomy or pneumonectomy
- Chemotherapy: drugs to kill cancer cells or slow their growth, often used in combination with surgery or radiation
- Radiation therapy: high-energy beams to destroy cancer cells, often used to shrink tumors before surgery or relieve symptoms
- Targeted therapy: drugs that target specific genetic mutations or pathways in cancer cells, with fewer side effects than chemotherapy. Some examples are Osimertinib for EGFR-mutated NSCLC, Alectinib for ALK-positive NSCLC, Crizotinib for ROS1-positive NSCLC.

- Immunotherapy: drugs that stimulate the immune system to recognize and attack cancer cells, particularly effective in certain subtypes of NSCLC.

15.3. Colorectal Cancer

> ➢ *Colorectal cancer is a malignancy that starts in the colon or rectum, often developing from benign polyps.*
>
> ➢ *It's the third most common cancer worldwide, with risk factors including age, family history, diet, and lifestyle. Early detection through screening tests like colonoscopy can improve outcomes.*
>
> ➢ *Treatment may involve surgery, chemotherapy, radiation, or targeted therapy depending on the stage and individual factors.*

Symptoms:

- Changes in bowel habits: persistent diarrhea, constipation, or changes in stool consistency, such as narrow or ribbon-like stools
- Blood in the stool: Bright red blood in the stool or dark, tarry stools may indicate bleeding from the rectum or lower digestive tract.
- Abdominal discomfort: persistent abdominal pain, cramping, or discomfort, such as gas pains, bloating, or feeling full even after a small meal
- Unexplained weight loss: Significant and unexplained weight loss may occur in some cases of colorectal cancer.
- Fatigue: generalized weakness, fatigue, or a sense of tiredness that does not improve with rest
- Anemia: Low red blood cell count may result from chronic bleeding in the digestive tract, leading to symptoms such as weakness, pale skin, or shortness of breath.
- Rectal bleeding: bleeding from the rectum or blood in the toilet bowl after a bowel movement

Causes and Risk Factors:

- Age: The risk of colorectal cancer increases with age, with the majority of cases diagnosed in patients over 50 years old.
- Family history: Having a first-degree relative (parent, sibling, or child) with colorectal cancer increases the risk of developing the disease.

- Personal history: Patients with a personal history of colorectal polyps, inflammatory bowel disease (such as Crohn's disease or ulcerative colitis), or previous colorectal cancer are at increased risk.
- Lifestyle factors: Poor diet (high in red or processed meats and low in fruits, vegetables, and fiber), sedentary lifestyle, obesity, smoking, and heavy alcohol consumption are associated with an increased risk of colorectal cancer.
- Genetic factors: Inherited genetic mutations, such as Lynch syndrome (hereditary nonpolyposis colorectal cancer) or familial adenomatous polyposis (FAP), can increase the risk of colorectal cancer.
- Race and ethnicity: African Americans have a higher risk of developing colorectal cancer compared to other racial or ethnic groups.
- Diabetes: Patients with diabetes have an increased risk of developing colorectal cancer, particularly if the diabetes is poorly controlled.
- Certain medical conditions: Conditions such as obesity, chronic inflammation of the colon, or a history of radiation therapy to the abdomen may increase the risk of colorectal cancer.

Epidemiology:

Colorectal cancer is one of the most common cancers worldwide, with an estimated 1.9 million new cases diagnosed annually. It is the third most commonly diagnosed cancer in both men and women, and the second leading cause of cancer-related deaths globally. The incidence and mortality rates of colorectal cancer vary by geographic region, with higher rates observed in developed countries.

Diagnosis:

- Screening:

    Colonoscopy, fecal occult blood test (FOBT), fecal immunochemical test (FIT), sigmoidoscopy, or virtual colonoscopy (CT colonography) may detect colorectal cancer or precancerous polyps in asymptomatic patients.

- Diagnostic tests:

    If colorectal cancer is suspected based on symptoms or screening results, colonoscopy, biopsy, or imaging studies (CT scan, MRI, PET scan) may be performed to confirm the diagnosis and evaluate the extent of the disease.

- **Staging:** Imaging studies or additional biopsies, may be performed to determine the stage of the cancer (extent of spread) and guide treatment decisions.

Treatment:

Treatment for colorectal cancer depends on several factors, including the stage of the cancer, the location of the tumor, the patient's overall health, and personal preferences.

- **Surgery:** Surgical removal of the tumor and surrounding tissues (colectomy, proctectomy) is the primary treatment for localized colorectal cancer.
- **Chemotherapy:** may be used before surgery (neoadjuvant therapy) to shrink tumors, after surgery (adjuvant therapy) to kill remaining cancer cells, or as the primary treatment for advanced or metastatic colorectal cancer
- **Radiation therapy:** may be used in combination with surgery and/or chemotherapy to treat colorectal cancer, particularly in cases where the tumor is located in the rectum or has spread to nearby tissues
- **Targeted therapy:** Monoclonal antibodies (e.g., Cetuximab, Panitumumab or Bevacizumab) or small molecule inhibitors (e.g., Sorafenib) may be used to target specific molecular pathways involved in colorectal cancer growth and progression.
- **Immunotherapy:** to boost the body's immune response against colorectal cancer cells, particularly in patients with mismatch repair deficient (dMMR) or microsatellite instability-high (MSI-H) metastatic colorectal cancer.

15.4. Prostate Cancer

> ➤ *Prostate cancer is a malignancy arising in the prostate gland, often asymptomatic in early stages but may cause urinary symptoms, blood in semen, or erectile dysfunction as it progresses.*
>
> ➤ *Screening methods include digital rectal exams and PSA tests. Early detection and individualized treatment plans are crucial for optimal outcomes.*
>
> ➤ *Treatment options range from active surveillance to surgery, radiation therapy, hormone therapy, chemotherapy, or immunotherapy depending on the stage and aggressiveness of the cancer.*

Symptoms:
- Urinary symptoms: changes in urinary habits, such as increased frequency, urgency, or difficulty starting or stopping urination
- Blood in the urine or semen: Blood in the urine or semen may be a sign of prostate cancer, although it can also be caused by other conditions.
- Erectile dysfunction: Difficulty achieving or maintaining an erection may occur in some cases of prostate cancer.
- Pain or discomfort: in the pelvic area, lower back, hips, or thighs in advanced stages of prostate cancer
- Bone pain: particularly in the spine, pelvis, or ribs if prostate cancer spreads to the bones

Causes and Risk Factors:
- Age: The risk of prostate cancer increases with age, particularly after age 50. The majority of prostate cancer cases are diagnosed in men over 65.
- Family history: Having a first-degree relative with prostate cancer increases the risk of developing the disease.
- Race and ethnicity: African American men have a higher risk of developing prostate cancer and are more likely to be diagnosed at an advanced stage compared to men of other racial or ethnic groups.
- Genetic factors: Inherited genetic mutations, such as mutations in the BRCA1 or BRCA2 genes, may increase the risk of prostate cancer.
- Dietary factors: High intake of red meat, processed meat, or dairy products, and low intake of fruits, vegetables, and fiber may be associated with an increased risk of prostate cancer.
- Obesity: Obesity and being overweight may increase the risk of developing aggressive or advanced prostate cancer.
- Smoking: Some studies suggest that smoking may be associated with an increased risk of death from prostate cancer.

Epidemiology:

Prostate cancer is one of the most common cancers among men worldwide. It is the second most commonly diagnosed cancer in men and the fifth leading cause of cancer-related deaths globally. The incidence and mortality rates of prostate cancer vary by geographic region, with higher rates observed in developed countries.

Diagnosis:
- Digital Rectal Examination (DRE):

    A urologist, PCP or APh inserts a lubricated, gloved finger into the rectum to feel for abnormalities in the prostate gland, such as lumps or enlargement.

- Prostate-Specific Antigen (PSA) test:

    A blood test measures the level of PSA, a protein produced by the prostate gland. Elevated PSA levels may indicate prostate cancer, although other conditions can also cause elevated PSA levels.

- Transrectal Ultrasound (TRUS): An ultrasound probe inserted into the rectum creates images of the prostate gland to evaluate its size, shape, and structure.

- Prostate biopsy:

    If prostate cancer is suspected based on DRE, PSA test results, or imaging studies, a biopsy may be performed to collect tissue samples from the prostate gland for examination under a microscope.

Treatment:
- Active Surveillance:

    For low-risk prostate cancer that is not causing symptoms or spreading, active surveillance involves closely monitoring the cancer with regular PSA tests, DREs, and periodic biopsies to detect any changes over time.

- Surgery: Surgical removal of the prostate gland may be recommended for localized or early-stage prostate cancer.

- Radiation Therapy: External beam radiation therapy or brachytherapy may be used to target and destroy cancer cells in the prostate gland.

- Hormone Therapy:

    Androgen deprivation therapy (ADT) or hormone therapy may be used to lower testosterone levels and slow the growth of prostate cancer cells, particularly in cases of advanced or metastatic prostate cancer.

- Chemotherapy: to kill cancer cells or slow the progression of advanced or metastatic prostate cancer, particularly if the cancer does not respond to hormone therapy. The key chemotherapeutics are Docetaxel, Cabazitaxel, Estramustine and Mitoxantrone.

- Immunotherapy: to boost the body's immune response against cancer cells, particularly in certain situations such as Sipuleucel-T for patients with asymptomatic or minimally symptomatic slowly progressive metastatic castration-resistant prostate cancer.

15.5. Melanoma

> ➤ *Melanoma is a potentially deadly form of skin cancer arising from melanocytes, often appearing as new or changing moles with irregular borders, asymmetry, color variation, and a diameter larger than a pencil eraser.*
>
> ➤ *Risk factors include UV exposure, fair skin, family history, and numerous moles. Early detection through regular skin checks and sun protection measures are critical for improving outcomes.*
>
> ➤ *Treatment involves surgical excision, immunotherapy, targeted therapy, chemotherapy, or radiation therapy depending on the stage and extent of the cancer.*

Symptoms:
- **C**hanges in moles: changes in the size, shape, color, or texture of existing moles or the development of new moles
- **A**symmetry: irregularly shaped moles or lesions that are asymmetrical
- **B**order irregularity: ragged, blurred, or notched edges of moles or lesions
- **C**olor variation: moles or lesions with uneven coloring or multiple colors, such as shades of brown, black, blue, red, or white
- **D**iameter: moles or lesions greater than 6 millimeters
- **E**volution: changes in the appearance, size, or elevation of moles or lesions over time, or symptoms such as itching, bleeding, or crusting

Causes and Risk Factors:
- Sun exposure: Overexposure to ultraviolet (UV) radiation from sunlight or artificial sources (such as tanning beds) is a major risk factor for melanoma.
- Fair skin: Patients with fair skin, light hair, and light eyes have a higher risk of developing melanoma.
- Family history: Having a first-degree relative with a history of melanoma increases the risk of developing the disease.

- Personal history: Patients with a personal history of melanoma or other types of skin cancer are at increased risk of developing additional melanomas.
- Genetic factors: Inherited genetic mutations, such as mutations in the CDKN2A or CDK4 genes, may increase the risk of melanoma.
- Moles: Having a large number of moles or atypical moles increases the risk of melanoma.
- Weakened immune system: Immunocompromised patients, such as organ transplant recipients or those with HIV/AIDS, have an increased risk of melanoma.
- Age: While melanoma can occur at any age, it is more common in older adults, with the highest incidence rates observed in patients over 65.

Epidemiology:

Melanoma is less common than other types of skin cancer but is more likely to grow and spread if not detected early. It accounts for a small percentage of skin cancer cases but causes the majority of skin cancer-related deaths. The incidence of melanoma varies by geographic region, with higher rates observed in regions with greater sun exposure and fair-skinned populations.

Diagnosis:

- Skin Examination: A PCP, APh or a dermatologist performs a thorough examination of the skin, including a visual inspection of moles, lesions, and other areas of concern.
- Dermoscopy: non-invasive imaging technique that allows for detailed examination of skin lesions and moles under magnification, helping to identify features suggestive of melanoma
- Skin Biopsy: If a suspicious mole or lesion is identified, a biopsy is collected and examined under a microscope by a dermatopathologist to confirm the diagnosis of melanoma and determine its characteristics, such as thickness, depth, and type.
- Sentinel Lymph Node Biopsy: In cases where melanoma has spread beyond the skin, sentinel lymph node biopsy may be performed to assess whether cancer cells have spread to nearby lymph nodes.

Treatment

- Surgery: Surgical removal of the melanoma and surrounding tissue (wide excision) is the primary treatment for early-stage melanoma.

- <u>Lymph Node Dissection:</u> If melanoma has spread to nearby lymph nodes, surgical removal of the affected lymph nodes may be performed.
- <u>Immunotherapy:</u> Immune checkpoint inhibitors (e.g., Pembrolizumab, Nivolumab+Ipilimumab) may be used to boost the body's immune response against melanoma cells.
- <u>Targeted therapy:</u> Drugs that target specific genetic mutations or pathways in cancer cells such as BRAF inhibitors and MEK inhibitors (e.g., Dabrafenib+Trametinib, Encorafenib+Binimetinib, Vemurafenib+Cobimetinib) for cancer with BRAF V600E mutation.
- <u>Chemotherapy:</u> to kill cancer cells or slow the progression of advanced or metastatic melanoma, particularly if the cancer does not respond to other treatments (e.g., Dacarbazine, Temozolomide, Carboplatin, Paclitaxel)
- <u>Radiation Therapy:</u> to target and destroy cancer cells in the skin, lymph nodes, or other areas of the body affected by melanoma

15.6. Basal Cell Carcinoma

> ➤ *Basal cell carcinoma (BCC) is the most common type of skin cancer, usually appearing as a pinkish or pearly bump with a rolled edge and often occurring on sun-exposed areas like the face and neck.*
>
> ➤ *It typically grows slowly and rarely metastasizes but can cause local tissue destruction if left untreated. Regular skin checks and sun protection are important for prevention and early detection.*
>
> ➤ *Treatment involves surgical removal, cryotherapy, photodynamic therapy, topical medications, targeted therapy or immunotherapy depending on the size, location, and depth of the lesion.*

Symptoms:
- Pearly or waxy bump: a translucent, flesh-colored, or pink bump with a pearly or shiny appearance
- Flat, flesh-colored or brown lesion: It may resemble a scar or be slightly raised.
- Pink growths: pink, red, or red-brown patches that may be slightly raised and have an elevated border
- Open sores or lesions: These may ooze, crust, or bleed intermittently and fail to heal, or they may heal and then reopen.
- Shiny or scaly patches: These may appear white, yellow, or waxy.

Causes and Risk Factors:
- Chronic sun exposure: Excessive exposure to ultraviolet (UV) radiation from the sun or tanning beds is the primary risk factor.
- Fair skin: Lighter skin types have less melanin, providing less protection against UV radiation.
- Age: Basal cell carcinoma is more common in older adults, although it can occur at any age.
- Gender: Men are more likely than women to develop basal cell carcinoma.
- Personal or family history: A personal history of skin cancer or a family history of skin cancer increases the risk.
- Immunosuppression: Patients with a weakened immune system, such as organ transplant recipients or those with HIV/AIDS, have an increased risk.
- Previous radiation exposure: Previous exposure to radiation therapy increases the risk of developing basal cell carcinoma.
- Certain genetic syndromes: Conditions such as basal cell nevus syndrome (Gorlin syndrome) increase the risk of developing multiple basal cell carcinomas.

Epidemiology:
- Basal cell carcinoma is the most common type of skin cancer, accounting for approximately 80% of all cases of skin cancer.
- It is more prevalent in regions with high levels of UV radiation, such as sunny climates and high altitudes.
- The incidence of basal cell carcinoma is increasing worldwide, particularly in fair-skinned populations.

Diagnosis:

Basal cell carcinoma is diagnosed through a combination of clinical examination and biopsy.
- <u>Clinical Examination:</u> A PCP, APh or a dermatologist typically evaluates suspicious skin lesions using dermoscopy and may perform a skin biopsy to confirm the diagnosis.
- <u>Biopsy:</u> The biopsy sample is examined under a microscope by a pathologist to identify characteristic features of basal cell carcinoma.

Treatment:
- <u>Surgical Excision:</u> surgical removal of the BCC tumor and surrounding tissue

- <u>Mohs Micrographic Surgery:</u> a specialized surgical technique that removes the tumor layer by layer while sparing healthy tissue
- <u>Curettage and Electrodesiccation:</u> scraping the BCC tumor followed by cauterization with an electric current
- <u>Cryotherapy:</u> freezing the BCC tumor with liquid nitrogen
- <u>Photodynamic therapy:</u> utilizing porphyrins-related cytotoxicity in the presence of oxygen after stimulation by a specific type of light.
- <u>Topical Therapies:</u> Prescription creams or gels containing medications such as imiquimod or 5-fluorouracil may be used for superficial basal cell carcinomas.
- <u>Radiation Therapy:</u> may be used to control BCC tumors that are not candidates for surgery.
- <u>Targeted Therapy:</u> Hedgehog pathway inhibitors such as vismodegib and sonidegib may be used for locally advanced or metastatic basal cell carcinoma.
- <u>Immunotherapy:</u> Cemiplimab is an option for patients who previously treated with or are not appropriate for a hedgehog pathway inhibitor.

15.7. Squamous Cell Carcinoma

> ➤ *Squamous cell carcinoma (SCC) is a common type of skin cancer characterized by scaly red patches, open sores, or elevated growths, often developing on sun-exposed areas.*
>
> ➤ *Prevention strategies include sun protection, regular skin examinations, and early treatment of precancerous lesions.*
>
> ➤ *It can metastasize to other parts of the body if left untreated, requiring prompt surgical removal, Mohs surgery, radiation therapy, chemotherapy, or immunotherapy depending on the stage and extent of the cancer.*

Symptoms:
- Persistent, firm, red nodules or lumps on the skin
- Rough, scaly, or crusty patches on the skin, often with an elevated border
- Ulcerated lesions or sores that fail to heal or recur
- Thickened or raised growths with central depression or crusting
- Lesions may be tender or painful, and they may bleed easily

Causes and Risk Factors:
- Chronic sun exposure: Long-term exposure to ultraviolet (UV) radiation from the sun is the primary risk factor for SCC.
- Fair skin: Lighter skin types are more susceptible to UV damage and have an increased risk of developing SCC.
- Age: SCC is more common in older adults, although it can occur at any age.
- Gender: Men are more likely than women to develop SCC.
- Personal or family history: A personal history of skin cancer or a family history of skin cancer increases the risk.
- Immunosuppression: Patients with a weakened immune system, such as organ transplant recipients or those with HIV/AIDS, have an increased risk.
- Previous radiation exposure: Previous exposure to radiation therapy increases the risk of developing SCC.
- Human papillomavirus (HPV) infection: Certain strains of HPV are associated with an increased risk of SCC, particularly in genital and oral lesions.

Epidemiology:
- Squamous cell carcinoma is the second most common type of skin cancer, accounting for approximately 20% of all cases of skin cancer.
- It is more prevalent in regions with high levels of UV radiation, such as sunny climates and high altitudes.
- The incidence of squamous cell carcinoma is increasing worldwide, particularly in fair-skinned populations.

Diagnosis:

Squamous cell carcinoma is diagnosed through a combination of clinical examination and skin biopsy.
- <u>Clinical Examination:</u> A PCP, APh or a dermatologist typically evaluates suspicious skin lesions using dermoscopy and may perform a skin biopsy to confirm the diagnosis.
- <u>Biopsy:</u> The biopsy sample is examined under a microscope by a pathologist to identify characteristic features of squamous cell carcinoma.

Treatment:
- <u>Surgical Excision:</u> surgical removal of the tumor and surrounding tissue

- <u>Mohs Micrographic Surgery:</u> a specialized surgical technique that removes the tumor layer by layer while sparing healthy tissue
- <u>Curettage and Electrodesiccation:</u> scraping the tumor followed by cauterization with an electric current
- <u>Cryotherapy:</u> freezing the tumor with liquid nitrogen
- <u>Radiation Therapy:</u> This may be recommended for tumors that are not candidates for surgical excision.
- <u>Topical Chemotherapies:</u> Prescription creams or gels containing medications such as 5-fluorouracil or imiquimod may be used for superficial squamous cell carcinomas.
- <u>Systemic Chemotherapy:</u> Anticancer agents such as Carboplatin and Paclitaxel may be used for advanced or metastatic squamous cell carcinoma.
- <u>Immunotherapy:</u> Cemiplimab, Pembrolizumab and Nivolumab are effective and less toxic than chemotherapeutic agents.

15.8. Bladder Cancer

> *Bladder cancer is a malignancy originating in the bladder lining, often presenting with blood in the urine, frequent urination, and pain during urination.*
>
> *Risk factors include smoking, exposure to certain chemicals, chronic bladder inflammation, and radiation therapy. Early detection through cystoscopy, urine cytology, and imaging tests improves prognosis and treatment outcomes.*
>
> *Treatment options vary depending on the stage of the cancer. For non-muscle invasive bladder cancer, TURBT is usually indicated with or without adjuvant intravesical therapy while radical cystectomy or trimodality therapy is needed for patients with muscle invasive disease. For advanced unresectable or metastatic disease, systemic treatment options include antibody-drug conjugates, chemotherapy, immune checkpoint inhibitors, and targeted therapies.*

Symptoms:
- Hematuria, which may be visible or detected during urinalysis
- Frequent urination or urgency to urinate
- Pain or burning sensation during urination
- Lower back pain or pelvic pain

- Difficulty urinating or weak urine stream
- Feeling the need to urinate but being unable to pass urine
- Urinary tract infections that recur or do not respond to treatment

Causes and Risk Factors:
- Smoking: Cigarette smoking is the most significant risk factor for bladder cancer, accounting for approximately half of all cases.
- Age: Bladder cancer is more common in older adults, with the risk increasing with age.
- Occupational exposure: Certain occupations involving exposure to chemicals such as aromatic amines (e.g., in the dye, rubber, and leather industries), as well as chemicals used in aluminum production and hairdressing, increase the risk.
- Chemical exposure: Exposure to certain chemicals, such as arsenic and chlorinated hydrocarbons, may increase the risk.
- Gender: Men are at higher risk of developing bladder cancer than women.
- Race and ethnicity: Caucasians have a higher incidence of bladder cancer than other racial and ethnic groups.
- Medical Conditions: Chronic bladder infections, bladder stones, and catheter use increase the risk.
- Previous cancer treatment: Previous radiation therapy or certain chemotherapy drugs increases the risk.
- Family history: patients with a family history of bladder cancer may have an increased risk.

Epidemiology:
- Bladder cancer is the sixth most common cancer in the United States, with an estimated 82,290 new cases expected in 2023.
- It is more common in men than women, with men being approximately three to four times more likely to develop bladder cancer.
- The incidence of bladder cancer increases with age, with the highest rates seen in patients over 65 years old.

Diagnosis:

Diagnosis of bladder cancer typically involves a combination of medical history, physical examination, imaging studies, and laboratory tests.
- <u>Urine Cytology:</u> microscopic examination of urine to detect cancer cells shed from the bladder lining

- Cystoscopy: a thin, flexible tube with a camera is inserted into the bladder to visualize the bladder lining and take a biopsy for further examination
- Imaging Tests: ultrasound, computed tomography (CT), magnetic resonance imaging (MRI), or retrograde ureteropyelography (UPRG) to assess the extent of the tumor and evidence of metastasis.

Treatment:
- Surgery: transurethral resection of the bladder tumor (TURBT) for early-stage tumors or radical cystectomy (removal of the bladder) for more advanced disease.
- Chemotherapy: intravesical chemotherapy (placement of chemotherapy drugs directly into the bladder) for localized disease or systemic chemotherapy for advanced or metastatic disease.
- Immunotherapy: Pembrolizumab, Nivolumab or Avelumab are common agents for advanced or metastatic disease. Pembrolizumab plus Enfortumab vedotin have become the first line treatment for patients with metastatic disease, but Nivolumab plus Gemcitabine and Cisplatin can be a reasonable alternative.
- Radiation therapy: may be used for curative or palliative purposes. Trimodality therapy, which incorporates maximal transurethral resection of bladder tumor (TURBT), radiation therapy, and concurrent chemotherapy, is an option for patients with muscle invasive urothelial bladder cancer who are not candidates for radical cystectomy or who desire to preserve their native bladder.
- Targeted therapy: Erdafitinib, a FGFR inhibitor, is an option for patients with advanced or metastatic bladder cancer with FGFR3 genetic alterations who progress on both platinum-based chemotherapy and immunotherapy.

15.9. Pancreatic Cancer

> ➤ *Pancreatic cancer is a highly aggressive malignancy arising from the cells of the pancreas, often asymptomatic in early stages but presenting with abdominal pain, jaundice, weight loss, and digestive issues as it progresses.*
>
> ➤ *Risk factors include smoking, obesity, family history, and certain genetic syndromes. Early detection remains challenging, emphasizing the importance of awareness and further research for improved screening methods and treatment strategies.*
>
> ➤ *Treatment options include surgery, chemotherapy, radiation therapy, targeted therapy depending on the stage and extent of the cancer.*

Symptoms:

- Abdominal pain or discomfort, often radiating to the back
- Jaundice (yellowing of the skin and eyes) due to obstruction of the bile duct by the tumor
- Unexplained weight loss and loss of appetite
- Nausea and vomiting
- New-onset diabetes or unexplained worsening of existing diabetes
- Changes in stool color (pale or clay-colored) and consistency (greasy or floating stools)
- Fatigue and weakness
- Enlargement of the gallbladder or liver (seen on imaging studies)
- Blood clots (deep vein thrombosis or pulmonary embolism) may occur in advanced cases

Causes and Risk Factors:

- Age: Pancreatic cancer is more common in older adults, with the majority of cases diagnosed after the age of 65.
- Smoking: Cigarette smoking is one of the most significant risk factors for pancreatic cancer, increasing the risk by two to three times compared to non-smokers.
- Family history: Patients with a family history of pancreatic cancer or certain genetic syndromes (e.g., hereditary pancreatitis, Lynch syndrome, familial atypical multiple mole melanoma syndrome) have an increased risk.
- Chronic pancreatitis: Long-standing inflammation of the pancreas increases the risk of pancreatic cancer.

- Obesity and poor diet: Obesity, a diet high in red meat and processed meats, and low consumption of fruits and vegetables may increase the risk.
- Diabetes: Patients with long-standing diabetes (especially if diagnosed after the age of 50) have an increased risk of pancreatic cancer.
- Alcohol consumption: Heavy alcohol consumption is associated with an increased risk, particularly in combination with smoking.
- Race and ethnicity: African Americans have a higher incidence of pancreatic cancer than other racial and ethnic groups.
- Occupational exposures: Exposure to certain chemicals, such as pesticides, benzene, or certain dyes, may increase the risk.

Epidemiology:
- Pancreatic cancer is relatively rare but has a high mortality rate, making it the fourth leading cause of cancer-related death in the United States.
- It accounts for approximately 3% of all cancers diagnosed in the United States and 7% of cancer deaths.
- The incidence of pancreatic cancer increases with age, with the highest rates seen in patients over 65 years old.

Diagnosis:

Diagnosis of pancreatic cancer typically involves a combination of medical history, physical examination, imaging studies, and laboratory tests.

- Imaging Tests: computed tomography (CT), magnetic resonance imaging (MRI), endoscopic ultrasound (EUS), or positron emission tomography (PET) to assess the size, location, and extent of the tumor
- Biopsy: A tissue sample obtained through EUS-guided fine needle aspiration (EUS-FNA) is necessary to confirm the diagnosis of pancreatic cancer and determine the histological subtype. Endoscopic retrograde cholangiopancreatography (ERCP)-based cytology is an alternative technique.
- Blood Tests: Tumor markers such as CA19-9 and CEA may be elevated in pancreatic cancer.

Treatment:
- Surgery: Surgical resection (removal) of the tumor, typically the Whipple procedure (pancreaticoduodenectomy) for tumors in the head of the pancreas or distal pancreatectomy for tumors in the body or tail of the pancreas.

- Chemotherapy: Systemic chemotherapy such as gemcitabine and nabpaclitaxel, FOLFIRINOX (combination of fluorouracil, leucovorin, irinotecan, and oxaliplatin), or other anticancer drugs may be used for advanced or metastatic disease. Some of them might be used before or after surgery as adjuvant therapy.
- Radiation Therapy: may be used to relieve symptoms or combined with chemotherapy for curative purposes.
- Targeted Therapy: Genetic testing is recommended for all patients with metastatic pancreatic cancer for personalized treatments. For example, platinum-based chemotherapy followed by maintenance therapy with PARP inhibitors is recommended for patients with pathogenic variants in BRCA1/2 or PALB2.

15.10. Ovarian Cancer

> ➤ *Ovarian cancer is a silent killer, often diagnosed at an advanced stage due to nonspecific symptoms like abdominal pain, bloating, and changes in bowel habits.*
>
> ➤ *Risk factors include family history, age, and certain genetic mutations. Early detection through screening tests like pelvic exams, ultrasound, and blood tests is crucial for improving outcomes.*
>
> ➤ *Treatment involving surgery, chemotherapy, targeted therapy, or immunotherapy depending on the stage and subtype of the cancer.*

Symptoms:
- Abdominal or pelvic pain or discomfort
- Bloating or feeling of fullness in the abdomen
- Difficulty eating or feeling full quickly
- Urinary urgency or frequency
- Changes in bowel habits, such as constipation or diarrhea
- Unexplained weight loss
- Fatigue or low energy
- Back pain
- Abnormal vaginal bleeding or discharge
- Enlargement or swelling of the abdomen

Causes and Risk Factors:
- Age: Ovarian cancer is more common in older women, with the majority of cases diagnosed in women over 50 years old.
- Family history: Women with a family history of ovarian cancer or certain genetic mutations, such as BRCA1 or BRCA2 mutations, have an increased risk.
- Personal history: Women who have had breast, uterine, or colorectal cancer have an increased risk of developing ovarian cancer.
- Inherited genetic syndromes: Certain genetic syndromes, such as Hereditary Breast and Ovarian Cancer Syndromes (HBOCs) and Hereditary Nonpolyposis Colorectal Cancer (HNPCC), also known as Lynch syndrome, increase the risk of ovarian cancer.
- Reproductive history: Factors such as never having been pregnant, early menstruation (before age 12), late menopause (after age 52), or nulliparity may increase the risk.
- Hormone replacement therapy: Long-term use of hormone replacement therapy (HRT) may increase the risk, particularly if estrogen-only therapy is used.
- Endometriosis: Endometriosis, a condition in which uterine tissue grows outside the uterus, may be slightly associated with some subtypes of ovarian cancer (e.g., endometrioid, clear cell).
- Obesity may increase the risk of developing certain types of ovarian cancer.
- Smoking has been associated with an increased risk of mucinous ovarian cancer.

Epidemiology:
- Ovarian cancer is the fifth most common cancer among women worldwide and the most lethal of all gynecological cancers.
- The incidence of ovarian cancer varies by geographic region and is highest in developed countries.
- The lifetime risk of developing ovarian cancer is approximately 1.37% for women in the United States.

Diagnosis:
Diagnosis of ovarian cancer typically involves a combination of medical history, physical examination, imaging studies, and laboratory tests.
- <u>Imaging Tests:</u> transvaginal ultrasound, computed tomography (CT), magnetic resonance imaging (MRI), or positron emission tomography (PET) to assess the size, location, and extent of the tumor.

- Blood tests: Tumor markers such as CA 125, HE4, and CA 19-9 may be elevated in ovarian cancer.
- Histological Evaluation: Tissue is obtained during surgical removal of an ovary or fallopian tube or biopsies of the peritoneum.

Treatment:

- Surgery: Surgical removal of the tumor and affected tissues, including the ovaries, fallopian tubes, uterus, and nearby lymph nodes (cytoreductive surgery).
- Chemotherapy: Systemic chemotherapy with platinum-based agents (e.g., carboplatin, cisplatin) and taxanes (e.g., paclitaxel) is the mainstay of treatment for ovarian cancer, often given after surgery (adjuvant chemotherapy) or as neoadjuvant therapy before surgery. Intravenous/intraperitoneal (IV/IP) chemotherapy as adjuvant treatment is an appropriate option for women with optimally cytoreduced disease.
- Targeted Therapy: Medications targeting specific molecular pathways involved in ovarian cancer, such as PARP inhibitors (e.g., olaparib, niraparib, rucaparib) and anti-angiogenic agent (bevacizumab), may be used for advanced or recurrent ovarian cancer, particularly in patients with BRCA mutations.
- Immunotherapy: Pembrolizumab may be used for advanced or recurrent ovarian cancer with mismatch repair deficient (dMMR) or microsatellite instability-high (MSI-H) features.

15.11. Cervical Cancer

> *Cervical cancer is a malignancy originating in the cells of the cervix, often caused by persistent human papillomavirus (HPV) infection, with risk factors including multiple sexual partners, smoking, and weakened immune system.*
>
> *Symptoms may include abnormal vaginal bleeding, pelvic pain, or pain during intercourse. Early detection and vaccination are key for reducing cervical cancer incidence and mortality.*
>
> *Prevention includes HPV vaccination, regular Pap smears, and HPV testing, while treatment involves surgery, radiation therapy, chemotherapy, or targeted therapy depending on the stage and extent of the cancer.*

Symptoms:
- Abnormal vaginal bleeding between periods, after intercourse, or after menopause
- Pelvic pain or pain during intercourse
- Vaginal discharge with an unpleasant odor
- Changes in menstrual cycle
- Unexplained weight loss
- Fatigue
- Pelvic mass or swelling

Causes and Risk Factors:
- Human papillomavirus (HPV) infection, particularly high-risk types such as HPV-16 and HPV-18
- Sexual activity at an early age
- Multiple sexual partners
- Smoking
- Immunosuppression (e.g., HIV infection, organ transplantation)
- History of sexually transmitted infections (e.g., chlamydia, gonorrhea)
- Long-term use of oral contraceptives
- Family history of cervical cancer
- Poor socioeconomic status
- Lack of access to cervical cancer screening and preventive healthcare

Epidemiology:

Cervical cancer is the fourth most common cancer in women globally, with an estimated 604,000 new cases and 342,000 deaths annually. The burden of cervical cancer is higher in low- and middle-income countries, where access to screening and preventive measures may be limited. In developed countries, widespread implementation of cervical cancer screening programs has led to a significant reduction in the incidence and mortality of the disease.

Diagnosis:
- <u>Pap Smear (Pap test):</u> screening test to detect abnormal cervical cells that may indicate precancerous or cancerous changes
- <u>HPV Testing:</u> molecular testing to detect high-risk HPV types in cervical cells, often performed in conjunction with Pap smear (co-testing)

- **Colposcopy:** visual examination of the cervix using a magnifying instrument (colposcope) after abnormal Pap smear results or HPV testing
- **Biopsy:** removal of tissue samples from the cervix for pathological examination to confirm the presence of cervical cancer or precancerous lesions
- **Imaging studies:** ultrasound, CT scan, or MRI to assess the extent of cancer spread (staging) and identify any metastasis

Treatment:
- **Surgery:**
  - cone biopsy or loop electrosurgical excision procedure (LEEP) for early-stage cervical cancer or precancerous lesions
  - hysterectomy (removal of the uterus) for more advanced or invasive cancers
- **Radiation Therapy:** external beam radiation or brachytherapy (internal radiation) for localized cervical cancer
- **Chemotherapy:** concurrent chemotherapy and radiation therapy (chemoradiation) for advanced or metastatic cervical cancer.
- **Targeted therapy:** Bevacizumab, a vascular endothelial growth factor (VEGF) inhibitor, can be incorporated in women with metastatic or recurrent cervical cancer.
- **Immunotherapy:** Immune checkpoint inhibitors such as Pembrolizumab or atezolizumab can be added to chemotherapy, depending on the expression of PD-L1 and the cost of treatment.

15.12. Thyroid Cancer

> *Thyroid cancer is a malignancy originating in the thyroid gland, typically presenting as a lump or nodule in the neck.*
>
> *Risk factors include radiation exposure, family history, and certain genetic syndromes. Prognosis is generally favorable as early detection and proper management usually lead to high survival rates.*
>
> *Treatment involves surgery, radioactive iodine therapy, thyroid hormone therapy, or targeted therapy depending on the cancer subtype and stage.*

Symptoms:
- Lump or nodule in the neck, often painless

- Swelling or enlargement of the thyroid gland
- Hoarseness or voice changes
- Dysphagia
- Persistent cough not associated with a cold or other respiratory condition
- Pain or discomfort in the neck or throat
- Enlarged lymph nodes in the neck

Causes and Risk Factors:
- Radiation exposure: particularly during childhood or adolescence, such radiation therapy for head and neck cancers or radiation fallout
- Family history of thyroid cancer or other thyroid conditions
- Genetic syndromes such as Familial adenomatous polyposis (FAP), Multiple endocrine neoplasia (MEN) or Cowden syndrome may associate with increased risk of thyroid cancer
- Gender: Thyroid cancer is more common in females
- Age: Thyroid cancer incidence increases with age, with most cases diagnosed between 20-55 years old
- History of Hashimoto's thyroiditis, goiter or benign thyroid nodules
- Iodine deficiency or excess in diet may possibly increase the risk of papillary thyroid cancer.
- Exposure to environmental toxins or pollutants

Epidemiology:

Thyroid cancer is relatively rare compared to other cancers, but its incidence has been increasing in recent decades, partially due to earlier detection with the widespread use of neck ultrasonography. It is the most common endocrine malignancy, accounting for approximately 1-2% of all cancers worldwide. The majority of thyroid cancers are papillary thyroid carcinoma, followed by follicular thyroid carcinoma, medullary thyroid carcinoma, and anaplastic thyroid carcinoma. Thyroid cancer is more common in females, with a peak incidence in the fourth to sixth decades of life.

Diagnosis:
- <u>Physical Examination:</u> assessment of the neck for palpable nodules or enlargement of the thyroid gland
- <u>Imaging Studies:</u> Ultrasound of the thyroid gland is done to evaluate the size, number, and characteristics of nodules. Other imaging

modalities such as CT scan or MRI may be used for staging and assessment of metastasis.

- <u>Fine-Needle Aspiration Biopsy (FNAB):</u> removal of tissue samples from thyroid nodules for cytological examination to determine if they are benign or malignant
- <u>Blood Tests:</u> measurement of thyroid function tests (TFTs) to assess thyroid hormone levels and thyroid-stimulating hormone (TSH) levels
- <u>Molecular testing:</u> genetic testing for specific mutations associated with thyroid cancer (e.g., BRAF, RAS, RET gene mutations) to aid in diagnosis and prognosis

Treatment:

- <u>Surgery:</u> Thyroidectomy, surgical removal of a part or all of the thyroid gland, may be performed depending on the extent and type of thyroid cancer.
- <u>Radioactive Iodine (RAI) Therapy:</u> adjuvant therapy following surgery to destroy any remaining thyroid tissue or cancer cells.
- <u>Thyroid Hormone Replacement Therapy:</u> Levothyroxine replaces thyroid hormone levels after thyroidectomy and suppresses TSH levels to prevent cancer recurrence.
- <u>External Beam Radiation Therapy (EBRT):</u> to treat advanced or recurrent thyroid cancer, particularly in patients who are not candidates for surgery or RAI therapy.
- <u>Systemic treatment:</u> Somatic mutation testing can be done to consider mutation-specific treatment options such as RET, TRK, or BRAF inhibitors. In the absence of a mutation, anti-angiogenic multikinase inhibitors such as lenvatinib, cabozantinib, sorafenib are available options.

15.13. Leukemia

> ➢ *Leukemia is a cancer of the blood and bone marrow, characterized by the overproduction of abnormal white blood cells.*
> ➢ *Symptoms include fatigue, frequent infections, easy bruising or bleeding, and enlarged lymph nodes or spleen. Prognosis varies depending on factors such as age, overall health, and specific characteristics of the leukemia.*
> ➢ *Treatment involves chemotherapy, radiation therapy, targeted therapy, immunotherapy, or stem cell transplantation depending on the type and subtype of leukemia.*

Symptoms:
- Fatigue and weakness
- Pale skin
- Easy bruising or bleeding
- Frequent infections
- Fever and night sweats
- Swollen lymph nodes, particularly in the neck, armpits, or groin
- Bone pain or tenderness
- Unexplained weight loss
- Hepatosplenomegaly
- Headaches, seizures, or other neurological symptoms

Causes and Risk Factors:
- Genetic predisposition or family history of leukemia
- Exposure to ionizing radiation or certain chemicals such as benzene or formaldehyde
- Previous history of chemotherapy or radiation therapy for other cancers
- Genetic syndromes: Down syndrome, Li-Fraumeni syndrome
- Smoking tobacco or exposure to secondhand smoke
- Viral infections: human T-cell leukemia virus, Epstein-Barr virus
- Exposure to high levels of electromagnetic fields (controversial association)
- Age: Risk increases with age, particularly in adults over 60.
- Gender: Some types of leukemia are more common in males.

- Previous history of myelodysplastic syndromes (MDS) or myeloproliferative neoplasms (MPNs)

Epidemiology:

Leukemia is a relatively common cancer of the blood and bone marrow, accounting for approximately 3-4% of all new cancer cases worldwide. It affects patients of all ages, with different types of leukemia having distinct age distributions. Acute lymphoblastic leukemia (ALL) is more common in children, while acute myeloid leukemia (AML) and chronic lymphocytic leukemia (CLL) are more common in adults. The exact incidence and prevalence of leukemia vary by geographic region and population demographics.

Diagnosis:

- Blood Tests:
    - Complete blood count (CBC): to evaluate the number and type of blood cells, including red blood cells, white blood cells, and platelets
        - Leukocytosis: an increased number of white blood cells (WBCs), particularly immature forms, which is common in acute leukemias
        - Anemia: a decrease in red blood cells (RBCs), leading to low hemoglobin levels, which can cause fatigue and weakness
        - Thrombocytopenia: a reduced platelet count, increasing the risk of bleeding and bruising
        - Abnormal differential: atypical presence of blast cells (immature WBCs) in the blood, a key indicator of acute leukemia
    - Peripheral blood smear: to examine blood cells under a microscope for abnormalities such as blasts (immature white blood cells)
- Bone Marrow Aspiration and Biopsy: collection of bone marrow samples from the hip bone for examination under a microscope to confirm the presence of leukemia cells and determine the type and subtype of leukemia
- Imaging Studies: X-rays, CT, or MRI may be performed to assess for enlarged lymph nodes, organ enlargement, or bone abnormalities associated with leukemia.
- Cytogenetic Testing: Analysis of leukemia cells for specific chromosomal abnormalities or genetic mutations that may influence prognosis and treatment decisions.

Treatment:

- Chemotherapy: may be given orally, intravenously, or directly into the cerebrospinal fluid (intrathecal chemotherapy) to kill leukemia cells and induce remission
- Targeted Therapy: use of drugs that target leukemia cells based on their molecular characteristics (e.g., tyrosine kinase inhibitors, monoclonal antibodies)
- Radiation Therapy: use of high-energy radiation to target and kill leukemia cells, particularly in localized disease or to prepare for stem cell transplantation
- Stem Cell Transplantation: Transplantation of healthy stem cells (either from a donor or the patient's own stem cells) to replace diseased bone marrow and restore normal blood cell production.
- Immunotherapy: use of immune-modulating drugs or cellular therapies (e.g., chimeric antigen receptor T-cell therapy) to enhance the body's immune response against leukemia cells

15.14. Lymphoma

> - *Lymphoma is a cancer of the lymphatic system, comprising Hodgkin lymphoma and non-Hodgkin lymphoma.*
> - *Symptoms may include swollen lymph nodes, fever, night sweats, weight loss, and fatigue. Prognosis varies but can be favorable with early diagnosis and appropriate treatment.*
> - *Treatment involves chemotherapy, radiation therapy, targeted therapy, immunotherapy, or stem cell transplantation depending on the type, stage, and subtype of lymphoma.*

Symptoms:

- Painless swelling of lymph nodes, usually in the neck, armpits, or groin
- Persistent fatigue
- Unexplained weight loss
- Night sweats
- Fever without an obvious cause (intermittent or persistent)
- Pruritus
- Splenomegaly or Hepatomegaly
- Difficulty breathing or chest pain (in cases of mediastinal lymphoma)

- Abdominal pain or swelling (in cases of abdominal lymphoma)
- Neurological symptoms, such as headaches, seizures, or weakness (less common)

Causes and Risk Factors:
- Age: The risk of lymphoma increases with age, with most cases diagnosed in patients over 60 years old.
- Gender: Certain types of lymphoma are more common in men than in women.
- Weakened immune system: Conditions or medications that suppress the immune system increase the risk of lymphoma, such as HIV/AIDS, organ transplantation, or immunosuppressive therapy.
- Infections: Chronic infections with certain viruses or bacteria, such as Epstein-Barr virus (EBV), human T-cell leukemia virus (HTLV-1), Helicobacter pylori (H. pylori), or human herpesvirus-8 (HHV-8), may increase the risk of lymphoma.
- Autoimmune diseases, such as rheumatoid arthritis, systemic lupus erythematosus (SLE), or Sjögren's syndrome, may slightly increase the risk of lymphoma.
- Family history: Having a first-degree relative (parent, sibling, or child) with lymphoma may increase the risk of developing the disease.
- Exposure to certain chemicals or pesticides may increase the risk of lymphoma, although the evidence is limited.
- Prior treatment with chemotherapy or radiation therapy for other cancers may slightly increase the risk of secondary lymphoma.

Epidemiology:

Lymphoma is one of the most common types of blood cancer, with two main subtypes: Hodgkin lymphoma (HL) and non-Hodgkin lymphoma (NHL). NHL is more common, accounting for about 90% of all lymphomas diagnosed. The incidence of NHL increases with age, peaking in older adults, while HL has a bimodal age distribution, with peaks in young adulthood (age 15-34) and older adulthood (age 55-74). The overall incidence and prevalence of lymphoma vary by geographic region, ethnicity, and other factors.

Diagnosis:
- <u>Physical Examination:</u> evaluation of lymph nodes, spleen, liver, and other organs for signs of enlargement or abnormalities

- Blood Tests: Complete blood count (CBC), blood chemistry, and lactate dehydrogenase (LDH) levels may be abnormal in patients with lymphoma.
    - Lymphocytosis: an increased number of lymphocytes, which can occur in some types of lymphoma
    - Anemia: a reduced number of red blood cells, leading to low hemoglobin levels, often due to the disease itself or as a side effect of treatment
    - Thrombocytopenia: low platelet counts, increasing the risk of bleeding, which can result from bone marrow involvement by lymphoma
    - Neutropenia: a decreased number of neutrophils, making patients more susceptible to infections, especially if the bone marrow is affected or as a side effect of treatments like chemotherapy
- Imaging Studies:

    Computed tomography (CT) scans, magnetic resonance imaging (MRI), positron emission tomography (PET) scans, or ultrasound may be used to visualize lymph nodes, organs, and other structures for signs of lymphoma.
- Biopsy: removal and examination of lymph node tissue or other affected tissue to confirm the diagnosis and determine the type and subtype of lymphoma
- Bone Marrow Biopsy: collection of bone marrow samples to assess for involvement of lymphoma cells in the bone marrow
- Immunophenotyping: testing of lymphoma cells for specific cell markers to classify the subtype of lymphoma and guide treatment decisions

Treatment:
- Chemotherapy: may be given alone or in combination with other treatments, such as radiation therapy or immunotherapy
    - Responsiveness to chemotherapy varies widely depending on the type and stage of lymphoma.
- Radiation Therapy: use of high-energy radiation to target and destroy lymphoma cells in localized areas, such as lymph nodes or organs
- Immunotherapy: treatment with monoclonal antibodies or immune checkpoint inhibitors to enhance the body's immune response against lymphoma cells

- **Targeted Therapy:** use of drugs that target specific molecular abnormalities or signaling pathways in lymphoma cells, such as tyrosine kinase inhibitors or proteasome inhibitors
- **Stem Cell Transplantation:** transplantation of healthy stem cells (either from a donor or the patient's own stem cells) to replace diseased bone marrow and restore normal blood cell production in certain cases of aggressive or refractory lymphoma
- **Watchful Waiting:** monitoring of asymptomatic or indolent lymphomas without immediate treatment, particularly in cases of low-grade NHL or HL with slow disease progression

15.15. Kidney Cancer

> ➤ Kidney cancer, or renal cell carcinoma, is a malignancy originating in the kidney cells, often asymptomatic in early stages but may present with blood in urine, abdominal pain, or a palpable mass.
>
> ➤ Risk factors include smoking, obesity, hypertension, and certain genetic syndromes. Early detection through imaging tests and removal of the tumor offers the best chance for cure.
>
> ➤ Treatment involves surgery, targeted therapy, immunotherapy, radiation therapy, or chemotherapy depending on the stage and extent of the cancer.

Symptoms:
- Blood in the urine
- Persistent back pain, usually below the ribs on one side
- Unintentional weight loss
- Fatigue
- Fever, typically low-grade
- Lump or mass in the abdomen
- Loss of appetite
- Anemia
- Swelling in the legs or ankles
- High blood pressure

Causes and Risk Factors:
- Smoking is a significant risk factor for kidney cancer, with smokers having a higher risk compared to nonsmokers.

- Obesity: Being overweight or obese increases the risk of developing kidney cancer, particularly in women.
- Hypertension is associated with an increased risk of kidney cancer.
- Family history: Having a first-degree relative (parent, sibling, or child) with kidney cancer increases the risk.
- Genetic factors: Hereditary conditions such as von Hippel-Lindau (VHL) syndrome, hereditary papillary renal cell carcinoma, and Birt-Hogg-Dubé syndrome increase the risk of kidney cancer.
- Gender: Men are at higher risk of developing kidney cancer than women.
- Age: The risk of kidney cancer increases with age, with most cases diagnosed in patients over 45 years old.
- Occupational exposure: Exposures to chemicals such as cadmium, organic solvents, or asbestos may increase the risk of kidney cancer.
- Chronic kidney disease: Patients with long-standing kidney disease, especially those on dialysis, have an increased risk of kidney cancer.
- Treatment for kidney failure: Kidney transplant recipients have a slightly higher risk of developing kidney cancer, particularly if they receive immunosuppressive medications.

Epidemiology:

Kidney cancer is among the top ten most common cancers worldwide, with renal cell carcinoma (RCC) being the most common type. The incidence of kidney cancer has been increasing globally over the past few decades, likely due to improved detection methods and changes in risk factors such as smoking and obesity. The majority of kidney cancers are diagnosed in patients between the ages of 50 and 70, although they can occur at any age.

Diagnosis:

- <u>Imaging Tests:</u> Computed tomography (CT) scan, magnetic resonance imaging (MRI), or ultrasound may be used to visualize the kidneys and detect any abnormalities or masses.
- <u>Blood and Urine Tests:</u>

    Blood tests may reveal elevated levels of certain substances, such as erythropoietin or calcium, which can indicate kidney cancer. Urine tests may detect blood or abnormal cells.
- <u>Biopsy:</u> removal and examination of a small sample of kidney tissue to confirm the presence of cancer cells and determine the type and subtype of kidney cancer

- Genetic Testing: for genetic mutations or markers associated with hereditary forms of kidney cancer, such as VHL gene mutations

Treatment:
- Surgery:

    The primary treatment for localized kidney cancer is surgical removal of the tumor and affected kidney (partial or radical nephrectomy). Minimally invasive techniques such as laparoscopic or robotic-assisted surgery may be used when appropriate.

- Targeted Therapy: drugs that target specific molecular pathways involved in the growth and spread of kidney cancer, such as tyrosine kinase inhibitors or mTOR inhibitors

- Immunotherapy:

    Drugs that stimulate the immune system to attack and destroy cancer cells, such as checkpoint inhibitors (e.g., nivolumab, pembrolizumab) or cytokines (e.g., interleukin-2, interferon-alpha).

- Radiation Therapy: to target and destroy cancer cells, particularly in cases of advanced or metastatic kidney cancer

- Chemotherapy: Systemic chemotherapy is not typically effective for kidney cancer, but may be used in certain cases of advanced or metastatic disease that are resistant to other treatments.

- Clinical Trials: participation in clinical trials evaluating novel therapies or treatment approaches for many types of cancer, including kidney cancer.

15.16. Liver Cancer

> ➤ *Liver cancer, or hepatocellular carcinoma, arises from liver cells and often develops in individuals with chronic liver disease or cirrhosis.*
>
> ➤ *Symptoms include abdominal pain, weight loss, jaundice, and enlarged liver, with risk factors including hepatitis B or C infection, alcohol abuse, obesity, and aflatoxin exposure. Early detection through surveillance programs in high-risk individuals can improve prognosis and treatment outcomes.*
>
> ➤ *Treatment involving surgery, liver transplantation, ablation therapy, chemotherapy, or targeted therapy depending on the stage and extent of the cancer.*

Symptoms:
- Abdominal pain or discomfort, especially in the upper right portion of the abdomen
- Unintentional weight loss
- Loss of appetite
- Feeling of fullness or bloating in the abdomen
- Nausea and vomiting
- Fatigue and weakness
- Hepatomegaly, felt as a mass under the ribs on the right side
- Jaundice
- Ascites
- Pruritus

Causes and Risk Factors:
- Chronic viral hepatitis: Chronic infection with hepatitis B virus (HBV) or hepatitis C virus (HCV) is the leading risk factor for liver cancer.
- Cirrhosis: Liver cirrhosis, often caused by chronic alcohol abuse, viral hepatitis, nonalcoholic fatty liver disease (NAFLD), or other liver diseases, significantly increases the risk of liver cancer.
- Heavy alcohol consumption: Excessive and long-term alcohol consumption can lead to liver damage and cirrhosis, increasing the risk of liver cancer.
- Nonalcoholic fatty liver disease (NAFLD) and nonalcoholic steatohepatitis (NASH): Conditions characterized by accumulation of fat in the liver, which can progress to cirrhosis and liver cancer.
- Obesity and metabolic syndrome: Obesity, diabetes, and metabolic syndrome are associated with an increased risk of liver cancer, particularly in the presence of NAFLD/NASH.
- Exposure to aflatoxins: Aflatoxins, produced by certain molds that grow on food crops such as peanuts, corn, and grains, are potent carcinogens associated with an increased risk of liver cancer in regions with aflatoxin contamination.
- Tobacco smoking: Smoking tobacco is a risk factor for liver cancer, particularly in patients with underlying liver disease.
- Family history: Having a first-degree relative (parent, sibling, or child) with liver cancer increases the risk.

- Genetic factors: Inherited genetic mutations or conditions such as hemochromatosis or alpha-1 antitrypsin deficiency may increase the risk of liver cancer.
- Exposure to certain chemicals: Occupational exposure to chemicals such as vinyl chloride, arsenic, or polychlorinated biphenyls (PCBs) may increase the risk of liver cancer.

Epidemiology:

Liver cancer is the sixth most common cancer worldwide and the fourth leading cause of cancer-related deaths. Hepatocellular carcinoma (HCC) accounts for approximately 75-85% of primary liver cancers. The incidence of liver cancer varies by geographic region, with the highest rates observed in regions with a high prevalence of chronic viral hepatitis, such as sub-Saharan Africa and Southeast Asia.

Men are at higher risk of liver cancer than women, and the disease typically affects patients over 40 years old, although the incidence is increasing in younger age groups due to rising rates of obesity and viral hepatitis.

Diagnosis:
- Imaging Tests: CT scans, MRI, or ultrasound may be used to visualize the liver and detect any abnormalities or masses.
- Blood Tests: may reveal elevated levels of certain liver enzymes (e.g., alanine aminotransferase, aspartate aminotransferase), alpha-fetoprotein (AFP), or other markers of liver function or damage
- Biopsy: removal and examination of a small sample of liver tissue to confirm the presence of cancer cells and determine the type and subtype of liver cancer
- Genetic Testing: testing for genetic mutations or markers associated with hereditary forms of liver cancer or underlying liver diseases

Treatment:
- Surgery:

    Surgical options for liver cancer may include partial hepatectomy, liver transplant, or ablative therapies such as radiofrequency ablation or microwave ablation to destroy cancerous tissue.

- Transarterial Chemoembolization (TACE): chemotherapy drugs are injected directly into the blood vessels supplying the liver tumor, followed by embolization to block blood flow to the tumor

- Targeted Therapy:

    use of drugs that target specific molecular pathways involved in the growth and spread of liver cancer, such as tyrosine kinase inhibitors (e.g., sorafenib, lenvatinib) or immune checkpoint inhibitors (e.g., atezolizumab, tremelimumab-durvalumab)

- Radiation Therapy: high-energy radiation to target and destroy cancer cells, particularly in localized or unresectable liver cancers
- Chemotherapy: may be used in certain cases of advanced or metastatic liver cancer, although its effectiveness is limited
- Palliative Care: symptom management and supportive care to improve quality of life and alleviate pain and discomfort in patients with advanced or terminal liver cancer

15.17. Esophageal Cancer

> *Esophageal cancer is a malignancy affecting the esophagus, often associated with smoking, excessive alcohol consumption, obesity, and acid reflux.*
>
> *Symptoms may include difficulty swallowing, chest pain, weight loss, and hoarseness. Prognosis is generally poor due to late diagnosis, highlighting the importance of early detection and risk factor modification.*
>
> *Treatment involves surgery, chemotherapy, radiation therapy, targeted therapy, or immunotherapy depending on the stage and location of the cancer.*

Symptoms:
- Dysphagia
- Persistent or worsening indigestion or heartburn
- Unintentional weight loss
- Chest pain or discomfort, particularly behind the breastbone
- Persistent cough or hoarseness
- Regurgitation of food or liquid
- Frequent hiccups
- Chronic cough or sore throat
- Difficulty breathing
- Vomiting blood or passing black, tarry stools

Causes and Risk Factors:
- Gastroesophageal reflux disease (GERD): Chronic acid reflux and Barrett's esophagus, a complication of GERD, significantly increases the risk of esophageal cancer.
- Smoking tobacco is a major risk factor for esophageal cancer, particularly squamous cell carcinoma.
- Excessive alcohol consumption, especially when combined with smoking, increases the risk of esophageal cancer.
- Obesity: Being overweight or obese is associated with an increased risk of esophageal adenocarcinoma.
- Barrett's esophagus: Chronic inflammation and damage to the lining of the esophagus due to GERD can lead to Barrett's esophagus, a precancerous condition that increases the risk of esophageal adenocarcinoma.
- Age: The risk of esophageal cancer increases with age, with most cases diagnosed in patients over 50 years old.
- Gender: Men are at higher risk of esophageal cancer than women, particularly for squamous cell carcinoma.
- Diet: Consumption of certain foods or beverages, such as processed meats, pickled foods, hot beverages, or very hot foods, may increase the risk of esophageal cancer.
- Occupational exposures: Exposure to certain chemicals or substances, such as asbestos, silica dust, or polycyclic aromatic hydrocarbons (PAHs), may increase the risk of esophageal cancer.
- Family history: Having a first-degree relative (parent, sibling, or child) with esophageal cancer increases the risk, although the genetic contribution to esophageal cancer risk is relatively low.

Epidemiology:

Esophageal cancer is the eighth most common cancer worldwide and the sixth leading cause of cancer-related deaths. The incidence of esophageal cancer varies by geographic region and histological subtype, with squamous cell carcinoma being more common in developing countries and adenocarcinoma more common in developed countries. Esophageal cancer is more common in men than women, with a peak incidence in patients over 50 years old.

Diagnosis:
- <u>Endoscopy:</u> visualization of the esophagus using a flexible tube with a camera (endoscope) to inspect for abnormalities or lesions

- Biopsy: removal and examination of a small sample of tissue from the esophagus to confirm the presence of cancer cells and determine the type and subtype of esophageal cancer
- Imaging Tests:

    Computed tomography (CT) scan, magnetic resonance imaging (MRI), positron emission tomography (PET) scan, or endoscopic ultrasound (EUS) may be used to assess the extent of tumor involvement and detect any spread to nearby lymph nodes or distant organs.
- Barium Swallow: X-ray examination of the esophagus after swallowing a barium contrast solution to detect abnormalities or blockages.
- Blood Tests:

    Blood tests may be performed to assess liver function, kidney function, and levels of tumor markers such as carcinoembryonic antigen (CEA) or squamous cell carcinoma antigen (SCC).

Treatment:
- Endoscopic Therapies: Minimally invasive techniques such as endoscopic mucosal resection (EMR) or endoscopic submucosal dissection (ESD) may be used to remove early-stage tumors without the need for surgery.
- Surgery: Removal of the tumor and affected portion of the esophagus (esophagectomy) may be performed for localized or early-stage esophageal cancer.
- Chemotherapy: to kill cancer cells and shrink tumors, either before surgery (neoadjuvant) or after surgery (adjuvant)
- Radiation therapy: to target and destroy cancer cells, often used in combination with chemotherapy (chemoradiotherapy) for locally advanced or unresectable esophageal cancer
- Palliative care: Symptom management and supportive care can improve quality of life and alleviate pain and discomfort in patients with advanced or terminal esophageal cancer.

15.18. Stomach Cancer

> ➢ *Stomach cancer, also known as gastric cancer, typically develops slowly over many years.*
> ➢ *Symptoms may include indigestion, stomach pain, vomiting, and weight loss.*
> ➢ *Treatment often involves surgery, chemotherapy, and radiation therapy, depending on the stage and location of the cancer cells.*

Symptoms:

- Early-stage symptoms: In the early stages, gastric cancer may not cause noticeable symptoms. However, as the cancer progresses, patients may experience:
    - Indigestion or discomfort in the upper abdomen
    - Persistent abdominal pain or discomfort
    - Nausea and vomiting
    - Loss of appetite or early satiety
    - Unexplained weight loss
    - Weakness or fatigue
- Advanced-stage symptoms: As gastric cancer advances, symptoms may become more pronounced and include:
    - Dysphagia
    - Hematemesis (blood in vomit) or melena (black, tarry stools) due to gastrointestinal bleeding
    - Ascites: abdominal swelling or fluid accumulation
    - Jaundice
    - Palpable mass in the abdomen
    - Enlarged lymph nodes in the abdomen or neck

Causes and Risk Factors:

- Helicobacter pylori infection: Chronic infection with H. pylori bacteria is a major risk factor for gastric cancer, particularly intestinal-type gastric adenocarcinoma.
- Chronic gastritis: Long-standing inflammation of the stomach lining, often associated with H. pylori infection, increases the risk of gastric cancer.

- Family history: Patients with a family history of gastric cancer or certain inherited genetic syndromes (e.g., hereditary diffuse gastric cancer syndrome) have an increased risk.
- Dietary factors: Consumption of smoked, salted, or pickled foods, processed meats, and low fruit and vegetable intake may elevate the risk of gastric cancer.
- Smoking tobacco and heavy alcohol consumption are associated with an increased risk of gastric cancer.
- Obesity: Overweight or obese patients have a higher risk of developing gastric cancer.
- Pernicious anemia: Chronic autoimmune gastritis and pernicious anemia are risk factors for gastric cancer, particularly of the gastric body and fundus.
- Surgical history: Patients who have undergone gastric surgery for benign conditions (e.g., peptic ulcer disease) have an increased risk of gastric cancer in the remaining stomach tissue.
- Medical conditions: Conditions such as Menetrier's disease, adenomatous gastric polyps, and Epstein-Barr virus infection increase the risk of gastric cancer.
- Age: Gastric cancer incidence increases with age, with the highest rates observed in patients over 65 years old.
- Gender: Men have a higher risk compared to women.

Epidemiology:

Gastric cancer is the fifth most common cancer worldwide and the third leading cause of cancer-related deaths. Its incidence varies geographically, with higher rates observed in East Asia, Eastern Europe, and parts of South America. In the United States, gastric cancer incidence has declined over the past several decades, but it remains a significant health concern, particularly among certain ethnic groups such as Asian Americans, Pacific Islanders, and Hispanics.

Diagnosis:

- <u>Upper Endoscopy:</u>

    Esophagogastroduodenoscopy (EGD) with biopsy is the gold standard for diagnosing gastric cancer, allowing direct visualization of the stomach lining and sampling of suspicious lesions for histopathological analysis.

- <u>Imaging Studies:</u>

    Computed tomography (CT) scans, magnetic resonance imaging (MRI), or positron emission tomography (PET) scans may be performed to assess the extent of disease spread (staging) and identify metastases.

- Endoscopic Ultrasound (EUS): EUS combines endoscopy with ultrasound imaging to evaluate the depth of tumor invasion into the stomach wall and assess nearby lymph nodes for metastasis.
- Blood Tests: to evaluate for anemia, liver function abnormalities, and tumor markers such as carcinoembryonic antigen (CEA) and carbohydrate antigen 19-9 (CA 19-9)

Treatment:

- Surgery: Surgical resection (partial or total gastrectomy) is the primary treatment for early-stage gastric cancer, aiming to remove the tumor and surrounding lymph nodes.
- Chemotherapy: Adjuvant or neoadjuvant chemotherapy may be recommended to shrink tumors, reduce the risk of recurrence, or improve surgical outcomes.
- Radiation Therapy: External beam radiation therapy may be used in combination with surgery and chemotherapy, particularly for locally advanced or unresectable gastric cancer.
- Targeted Therapy:

    Molecularly targeted drugs, such as trastuzumab (Herceptin) for HER2-positive gastric cancer or ramucirumab (Cyramza) for advanced gastric adenocarcinoma, may be used in combination with chemotherapy.

- Immunotherapy:

    Immune checkpoint inhibitors, such as pembrolizumab (Keytruda) or nivolumab (Opdivo), may be used in certain cases of advanced or metastatic gastric cancer that express programmed death-ligand 1 (PD-L1).

15.19. Endometrial Cancer

> ➤ *Endometrial cancer, the most common type of uterine cancer, begins in the lining of the uterus (endometrium).*
>
> ➤ *Symptoms include abnormal vaginal bleeding, pelvic pain, and abnormal vaginal discharge.*
>
> ➤ *Treatment often involves surgery, chemotherapy, radiation therapy, or hormone therapy depending on the stage and patient's factors.*

Symptoms:
- Abnormal vaginal bleeding, such as postmenopausal bleeding or intermenstrual bleeding
- Pelvic pain or discomfort
- Pelvic pressure or feeling of fullness
- Unintended weight loss
- Fatigue or weakness
- Changes in bowel or bladder habits

Causes and Risk Factors:
- Hormonal factors: Increased exposure to estrogen without progesterone, such as in women with obesity, polycystic ovary syndrome (PCOS), or estrogen hormone therapy, raises the risk of endometrial cancer.
- Age: Endometrial cancer incidence increases with age, particularly in postmenopausal women.
- Obesity is a significant risk factor for endometrial cancer due to increased estrogen levels from adipose tissue.
- Hormone replacement therapy (HRT): Estrogen-only HRT, without progesterone, increases endometrial cancer risk in postmenopausal women.
- Reproductive factors: Nulliparity (never giving birth), early menarche, late menopause, or infertility may elevate the risk.
- Tamoxifen use: Tamoxifen, a medication used for breast cancer treatment or prevention, can increase the risk of endometrial cancer.
- Hereditary factors: Lynch syndrome (hereditary nonpolyposis colorectal cancer) and other genetic syndromes increase the risk of endometrial cancer.
- Women with diabetes, particularly type 2 diabetes, have a higher risk of endometrial cancer.
- Personal history: Previous diagnosis of endometrial hyperplasia, endometrial polyps, or breast cancer increases the risk.
- Race and ethnicity: White women are at higher risk than African American or Asian women, although rates vary by ethnicity.

Epidemiology:

Endometrial cancer is the most common gynecologic malignancy in developed countries. It primarily affects postmenopausal women, but approximately 25% of cases occur in premenopausal women. The incidence of endometrial cancer has been increasing, partly due to rising obesity rates and hormonal factors.

Diagnosis:
- Transvaginal Ultrasound: used to assess endometrial thickness and detect abnormalities
- Endometrial Biopsy: gold standard for diagnosing endometrial cancer, often performed in the office setting
- Hysteroscopy: minimally invasive procedure that allows direct visualization of the uterine cavity and biopsy of suspicious lesions
- Imaging Studies: Computed tomography (CT) scans, magnetic resonance imaging (MRI), or positron emission tomography (PET) scans may be performed for disease staging.

Treatment:
- Surgery: Total hysterectomy with bilateral salpingo-oophorectomy is the primary treatment for endometrial cancer.
- Radiation Therapy: External beam radiation therapy or brachytherapy may be used as adjuvant therapy following surgery.
- Chemotherapy: Systemic chemotherapy may be recommended for advanced or metastatic endometrial cancer.
- Hormonal Therapy: Progestin therapy may be used for early-stage or low-grade endometrial cancer in women who wish to preserve fertility or are poor surgical candidates.
- Targeted Therapy: Molecularly targeted drugs, such as progesterone receptor modulators or antiangiogenic agents, may be used in certain cases, particularly for advanced or recurrent endometrial cancer.

15.20. Brain Cancer

> ➤ *Brain cancer refers to abnormal growths of cells within the brain or nearby structures.*
>
> ➤ *Symptoms may include headaches, seizures, cognitive changes, or motor deficits. Early diagnosis and comprehensive treatment plans are crucial for improving outcomes and quality of life.*
>
> ➤ *Treatment often involves surgery, radiation therapy, chemotherapy, targeted therapy, or immunotherapy, depending on the type, location, and stage of the cancer, with prognosis varying widely depending on factors such as tumor type, size, and patient's overall health.*

Symptoms:
- Headaches: persistent or severe headaches that may worsen over time, especially in the morning
- Seizures: new onset or changes in seizure patterns
- Neurological deficits: weakness, numbness, or tingling in one side of the body, changes in coordination, balance difficulties, or cognitive impairment
- Nausea and vomiting: often accompanied by headaches or changes in mental status.
- Visual changes: blurred vision, double vision (diplopia), or loss of vision in one eye
- Personality or behavioral changes: mood swings, irritability, depression, or personality changes
- Speech difficulties: slurred speech, difficulty finding words, or changes in speech patterns

Causes and Risk Factors:
- Age: Brain cancer incidence increases with age, with higher rates observed in older adults.
- Genetics: Certain genetic syndromes, such as neurofibromatosis type 1 (NF1), Li-Fraumeni syndrome, or familial adenomatous polyposis (FAP), increase the risk of brain tumors.
- Radiation exposure: Previous exposure to ionizing radiation, such as radiation therapy for other cancers or radiation exposure during childhood, raises the risk.
- Family history: A family history of brain tumors or certain genetic conditions may increase the risk.
- Immune system disorders: Conditions that weaken the immune system, such as HIV/AIDS or organ transplantation, may elevate the risk.
- Environmental factors: Exposure to certain chemicals, such as vinyl chloride or pesticides, has been associated with an increased risk of brain cancer, although evidence is limited.
- Cell phone use: While controversial, some studies suggest a potential link between long-term cell phone use and an increased risk of brain cancer, although further research is needed to confirm this association.

Epidemiology:
Brain cancer is relatively rare compared to other types of cancer, accounting for about 1.4% of all new cancer cases in the United States. Glioblastoma, the most aggressive and common type of primary brain tumor, has an incidence of approximately 3 cases per 100,000 patients per year. While brain tumors can occur at any age, they are more common in older adults, with the highest incidence observed in patients over 65 years old.

Primary Brain Tumors:
- Gliomas: These are the most common type of primary brain tumor, which originate in the glial cells. Gliomas are further subdivided based on the specific glial cells involved, including:
    - Astrocytomas (including glioblastoma, the most aggressive type)
    - Oligodendrogliomas
    - Ependymomas
- Meningiomas: These arise from the meninges, the membranes that surround the brain and spinal cord, and are often benign but can be malignant in rare cases.
- Pituitary Adenomas: formed in the pituitary gland and can affect hormonal balance and have various physiological effects
- Medulloblastomas: These are malignant tumors that originate in the cerebellum. They are most common in children but can occur in adults.
- Schwannomas: Also known as acoustic neuromas, these are benign tumors that develop from the Schwann cells that cover nerves. The most common type affects the vestibular nerve, leading to hearing loss and balance problems.
- Primary Central Nervous System (CNS) Lymphomas: malignant tumors that arise from lymphocytes in the brain or spinal cord

Secondary (Metastatic) Brain Tumors

These tumors originate from cancer cells that have spread to the brain from other parts of the body, such as the lungs, breasts, skin, or kidneys. Metastatic brain tumors are more common than primary brain tumors and are named after the site of the original cancer (e.g., metastatic lung cancer).

Diagnosis:

- Neurological Examination: assessment of neurological function, including reflexes, muscle strength, coordination, and sensory perception
- Imaging Studies: MRI and CT scans are used to visualize brain tumors and assess their size, location, and extent of spread.
- Biopsy: Surgical removal of a sample of tumor tissue for histopathological analysis is essential for confirming the diagnosis and determining the tumor's grade and subtype.
- Cerebrospinal Fluid Analysis: Examination of cerebrospinal fluid obtained by lumbar puncture may be performed to detect cancer cells or tumor markers in cases of leptomeningeal metastasis.

Treatment:

- Surgery: Surgical resection of the tumor is often the initial treatment for accessible brain tumors, aiming to remove as much tumor tissue as possible while preserving neurological function.
- Radiation Therapy:

    External beam radiation therapy or stereotactic radiosurgery may be used to target and kill remaining tumor cells after surgery or as a primary treatment for inoperable tumors.

- Chemotherapy: Systemic chemotherapy or intrathecal chemotherapy may be administered to shrink tumors, control tumor growth, or manage metastatic disease.
- Targeted Therapy:

    Molecularly targeted drugs, such as bevacizumab (Avastin) or temozolomide (Temodar), may be used in combination with standard treatments for certain types of brain tumors, including glioblastoma.

- Immunotherapy: Immunotherapeutic approaches, such as immune checkpoint inhibitors or cancer vaccines, are being investigated in clinical trials for the treatment of brain tumors.

15.21. Testicular Cancer

> ➤ Testicular cancer is a malignancy originating in the testicles, typically presenting as a painless lump or swelling in the scrotum.
>
> ➤ Risk factors include undescended testicles, family history, and prior history of testicular cancer. Prognosis is generally excellent, especially when diagnosed early, with high survival rates even in advanced stages.
>
> ➤ Treatment involves surgery, chemotherapy, radiation therapy, or targeted therapy depending on the stage and type of cancer.

Symptoms:

- Lump or swelling: A painless lump or enlargement in the testicle is the most common symptom of testicular cancer.
- Testicular pain: Discomfort, heaviness, or pain in the testicle or scrotum may occur, although it is less common.
- Changes in testicular size or shape: Alterations in the size, shape, or consistency of the testicle may indicate underlying pathology.
- Heaviness or discomfort in the lower abdomen or groin: Some patients may experience a sense of fullness, pressure, or discomfort in the lower abdomen or groin area.
- Back pain: In advanced cases, testicular cancer may spread to nearby lymph nodes or distant organs, leading to back pain or discomfort.

Causes and Risk Factors:

- Cryptorchidism: Men with a history of cryptorchidism have an increased risk of testicular cancer, particularly if the condition was not corrected in early childhood.
- Family history: Patients with a family history of testicular cancer, especially in first-degree relatives, have a higher risk.
- Personal history: Previous diagnosis of testicular cancer in one testicle increases the risk of developing cancer in the other testicle.
- Age: Testicular cancer is most common in young and middle-aged men, with the highest incidence observed in patients between 15 and 35 years old.
- Race and ethnicity: Testicular cancer is more common in Caucasian men compared to men of other racial or ethnic backgrounds.

- Genetic factors: Certain genetic conditions, such as Klinefelter syndrome or familial testicular germ cell tumors, may predispose patients to testicular cancer.
- Testicular microlithiasis: The presence of calcifications within the testicle detected by ultrasound may increase the risk of testicular cancer.
- HIV infection: Men with human immunodeficiency virus (HIV) have a slightly higher risk of developing testicular cancer.

Epidemiology:

Testicular cancer is relatively rare compared to other cancers, accounting for approximately 1% of all male cancers. However, it is the most common cancer in young men aged 15 to 35 years. The incidence of testicular cancer has been increasing globally, with the highest rates reported in Northern Europe and North America.

Diagnosis:

- Physical Examination: A thorough physical examination, including palpation of the testicles, groin, and abdomen, is performed to assess for abnormalities.
- Ultrasound: Scrotal ultrasound is the primary imaging modality used to evaluate testicular masses, distinguish between benign and malignant lesions, and assess for metastasis to nearby lymph nodes.
- Tumor Markers:

    Blood tests for tumor markers, including alpha-fetoprotein (AFP), beta-human chorionic gonadotropin (β-hCG), and lactate dehydrogenase (LDH), are performed to aid in diagnosis and monitoring treatment response.

- Biopsy:

    In most cases, a biopsy is not necessary for diagnosing testicular cancer. However, if imaging and tumor marker tests are inconclusive, or if a non-germ cell tumor is suspected, a biopsy may be performed to obtain tissue for histopathological analysis.

Treatment:

- Surgery: Radical inguinal orchiectomy, the surgical removal of the affected testicle through an incision in the groin, is the primary treatment for testicular cancer.
- Radiation Therapy: External beam radiation therapy may be used in select cases, particularly for seminomas or as adjuvant therapy after surgery to prevent recurrence.

- Chemotherapy: Chemotherapy, often based on platinum-based regimens such as BEP (bleomycin, etoposide, cisplatin), is the mainstay of treatment for metastatic or advanced testicular cancer.
- Stem Cell Transplant: High-dose chemotherapy followed by autologous stem cell transplantation may be considered for refractory or relapsed disease.
- Surveillance: Regular follow-up appointments with physical examinations, imaging studies, and tumor marker tests, may be appropriate for select cases of stage I testicular cancer with low-risk features.

15.22. Anemia

> *Anemia is a condition characterized by a deficiency in red blood cells or hemoglobin, leading to reduced oxygen-carrying capacity in the blood.*
>
> *Symptoms may include fatigue, weakness, pale skin, shortness of breath, dizziness, and irregular heartbeat, with causes ranging from nutritional deficiencies to chronic diseases or blood loss.*
>
> *Treatment involves addressing the underlying cause, iron supplementation, blood transfusions, or medication depending on the severity and type of anemia.*

Symptoms:
- Fatigue: feeling tired or weak, even with adequate rest
- Weakness: reduced strength or stamina for physical activities
- Pale skin: skin, lips, or nail beds appearing pale or whitish
- Shortness of breath: difficulty breathing or feeling breathless, especially during physical exertion
- Dizziness or lightheadedness: sensation of feeling faint or dizzy, particularly when standing up quickly
- Cold hands and feet: reduced circulation may lead to cold extremities
- Persistent or frequent headaches
- Chest pain or palpitations: in severe cases

Causes and Risk Factors:
- Nutritional deficiencies: inadequate intake of iron, vitamin B12, folate, or other essential nutrients necessary for red blood cell production

- Gastrointestinal bleeding: Conditions such as peptic ulcers, gastritis, inflammatory bowel disease, or gastrointestinal cancers may lead to chronic blood loss.
- Menstrual blood loss: Heavy menstrual bleeding, particularly in women with conditions such as menorrhagia or uterine fibroids.
- Chronic diseases: Chronic kidney disease, cancer, autoimmune disorders, or chronic inflammatory conditions may impair red blood cell production or lead to hemolysis.
- Genetic disorders: Inherited conditions such as sickle cell anemia, thalassemia, or hereditary spherocytosis may cause chronic anemia.
- Pregnancy: Increased demand for iron and other nutrients during pregnancy may lead to anemia if dietary intake is insufficient.
- Age: Infants, children, and older adults may be at increased risk of anemia due to dietary factors, chronic diseases, or other medical conditions.

Epidemiology:

Anemia is a global health concern affecting patients of all ages and socioeconomic backgrounds. The prevalence of anemia varies depending on factors such as geographic location, age, gender, and underlying health conditions. Iron deficiency anemia is the most common type of anemia worldwide, particularly in developing countries, while anemia of chronic disease is more prevalent in industrialized nations, affecting patients with chronic illnesses such as chronic kidney disease or inflammatory disorders.

Anemia subtypes:
- Iron deficiency anemia: caused by inadequate iron intake, blood loss, or poor absorption
- Vitamin deficiency anemia: resulting from insufficient levels of vitamins like B12, folate, or vitamin C
- Hemolytic anemia: occurs when red blood cells are destroyed faster than they're produced, often due to autoimmune disorders or genetic conditions
- Aplastic anemia: stem cells fail to produce enough red blood cells, typically due to bone marrow disorders or exposure to toxic substances
- Sickle cell anemia: inherited disorder where red blood cells become sickle-shaped, leading to blockages and reduced oxygen delivery
- Thalassemia: genetic disorder causing abnormal hemoglobin production, resulting in reduced oxygen-carrying capacity

Diagnosis:

- Complete Blood Count (CBC):

    CBC measures hemoglobin levels, hematocrit, red blood cell count, and other indices to assess for anemia. Anemia is diagnosed when hemoglobin value of less than 13.5 gm/dl in a man or less than 12.0 gm/dl in a woman

- Peripheral Blood Smear: Examination of a blood smear under a microscope can provide information about red blood cell morphology and identify abnormalities.

- Serum ferritin: Measurement of serum ferritin levels helps evaluate iron stores and diagnose iron deficiency anemia.

- Serum Vitamin B12 and Folate Levels: Testing for vitamin B12 and folate levels is essential for diagnosing megaloblastic anemia due to deficiencies.

- Additional Tests: Depending on the suspected cause of anemia, additional tests such as reticulocyte count, serum erythropoietin levels, stool occult blood test, or bone marrow biopsy may be performed.

Treatment:

Treatment depends on the specific subtype and underlying cause of anemia.

- Iron Supplementation: Oral iron supplements are the first-line treatment for iron deficiency anemia, with adjustments in dosage based on severity and response to therapy.

- Dietary Modifications: Increasing dietary intake of iron-rich foods such as red meat, poultry, fish, beans, lentils, leafy green vegetables, and fortified cereals.

- Vitamin Supplementation:

    Vitamin B12 injections or oral supplements may be prescribed for megaloblastic anemia due to vitamin B12 deficiency, while folate supplementation is recommended for folate deficiency anemia.

- Treatment of Underlying Conditions:

    Management of underlying medical conditions contributing to anemia, such as gastrointestinal bleeding, chronic kidney disease, or autoimmune disorders.

- Blood Transfusion: may be necessary for severe anemia or in cases where rapid correction of hemoglobin levels is required

- Erythropoiesis-stimulating agents (ESA):

    Erythropoietin can stimulate red blood cell production in cases of anemia associated with chronic kidney disease or chemotherapy-induced anemia.

- Lifestyle Modifications:

    Regular exercise, adequate sleep, stress management, and avoidance of tobacco and excessive alcohol consumption can help improve overall health and support anemia treatment.

15.23. Pancytopenia

> ➤ *Pancytopenia is a condition characterized by low levels of all three blood cell types: red blood cells, white blood cells, and platelets.*
>
> ➤ *It can result from bone marrow disorders, chemotherapy, infections, autoimmune diseases, or nutritional deficiencies, leading to symptoms such as fatigue, infections, easy bruising, and bleeding tendencies.*
>
> ➤ *Treatment involves addressing the underlying cause, supportive care like blood transfusions or growth factors, and sometimes bone marrow transplantation in severe cases.*

Symptoms:

- Fatigue: persistent tiredness or weakness, even with adequate rest
- Shortness of breath: difficulty breathing, especially during physical activity
- Pale skin: skin, lips, or nail beds appearing pale or whitish
- Easy bruising or bleeding: increased susceptibility to bruising or bleeding from minor injuries or mucosal surfaces
- Frequent infections: Due to decreased production of white blood cells, patients with pancytopenia may experience recurrent or severe infections.
- Petechiae or purpura: small red or purple spots on the skin caused by bleeding under the skin
- Enlarged spleen or liver: In some cases, the spleen or liver may become enlarged due to increased workload or underlying disease.

Causes and Risk Factors:

- Bone marrow disorders: Conditions that affect the bone marrow, such as aplastic anemia, myelodysplastic syndromes (MDS), or leukemia, are common causes of pancytopenia.

- Chemotherapy or radiation therapy: Cancer treatments can suppress bone marrow function and lead to pancytopenia.
- Autoimmune disorders: Systemic lupus erythematosus (SLE), rheumatoid arthritis, or autoimmune hepatitis may cause pancytopenia due to immune-mediated destruction of blood cells.
- Infections: Certain viral infections, such as HIV, Epstein-Barr virus (EBV), or hepatitis viruses, can affect bone marrow function and cause pancytopenia.
- Medications: Some medications, including certain antibiotics, antiepileptic drugs, and immunosuppressants, may induce bone marrow suppression and pancytopenia as adverse effects.
- Chemical exposure: Exposure to toxins or chemicals such as benzene, pesticides, or heavy metals can damage bone marrow cells and lead to pancytopenia.
- Malnutrition: Severe nutritional deficiencies, particularly deficiencies of vitamin B12, folate, or certain minerals, may impair hematopoiesis and result in pancytopenia.

Epidemiology:

Pancytopenia is relatively uncommon but can occur at any age and affect patients of all demographics. The exact prevalence of pancytopenia varies depending on geographic location, underlying etiology, and patient population. While certain conditions such as aplastic anemia or myelodysplastic syndromes are more frequently associated with pancytopenia, it can also occur as a complication of other diseases or medical treatments.

Diagnosis:

- <u>Complete Blood Count:</u> A CBC with differential is the initial laboratory test used to diagnose pancytopenia, revealing anemia, leukopenia, and thrombocytopenia.
- <u>Peripheral Blood Smear:</u> Examination of a blood smear under a microscope can provide additional information about the morphology of blood cells and identify any abnormalities.
- <u>Bone Marrow Biopsy:</u>

    A bone marrow biopsy may be performed to assess the cellular composition of the bone marrow, evaluate for infiltration by abnormal cells, and determine the underlying cause of pancytopenia.

- Serum Chemistry:

    Additional laboratory tests, such as liver function tests, kidney function tests, and assessment of serum electrolytes, may be performed to evaluate for associated organ dysfunction or underlying metabolic abnormalities.

Treatment:

- Identifying and Treating Underlying Causes:

    The treatment approach for pancytopenia depends on the underlying etiology. Addressing the underlying condition, such as bone marrow disorders, infections, autoimmune diseases, or medication-related causes, is essential for managing pancytopenia.

- Supportive Care: Blood transfusions to correct anemia or thrombocytopenia, administration of growth factors to stimulate blood cell production, and antimicrobial therapy for infections.

- Immunosuppressive Therapy:

    In cases of immune-mediated pancytopenia, immunosuppressive medications such as corticosteroids, immunoglobulins, or other immunomodulatory agents may be used to suppress the immune response and improve blood cell counts.

- Bone Marrow Transplantation:

    For severe or refractory cases of pancytopenia, particularly those associated with bone marrow failure syndromes or hematologic malignancies, allogeneic or autologous bone marrow transplantation may be considered as a definitive treatment option.

- Symptom Management: Pain management, management of bleeding or infection, and nutritional support, are important aspects of comprehensive care for patients with pancytopenia.

15.24. Thrombocytopenia

> ➢ Thrombocytopenia is a condition characterized by an abnormally low number of platelets in the blood, leading to increased bleeding and bruising risks.
>
> ➢ It can result from various factors, including autoimmune diseases, bone marrow disorders, and certain medications.
>
> ➢ Diagnosis involves blood tests and sometimes bone marrow biopsy, with treatment depending on the underlying cause.

Symptoms:
- Easy or excessive bruising (purpura) on skin
- Superficial bleeding into the skin that appears as a rash of pinpoint-sized reddish-purple spots (petechiae), usually on the lower legs
- Prolonged bleeding from cuts
- Spontaneous bleeding from the gums or nose
- Blood in urine or stools
- Unusually heavy menstrual flows
- Fatigue
- Enlarged spleen

Causes and Risk Factors
- Autoimmune diseases: Conditions like lupus and rheumatoid arthritis can lead to the destruction of platelets.
- Bone marrow disorders: Diseases such as leukemia or myelodysplastic syndromes can affect the bone marrow's ability to produce platelets.
- Chemotherapy and radiation therapy: These cancer treatments can damage the bone marrow.
- Certain medications: Some drugs, including heparin, quinine, sulfa-containing antibiotics, and anticonvulsants, can reduce platelet counts.
- Chronic liver disease: Liver disorders can lead to decreased production of clotting factors, including platelets.
- Viral infections: HIV, hepatitis C, and other viral infections can lower platelet count.

Epidemiology

The prevalence of thrombocytopenia can vary widely depending on the underlying cause, age group, and other demographic factors. It is more common in individuals with certain conditions, such as chronic liver disease, HIV, and those undergoing cancer treatment.

Subtypes of thrombocytopenia

- Immune Thrombocytopenic Purpura (ITP): This is one of the most common types of thrombocytopenia. It occurs when the immune system mistakenly attacks and destroys platelets, leading to a low platelet count. ITP can be acute (short-term) or chronic (long-term).

- Drug-Induced Thrombocytopenia: Certain medications can cause thrombocytopenia by either directly damaging platelets or inducing an immune reaction against them. Examples include heparin-induced thrombocytopenia (HIT) and drug-induced immune thrombocytopenia.

- Thrombotic Thrombocytopenic Purpura (TTP): TTP is a rare but serious condition characterized by the formation of blood clots in small blood vessels throughout the body. These clots can lead to a low platelet count, resulting in symptoms such as bruising, petechiae, and organ damage.

- Hemolytic Uremic Syndrome (HUS): HUS is a disorder that involves the formation of blood clots in small blood vessels, leading to the destruction of red blood cells, low platelet count, and kidney failure. It can be caused by infections, certain medications, or genetic factors.

Diagnosis

- Medical History and Physical Examination: to identify any underlying conditions or factors

- Complete Blood Count (CBC):
    - Low Platelet Count: platelets below the normal range (typically less than 150,000 to 100,000 per microliter of blood), which is the hallmark of thrombocytopenia
    - Normal Red Blood Cell (RBC) Count and Hemoglobin: unless the thrombocytopenia is part of a broader hematological disorder or caused by bone marrow suppression, in which case anemia might also be present
    - Normal White Blood Cell (WBC) Count: unless thrombocytopenia is due to a condition affecting the bone marrow or the immune system

- **Blood Smear:** a sample of blood is examined under a microscope to look at platelet size and activity
- **Bone Marrow Biopsy:** to examine the bone marrow's health and functioning
- **Additional Tests:** to identify specific causes or associated conditions

Treatment

Treatment of thrombocytopenia depends on its cause and severity:

- **Observation:** Mild cases may not require treatment and only regular monitoring.
- **Medications:** Drugs may be used to treat underlying conditions, boost platelet production, or suppress the immune system (e.g., corticosteroids, IVIG).
- **Platelet Transfusions:** for severe bleeding or before surgery
- **Splenectomy:** surgical removal of the spleen
- **Treatments for Underlying Conditions:** addressing liver disease, infections, or autoimmune diseases that may be causing the thrombocytopenia

References

- DeSantis, C. E., Ma, J., & et al. (2019). Breast cancer statistics, 2019. CA: A Cancer Journal for Clinicians, 69(6), 438-451.
- Siegel, R. L., Miller, K. D., & et al. (2019). Cancer statistics, 2019. CA: A Cancer Journal for Clinicians, 69(1), 7-34.
- Dekker, E., Tanis, P. J., & et al. (2019). Colorectal cancer. The Lancet, 394(10207), 1467-1480.
- Litwin, M. S., Tan, H. J., & et al. (2017). Long-term follow-up of health-related quality of life among prostate cancer survivors treated with radical prostatectomy, prostatectomy in older men, and watchful waiting. JAMA, 317(11), 1126-1140.
- Tsao, H., Chin, L., & et al. (2012). Melanoma: from mutations to medicine. Genes & Development, 26(11), 1131-1155.
- Rubin, A. I., Chen, E. H., & et al. (2005). Basal-cell carcinoma. New England Journal of Medicine, 353(21), 2262-2269.
- Brantsch, K. D., Meisner, C., & et al. (2008). Analysis of risk factors determining prognosis of cutaneous squamous-cell carcinoma: a prospective study. The Lancet Oncology, 9(8), 713-720.
- Babjuk, M., Böhle, A., & et al. (2017). EAU guidelines on non–muscle-invasive urothelial carcinoma of the bladder: update 2016. European Urology, 71(3), 447-461.

- Neoptolemos, J. P., Kleeff, J., & et al. (2018). Therapeutic developments in pancreatic cancer: current and future perspectives. Nature Reviews Gastroenterology & Hepatology, 15(6), 333-348.
- Jayson, G. C., Kohn, E. C., & et al. (2014). Ovarian cancer. The Lancet, 384(9951), 1376-1388.
- Walboomers, J. M., Jacobs, M. V., & et al. (1999). Human papillomavirus is a necessary cause of invasive cervical cancer worldwide. The Journal of Pathology, 189(1), 12-19.
- La Vecchia, C., Malvezzi, M., & et al. (2015). Thyroid cancer mortality and incidence: a global overview. International Journal of Cancer, 136(9), 2187-2195.
- Estey, E. H. (2013). Acute myeloid leukemia: 2013 update on risk-stratification and management. American Journal of Hematology, 88(4), 318-327.
- Swerdlow, S. H., Campo, E., & et al. (2016). The 2016 revision of the World Health Organization classification of lymphoid neoplasms. Blood, 127(20), 2375-2390.
- Capitanio, U., & Montorsi, F. (2016). Renal cancer. The Lancet, 387(10021), 894-906.
- Forner, A., Reig, M., & et al. (2018). Current strategy for staging and treatment: the BCLC update and future prospects. Seminars in Liver Disease, 40(03), 215-231.
- Pennathur, A., Gibson, M. K., & et al. (2013). Oesophageal carcinoma. The Lancet, 381(9864), 400-412.
- Smyth, E. C., & Nilsson, M. (2017). Gastric cancer: available therapies and future directions. World Journal of Gastroenterology, 23(28), 4999-5016.
- Lortet-Tieulent, J., Ferlay, J., & et al. (2018). International patterns and trends in endometrial cancer incidence, 1978–2013. Journal of the National Cancer Institute, 110(4), 354-361.
- Stupp, R., Mason, W. P., & et al. (2005). Radiotherapy plus concomitant and adjuvant temozolomide for glioblastoma. New England Journal of Medicine, 352(10), 987-996.
- Chovanec, M., Abu Zaid, M., & et al. (2018). Long-term toxicity of cisplatin in germ-cell tumor survivors. Annals of Oncology, 29(11), 2090-2097.
- Guralnik, J. M., Eisenstaedt, R. S., & et al. (2004). Prevalence of anemia in persons 65 years and older in the United States: evidence for a high rate of unexplained anemia. Blood, 104(8), 2263-2268.
- Geary, J. (2010). Management of pancytopenia. Hematology/Oncology Clinics, 24(2), 287-295.

Chapter 16. Obstetric and Gynecologic Disorders

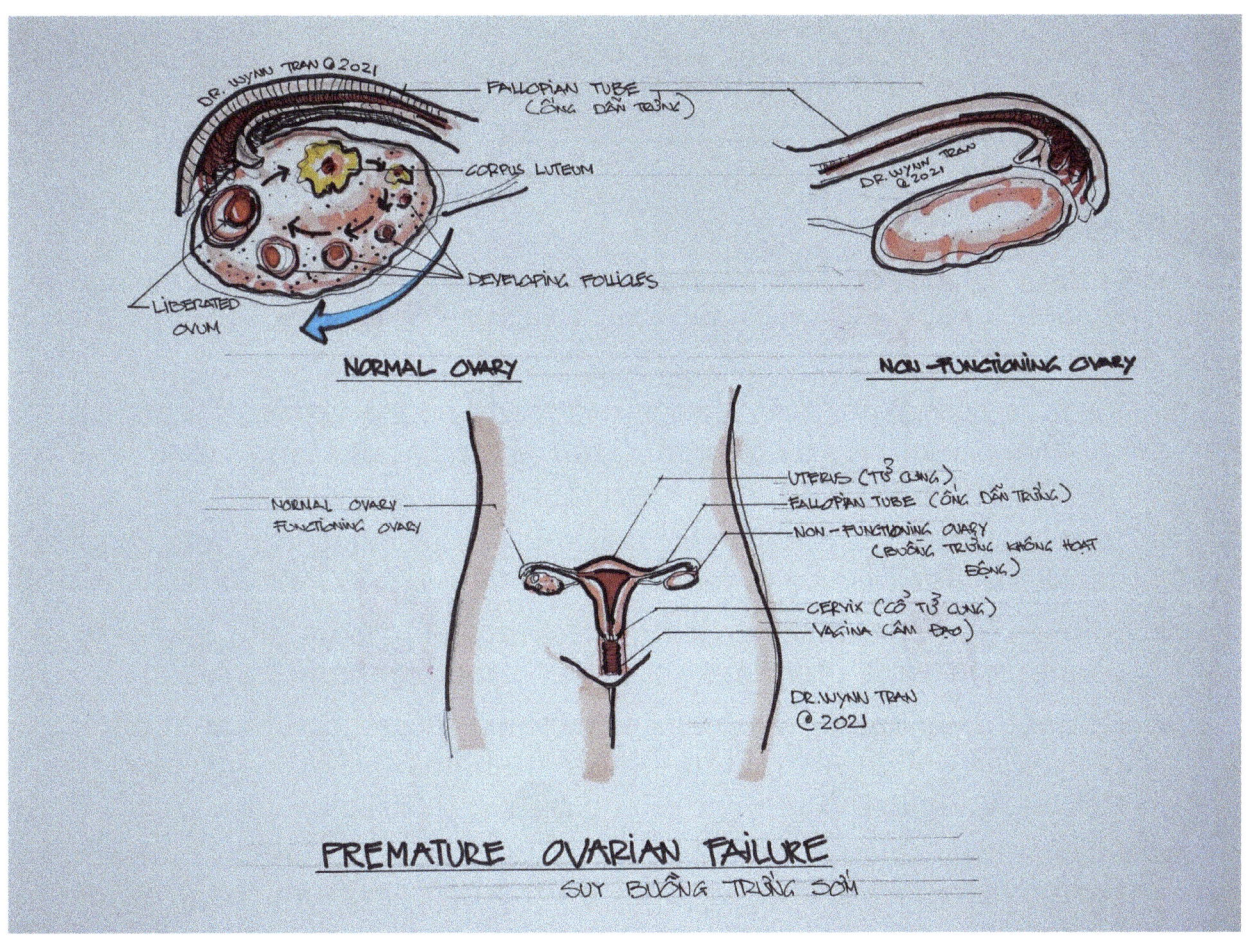

The APh should be familiar with the presentation, diagnosis, and management of these common OB/GYN disorders to provide appropriate care and referral to the obstetrician/gynecologist when necessary.

16.1. Intrauterine Pregnancy

> ➢ *Intrauterine pregnancy refers to a pregnancy where the fertilized egg implants and develops inside the uterus.*
> ➢ *It is the normal and desired location for fetal development.*
> ➢ *Intrauterine pregnancies are typically confirmed through ultrasound imaging and are associated with the most favorable outcomes for both the mother and the baby.*

Symptoms:

- Missed period: One of the earliest signs of pregnancy is a missed menstrual period, although other causes of missed periods should also be considered.
- Positive pregnancy test: Home pregnancy tests or blood tests can confirm pregnancy by detecting the presence of human chorionic gonadotropin (hCG).
- Breast changes: Tenderness, swelling, or changes in nipple color or sensitivity may occur in early pregnancy.
- Nausea and vomiting: Morning sickness, or nausea and vomiting, is common in early pregnancy due to hormonal changes.
- Fatigue: Feelings of tiredness or exhaustion are common in early pregnancy, often attributed to hormonal changes and increased metabolic demands.
- Frequent urination: Increased urination frequency may occur due to hormonal changes and pressure on the bladder from the growing uterus.
- Food cravings or aversions: Some pregnant patients may experience changes in appetite, including cravings for certain foods or aversions to others.
- Mood changes: Hormonal fluctuations during pregnancy can lead to mood swings, irritability, or emotional sensitivity.
- Abdominal bloating or discomfort: Some pregnant patients may experience abdominal bloating, cramping, or discomfort, similar to premenstrual symptoms.
- Vaginal bleeding: Light spotting or implantation bleeding may occur around the time of expected menstruation, although heavy or persistent bleeding should be evaluated.

Epidemiology:

Intrauterine pregnancies are the most common type of pregnancies and occur in the majority of cases where pregnancy is desired. The incidence of intrauterine pregnancies varies by geographic region, population demographics, and access to reproductive healthcare services.

Diagnosis:

- Physical Examination: Examination of the abdomen and pelvis may reveal signs of pregnancy, such as uterine enlargement, softening of the cervix, or changes in the breasts.
- Pregnancy Tests: Home pregnancy tests, urine tests, or blood tests can detect the presence of hCG, confirming pregnancy.
- Ultrasound:

    Transabdominal or transvaginal ultrasound imaging can visualize the uterus and confirm the presence of an intrauterine pregnancy, assess fetal development and viability, and evaluate for signs of complications such as ectopic pregnancy or miscarriage.

Treatment:

- Prenatal Care Visits:

    Regular visits with a healthcare provider are essential for monitoring pregnancy progress, assessing fetal growth and development, and addressing any concerns or complications.

- Nutritional Counseling:

    Maintaining a healthy diet, taking prenatal vitamins, and avoiding harmful substances such as alcohol, tobacco, and illicit drugs is important for promoting a healthy pregnancy.

- Screening Tests:

    Routine screening tests such as blood tests, ultrasounds, and genetic screening may be recommended to assess the risk of genetic conditions or birth defects and guide prenatal care.

- Management of Pregnancy Symptoms:

    Symptomatic relief for common pregnancy symptoms such as nausea, fatigue, and discomfort may include dietary modifications, lifestyle changes, and medications as appropriate.

- Education and Support:

    Providing education and support to the pregnant patient and their family regarding pregnancy, childbirth, breastfeeding, newborn care, and postpartum recovery can help promote a positive pregnancy experience and optimal outcomes.

16.2. Ectopic Pregnancy

> ➢ Ectopic pregnancy occurs when a fertilized egg implants outside the uterus, commonly in the fallopian tubes.
>
> ➢ This can lead to serious complications such as rupture of the fallopian tube and internal bleeding.
>
> ➢ Prompt medical attention is essential to manage ectopic pregnancies, often through medication or surgery.

Symptoms:

- Abdominal pain: sharp, stabbing pain in the pelvis, abdomen, or lower back, which may vary in intensity and duration
- Vaginal bleeding: light vaginal bleeding may occur, often lighter or different from normal menstrual bleeding
- Shoulder pain: may occur due to irritation of the diaphragm from internal bleeding
- Pelvic pain: Pain during intercourse or during bowel movements may occur.
- Weakness, dizziness, or fainting: These symptoms may occur if there is significant internal bleeding.

Causes and Risk Factors:

- Previous ectopic pregnancy: Patients who have had an ectopic pregnancy in the past are at increased risk of having another.
- History of pelvic inflammatory disease (PID), particularly those caused by sexually transmitted infections (STD) like chlamydia or gonorrhea, increase the risk of ectopic pregnancy.
- Previous pelvic or abdominal surgery, such as tubal ligation or surgery for appendicitis, can increase the risk of ectopic pregnancy.
- Smoking: Tobacco use increases the risk of ectopic pregnancy.
- In vitro fertilization (IVF) increases the risk of ectopic pregnancy.
- Age: Ectopic pregnancy is more common in patients of reproductive age, particularly those between 20 and 40 years old.
- Contraceptive use: While contraceptives like intrauterine devices (IUDs) are highly effective at preventing pregnancy, they carry a small risk of ectopic pregnancy if pregnancy does occur.

Epidemiology:

Ectopic pregnancy accounts for approximately 1-2% of all pregnancies. It is a significant cause of maternal morbidity and mortality, especially if not diagnosed and treated promptly.

Diagnosis:

- Pelvic Exam: A physical examination may reveal tenderness or mass in the pelvis.
- Ultrasound: Transvaginal ultrasound imaging can visualize the uterus and fallopian tubes and detect the presence of an ectopic pregnancy.
- Blood Tests:

  Measurement of serum beta-human chorionic gonadotropin (β-hCG) levels can help confirm pregnancy and monitor its progression. In ectopic pregnancy, β-hCG levels may rise more slowly than in a normal pregnancy or may plateau or decline.

Treatment:

- Medication: Methotrexate, a medication that stops the growth of the pregnancy tissue, may be given to patients with early, unruptured ectopic pregnancies and stable conditions.
- Surgery:

  Laparoscopic surgery may be performed to remove the ectopic pregnancy and repair any damage to the fallopian tube. In some cases, laparotomy may be necessary, especially if there is significant bleeding or damage to the tube.

- Expectant Management:

  In select cases where the ectopic pregnancy is very early, small, and not causing symptoms, close monitoring without immediate intervention may be an option. However, this approach carries a risk of rupture and requires careful observation.

- Supportive Care: Pain management, intravenous fluids, and emotional support are essential for patients undergoing treatment for ectopic pregnancy.

16.3. Back Pain in Pregnancy

> ➤ *Back pain during pregnancy is common due to hormonal changes, weight gain, and shifts in posture.*
>
> ➤ *It typically occurs in the lower back and can range from mild discomfort to severe pain.*
>
> ➤ *Gentle exercises, proper posture, and supportive devices like maternity belts can help alleviate symptoms.*

Symptoms:

- Pain in the lower back or pelvis: may range from mild discomfort to severe pain
- Muscle stiffness: feeling of tightness or stiffness in the back muscles, particularly after prolonged standing or sitting
- Radiating pain: pain that radiates from the lower back down the legs, often due to pressure on the sciatic nerve
- Difficulty standing or walking: Some pregnant patients may experience difficulty standing up straight or walking due to back pain.
- Worsening with activity: such as lifting, bending, or prolonged sitting or standing
- Improvement with rest: Symptoms may improve with rest, lying down, or changing positions.

Causes and Risk Factors:

- Weight gain: Excessive weight gain during pregnancy can increase strain on the back and contribute to back pain.
- Posture changes: Changes in posture and spinal alignment due to the growing uterus and shifting center of gravity can lead to back pain.
- Hormonal changes: Hormonal changes during pregnancy, particularly increased levels of relaxin, can relax ligaments and joints, leading to instability and back pain.
- Previous history of back pain: Patients with a history of back pain or spinal conditions may be more prone to experiencing back pain during pregnancy.
- Occupational factors or activities that involve heavy lifting, prolonged standing, or repetitive bending can increase the risk of back pain during pregnancy.

- Multiple pregnancies: Pregnant patients carrying twins or multiples may experience increased strain on the back due to the additional weight and pressure on the spine.

Epidemiology:

Back pain is a common complaint during pregnancy, with prevalence rates ranging from 50% to 70%. It typically occurs in the second half of pregnancy and may persist or worsen as the pregnancy progresses.

Diagnosis:

Diagnosis of back pain during pregnancy is typically based on a clinical evaluation of symptoms reported by the pregnant patient. Laboratory tests or imaging studies are not usually necessary unless there are concerns about underlying medical conditions or complications.

Treatment:
- Physical Therapy: Gentle stretching exercises, pelvic tilts, and strengthening exercises can help improve posture, stabilize the spine, and relieve back pain.
- Prenatal Yoga or Pilates: Low-impact exercises and relaxation techniques can help improve flexibility, reduce muscle tension, and promote relaxation.
- Supportive Garments: Maternity support belts or abdominal binders can provide support to the lower back and abdomen, reducing strain on the spine.
- Posture Modification: Practicing good posture, avoiding prolonged standing or sitting, and using proper body mechanics when lifting or carrying objects can help prevent or reduce back pain.
- Heat or Cold Therapy: Applying heat packs or cold compresses to the affected area can help alleviate muscle tension and reduce pain and inflammation.
- Massage Therapy: Gentle massage techniques performed by a qualified therapist can help relieve muscle tension and promote relaxation.
- Acupuncture or Acupressure: Some pregnant patients find relief from back pain with acupuncture or acupressure treatments performed by a licensed practitioner.
- Medications: Acetaminophen may be recommended to help relieve mild to moderate back pain during pregnancy. **Avoid** nonsteroidal anti-inflammatory drugs (NSAIDs) due to potential risks to the fetus.

- Sleep Support: Using pregnancy pillows or additional pillows for support while sleeping can help maintain proper spinal alignment and reduce back pain.

16.4. Morning Sickness

> ➢ *Morning sickness, common in early pregnancy, involves nausea and vomiting, often occurring in the morning but can happen at any time of day.*
>
> ➢ *It is thought to be caused by hormonal changes and typically improves after the first trimester.*
>
> ➢ *Management may include dietary adjustments, ginger supplements, and medication in severe cases.*

Symptoms:

- Nausea: feeling queasy or unsettled in the stomach, often accompanied by an urge to vomit
- Vomiting: expelling the contents of the stomach through the mouth, which may occur occasionally or frequently
- Sensitivity to odors: can trigger nausea and vomiting
- Loss of appetite: Nausea and vomiting can lead to a decreased desire to eat, resulting in a loss of appetite.

Causes and Risk Factors:

- Hormonal changes: Fluctuations in hormone levels, particularly human chorionic gonadotropin (hCG) and estrogen, play a significant role in the development of morning sickness.
- History of morning sickness: Pregnant patients who experienced morning sickness in previous pregnancies are more likely to experience it again in subsequent pregnancies.
- Multiple pregnancies: Morning sickness may be more severe in pregnancies with twins or multiples due to higher hormone levels.
- Certain medical conditions: Women with a history of motion sickness, migraines, or gastrointestinal disorders may be more prone to experiencing nausea and vomiting during pregnancy.

Epidemiology:

Morning sickness is extremely common during pregnancy, with the majority of pregnant patients experiencing some degree of nausea and vomiting, particularly during the first trimester. While it's commonly referred to as "morning sickness," symptoms can occur at any time of day and may vary in severity among patients.

Diagnosis:

Diagnosis of morning sickness is typically based on a clinical evaluation of symptoms reported by the pregnant patient. Laboratory tests or imaging studies are not usually necessary unless there are concerns about dehydration or underlying medical conditions.

Treatment:

- Dietary Modifications: Eating small, frequent meals throughout the day, avoiding spicy or greasy foods, and consuming bland, easily digestible foods may help reduce nausea and vomiting.
- Ginger: Ginger supplements, ginger tea, or ginger ale may help alleviate nausea and vomiting in some pregnant patients.
- Acupressure Wristbands: Wearing acupressure wristbands, which apply pressure to specific points on the wrist, may help reduce nausea and vomiting.
- Vitamin B6 Supplementation: May help alleviate nausea and vomiting in some pregnant patients, although it's important to consult with a healthcare provider before starting any new supplements.
- Prescription Medications: In severe cases of morning sickness, antihistamines (doxylamine) or antiemetics (ondansetron) may be prescribed to help control symptoms.
- Intravenous Fluids: In cases of severe dehydration or inability to tolerate oral fluids, intravenous fluids may be administered in a hospital setting to restore hydration and electrolyte balance.

16.5. Gestational Diabetes Mellitus

> ➤ *Gestational diabetes mellitus (GDM) develops during pregnancy when the body cannot produce enough insulin to meet the increased demands.*
>
> ➤ *It can lead to complications for both mother and baby if not properly managed.*
>
> ➤ *Treatment often involves dietary changes, regular exercise, blood sugar monitoring, and in some cases, insulin therapy.*

Symptoms:

- Often asymptomatic: Gestational diabetes may not present with noticeable symptoms in some cases.

- Increased thirst: Polydipsia may occur due to elevated blood sugar levels.
- Frequent urination: Polyuria, or increased urination, may result from the body's attempt to eliminate excess glucose through urine.
- Fatigue: Generalized fatigue or feeling tired may occur, often attributed to hormonal changes and increased metabolic demands during pregnancy.
- Increased hunger: Polyphagia may occur due to insulin resistance and difficulty regulating blood sugar levels.
- Blurred vision: Changes in vision or blurred vision may occur, particularly if blood sugar levels are poorly controlled.

Causes and Risk Factors:
- Obesity or overweight: Pregnant patients with a body mass index (BMI) above normal range have a higher risk of developing gestational diabetes.
- Advanced maternal age: Pregnant patients over the age of 35 are at increased risk of gestational diabetes.
- Family history: A personal or family history of diabetes (type 1 or type 2) increases the risk of gestational diabetes.
- Previous history of gestational diabetes: Patients who have had gestational diabetes in previous pregnancies are at increased risk of developing it again.
- Ethnicity: Certain ethnic groups, including African American, Hispanic/Latino, Native American, Asian American, and Pacific Islander, have a higher prevalence of gestational diabetes.
- Polycystic ovary syndrome (PCOS): Women with PCOS have an increased risk of insulin resistance and gestational diabetes.
- Hypertension: increases the risk of gestational diabetes
- Previous history of delivering a large baby: Previous delivery of a baby weighing 9 pounds (4,000 grams) or more increases the risk of gestational diabetes in subsequent pregnancies.

Epidemiology:

Gestational diabetes mellitus affects approximately 2-10% of pregnancies, depending on the population and diagnostic criteria used. Its prevalence is increasing globally due to rising rates of obesity, sedentary lifestyles, and changes in maternal age.

Diagnosis:
- <u>One-Step Approach (75-Gram Oral Glucose Tolerance Test):</u>

After an overnight fast, the pregnant patient drinks a glucose solution, and blood samples are taken at specific intervals to measure blood sugar levels. Diagnosis is based on predetermined cutoff values for fasting, one-hour, two-hour, and three-hour blood glucose levels.

- Two-Step Approach (50-Gram Glucose Challenge Test Followed by 100-Gram Oral Glucose Tolerance Test):

    In the first step, the pregnant patient drinks a glucose solution, and blood sugar levels are measured one hour later. If the result is above a certain threshold, a diagnostic oral glucose tolerance test (OGTT) is performed, involving fasting overnight followed by blood samples taken at specific intervals after drinking a larger glucose solution.

Treatment:

- Dietary Modifications: following a well-balanced diet with controlled carbohydrate intake, spacing meals evenly throughout the day, and avoiding sugary foods and beverages
- Regular Physical Activity: walking, swimming, or prenatal yoga to help lower blood sugar levels and improve insulin sensitivity
- Blood Glucose Monitoring: using a glucometer at home to track levels and adjust treatment as needed
- Insulin Therapy: Insulin injections may be necessary if blood sugar levels remain elevated despite dietary and lifestyle modifications.
- Oral Medications: In some cases, oral medications such as metformin or glyburide may be prescribed to help lower blood sugar levels.
- Fetal Monitoring: Regular monitoring of fetal growth and well-being through ultrasound scans and non-stress tests to detect and manage any potential complications.

16.6. Preeclampsia

> ➤ *Preeclampsia is a pregnancy complication characterized by hypertension and signs of damage to other organ systems, often developing after the 20th week.*
> ➤ *It can lead to serious complications for both the mother and the baby, including seizures (eclampsia) and organ failure.*
> ➤ *Management typically involves close monitoring, medication to control blood pressure, and delivery of the baby, depending on the severity.*

Symptoms:
- Hypertension: blood pressure reading consistently higher than 140/90 mm Hg
- Proteinuria: detected through a urine test
- Edema: particularly in the hands and face, although generalized swelling can occur
- Persistent headaches, often severe and not relieved by usual remedies
- Vision changes: blurred vision, flashing lights, or temporary loss of vision
- Upper abdominal pain: typically under the ribs on the right side
- Nausea or vomiting: especially in combination with other symptoms

Causes and Risk Factors:
- First pregnancy: Preeclampsia is more common in first pregnancies.
- History of preeclampsia: Previous history of preeclampsia increases the risk in subsequent pregnancies.
- Chronic hypertension: Women with pre-existing hypertension have a higher risk of developing preeclampsia.
- Multiple pregnancies: Pregnant patients carrying twins or multiples are at increased risk.
- Age: Both very young (<20 years old) and older (>35 years old) pregnant patients are at higher risk.
- Obesity: Being overweight or obese increases the risk of developing preeclampsia.
- Medical Conditions: Conditions such as diabetes, kidney disease, autoimmune diseases, and certain clotting disorders increase the risk.
- Family history: Having a mother or sister who had preeclampsia increases the risk.
- Assisted reproductive technology (ART): The use of ART, such as in vitro fertilization (IVF), is associated with a higher risk.
- Race: African American patients have a higher risk compared to patients of other racial or ethnic backgrounds.

Epidemiology:

Preeclampsia affects approximately 2-8% of pregnancies worldwide. It is a leading cause of maternal and fetal morbidity and mortality, particularly in developing countries where access to prenatal care and medical interventions may be limited.

Diagnosis:
- Hypertension: blood pressure reading consistently higher than 140/90 mm Hg, measured at least twice, at least 4 hours apart, after 20 weeks of pregnancy
- Proteinuria: typically measured through a 24-hour urine collection or a spot urine test
- Organ Dysfunction: Evidence of damage to other organs, such as elevated liver enzymes, low platelet count (thrombocytopenia), kidney dysfunction, pulmonary edema, or visual disturbances.

Treatment:
- Close Monitoring: regular prenatal visits with frequent blood pressure monitoring, urine testing, and assessment of fetal well-being through ultrasound and non-stress tests
- Blood Pressure Management: Antihypertensive medications may be prescribed to lower blood pressure and reduce the risk of complications.
- Hospitalization: Severe cases of preeclampsia may require hospitalization for close monitoring and management of complications.
- Magnesium Sulfate: Administration of magnesium sulfate may be indicated to prevent seizures (eclampsia) in patients with severe preeclampsia.
- Delivery:
    Delivery is the only definitive treatment for preeclampsia, and the timing and mode of delivery depend on various factors, including gestational age, severity of symptoms, and fetal well-being.
- Corticosteroids: In some cases, corticosteroids may be given to help accelerate fetal lung maturity if delivery is imminent.
- Supportive Care: Adequate hydration, rest, and nutritional support are essential components of supportive care for patients with preeclampsia.

16.7. Iron-Deficiency Anemia

> ➢ Iron-deficiency anemia in pregnancy occurs when there's a shortage of red blood cells due to insufficient iron levels, often exacerbated by increased demands during pregnancy.
>
> ➢ Symptoms may include fatigue, weakness, and shortness of breath.
>
> ➢ Treatment involves iron supplementation and dietary changes to prevent complications for both the mother and the baby.

Symptoms:
- Fatigue and weakness
- Pale skin and mucous membranes
- Shortness of breath
- Dizziness or lightheadedness
- Rapid or irregular heartbeat
- Cold hands and feet
- Brittle nails
- Headaches
- Cravings for non-nutritive substances (pica), such as ice or dirt

Causes and Risk Factors:
- Inadequate dietary intake of iron-rich foods
- Increased iron requirements during pregnancy, especially in the second and third trimesters
- Multiple pregnancies
- History of heavy menstrual bleeding or bleeding disorders
- Previous pregnancies with iron-deficiency anemia
- Poor absorption of iron due to gastrointestinal disorders
- Teenage pregnancy
- Low socioeconomic status

Epidemiology:
- Iron-deficiency anemia is one of the most common nutritional deficiencies worldwide, affecting pregnant women, infants, and young children disproportionately.

- Pregnant women are particularly susceptible to iron deficiency due to increased iron requirements for fetal growth and placental development.

Diagnosis:

Screening for anemia is a routine part of prenatal care, typically performed during the first trimester and repeated periodically throughout pregnancy.

Diagnosis of iron-deficiency anemia is based on laboratory tests, including:

- Hemoglobin level: below 11 g/dL during the first and third trimesters, below 10.5 g/dL during the second trimester
- Serum ferritin level: below 15 ng/mL is indicative of depleted iron stores
- Mean corpuscular volume (MCV): may be decreased in iron-deficiency anemia

Treatment:

- <u>Oral Iron Supplementation:</u> This is the first-line treatment for iron-deficiency anemia during pregnancy.
    - The recommended daily dose of elemental iron is typically 30-60 mg/day, taken in divided doses.
    - Iron supplements should be taken with vitamin C to enhance absorption and should be separated from calcium-rich foods or supplements to prevent interference with iron absorption.
- <u>Intravenous Iron Therapy:</u> In severe cases of iron-deficiency anemia or when oral supplementation is not tolerated, intravenous iron therapy may be considered.
- <u>Dietary Counseling:</u>

    In addition to iron supplementation, dietary counseling to increase intake of iron-rich foods (e.g., red meat, poultry, fish, legumes, fortified cereals, leafy green vegetables) is essential.

16.8. Pruritus Gravidarum

> ➤ *Pruritus gravidarum, or pregnancy-related itching, is a common condition characterized by itching of the skin during pregnancy, particularly on the abdomen, arms, legs, and palms.*
>
> ➤ *While the exact cause is unclear, hormonal changes and stretching of the skin are believed to contribute.*
>
> ➤ *Management typically involves moisturizing the skin, wearing loose clothing, and avoiding hot baths or showers.*

Symptoms:

- Generalized itching, often without a visible rash
- Itching may be mild to severe and may occur on various parts of the body, including the abdomen, breasts, arms, legs, and palms of the hands.
- Itching may worsen at night and interfere with sleep.
- Some women may develop scratch marks or secondary skin infections due to scratching.

Causes and Risk Factors:

Pruritus gravidarum can occur in any pregnant woman, but certain factors may increase the risk or severity of symptoms, including:

- Previous history of skin conditions such as eczema or dermatitis
- Multiple pregnancies
- Pre-existing liver conditions such as cholestasis or hepatitis
- Family history of pruritus gravidarum or cholestasis of pregnancy
- Certain medications or supplements

Epidemiology:

- Pruritus gravidarum is estimated to affect up to 20% of pregnant women, although the prevalence may vary depending on the population studied.
- It is most commonly reported in the third trimester of pregnancy but may occur at any stage.

Diagnosis:

- <u>Clinical Assessment:</u> Diagnosis of pruritus gravidarum is based on clinical evaluation, including a thorough medical history and physical examination.

- **Laboratory Tests:** may be performed to rule out underlying conditions that can cause itching during pregnancy, such as intrahepatic cholestasis of pregnancy (ICP) or other liver disorders
    - Blood tests may include liver function tests, bile acid levels, and other markers of liver function.
- **Other Tests:** Ultrasound imaging or fetal monitoring, may be performed if there are concerns about potential complications related to liver or placental function.

Treatment:

Treatment for pruritus gravidarum aims to relieve symptoms and minimize discomfort, while also addressing any underlying causes if present.

- **Topical Treatments:** Moisturizers, emollients, and anti-itch creams or lotions containing ingredients such as menthol, camphor, or oatmeal may provide relief from itching.
- **Avoiding Irritants:** Women with pruritus gravidarum should avoid hot baths or showers, harsh soaps, and tight-fitting clothing that can exacerbate itching.
- **Cool Compresses:** Applying cool, damp compresses to the affected areas can help soothe itching and reduce inflammation.
- **Oral Medications:**

    In severe cases, oral antihistamines or corticosteroids may be prescribed to help relieve itching and inflammation. However, these medications should be used with caution during pregnancy and under medical supervision.

- **Monitoring and Follow-Up:** Pregnant women with pruritus gravidarum should be closely monitored to assess symptoms, monitor liver function, and ensure the well-being of both the mother and baby.

16.9. Striae Gravidarum

> ➢ *Striae gravidarum, or stretch marks, are common during pregnancy due to rapid stretching of the skin, particularly in the abdomen, breasts, hips, and thighs.*
> ➢ *They appear as reddish or purplish streaks that fade to a lighter color over time.*
> ➢ *Prevention methods include moisturizing the skin and maintaining a healthy weight, but they often cannot be completely avoided.*

Symptoms:

- Pink, red, purple, or dark brown streaks or lines on the skin

- Initially, stretch marks may appear slightly raised and may feel itchy or sensitive.
- Over time, they often fade to a lighter color and become less noticeable, although they may remain slightly indented or wrinkled.

Causes and Risk Factors:
- Rapid weight gain and stretching of the skin during pregnancy are the primary risk factors for developing stretch marks.
- Genetics: A family history of stretch marks may increase the likelihood of developing them.
- Skin type: Patients with certain skin types, including fair skin, are more prone to developing stretch marks.
- Multiple pregnancies: Women carrying twins or triplets, or those who have had multiple pregnancies, may be at higher risk.
- Excessive weight gain: Rapid or excessive weight gain, whether during pregnancy or due to other factors, can increase the risk of developing stretch marks.
- Hormonal factors: Increased levels of cortisol and other hormones during pregnancy may contribute to the development of stretch marks.

Epidemiology:

Stretch marks are extremely common during pregnancy, with the majority of women experiencing them to some degree. It is estimated that up to 90% of pregnant women develop stretch marks, typically during the later stages of pregnancy.

Diagnosis:

Diagnosis of stretch marks is typically based on clinical examination and observation of characteristic skin changes. Stretch marks are usually identified based on their appearance, location (commonly occurring on the abdomen, breasts, hips, thighs, and buttocks), and history of rapid weight gain or stretching of the skin.

Treatment:
- <u>Prevention:</u> While it may not be possible to completely prevent stretch marks, certain measures may help minimize their development or severity, including:
    - Maintaining a healthy weight during pregnancy
    - Staying hydrated by drinking plenty of water
    - Eating a balanced diet rich in vitamins and nutrients
    - Regular exercise to promote skin elasticity

- o Using moisturizers and oils to keep the skin hydrated and supple
- **Topical Treatments:**

    Various creams, lotions, and oils containing ingredients such as cocoa butter, shea butter, vitamin E, hyaluronic acid, or retinoids may be used to moisturize the skin and improve its appearance. However, the effectiveness of these treatments in preventing or reducing stretch marks is limited, and results may vary.

- **Laser Therapy:** Fractional laser therapy or pulsed dye laser therapy may be used to improve the appearance of stretch marks by stimulating collagen production and reducing redness.
- **Microneedling:** This procedure creates tiny punctures in the skin with fine needles and may help improve the appearance of stretch marks by promoting collagen remodeling and skin regeneration.
- **Cosmetic Procedures:**

    Abdominoplasty (tummy tuck) or dermabrasion may be considered for severe or persistent stretch marks, although they are typically not recommended during pregnancy or breastfeeding.

16.10. Melasma of Pregnancy

> ➢ *Melasma, commonly known as "pregnancy mask," is a skin condition characterized by dark patches or hyperpigmentation, typically on the face, during pregnancy.*
> ➢ *It is caused by hormonal changes and increased melanin production.*
> ➢ *Sun protection, topical treatments, and avoiding sun exposure can help manage melasma, which often fades after pregnancy.*

Symptoms:
- Brown or grayish patches of pigmentation on the face, typically symmetrical in appearance
- Patches may vary in size and shape and may darken or lighten over time.
- Melasma most commonly affects areas of the face that are exposed to sunlight, such as the cheeks, forehead, nose, and upper lip.
- In some cases, melasma may also occur on other sun-exposed areas of the body, such as the neck and arms.

Risk Factors:
- Pregnancy: Melasma is often triggered or exacerbated by hormonal changes during pregnancy, particularly increased levels of estrogen and progesterone.
- Sun exposure: Ultraviolet (UV) radiation from the sun is a significant risk factor for melasma, as it can stimulate the production of melanin (pigment) in the skin and darken existing patches.
- Hormonal factors: Hormonal fluctuations associated with pregnancy, oral contraceptives, hormone replacement therapy, or hormonal imbalances may increase the risk of melasma.
- Genetic predisposition: Patients with a family history of melasma or a personal history of other pigmentary disorders may have an increased risk.
- Skin type: Melasma is more common in patients with darker skin types, particularly those of Hispanic, Asian, African, or Middle Eastern descent.
- Certain medications (e.g., phenytoin, hormonal medications) or cosmetics containing ingredients such as fragrances or dyes may increase the risk of developing melasma or exacerbate existing patches.

Epidemiology:
- Melasma is a common condition, particularly among women of reproductive age.
- It is estimated to affect up to 50-70% of pregnant women, with the highest prevalence observed in patients with darker skin types.
- Melasma typically develops or worsens during pregnancy and may improve or resolve after delivery, although it may persist for months or years in some cases.

Diagnosis:
- <u>Clinical Assessment:</u> Diagnosis of melasma is usually based on clinical evaluation and observation of characteristic skin changes.
- <u>Physical Examination:</u> The APh may perform a physical examination and take a thorough medical history to assess risk factors and rule out other possible causes of hyperpigmentation.
- <u>Others:</u> In some cases, a Wood's lamp examination or skin biopsy may be performed to aid in diagnosis or rule out other pigmentation disorders.

Treatment:
- Sun Protection:

    Sunscreen is the cornerstone of melasma treatment, as sun exposure can exacerbate pigmentation and darken existing patches. Broad-spectrum sunscreen with a high sun protection factor (SPF) should be applied daily, even on cloudy days, and reapplied every two hours when outdoors.

- Topical Treatments: Various topical medications and skincare products may be used to lighten or reduce the appearance of melasma, including:
    - Hydroquinone: A bleaching agent that inhibits melanin production. It is available over-the-counter or by prescription in concentrations up to 4%.
    - Topical retinoids: Vitamin A derivatives such as tretinoin or adapalene may help improve skin texture and reduce pigmentation.
    - Corticosteroids: Topical corticosteroids may be used in combination with other medications to reduce inflammation and lighten pigmentation.
    - Azelaic acid: A naturally occurring acid that inhibits melanin production and has anti-inflammatory properties.
    - Kojic acid, licorice extract, and alpha hydroxy acids (AHAs) may also be used in topical formulations to lighten pigmentation.

- Chemical Peels:

    Superficial chemical peels containing ingredients such as glycolic acid, salicylic acid, or trichloroacetic acid (TCA) may help improve melasma by exfoliating the outer layers of the skin and promoting skin renewal.

- Laser Therapy:

    Various laser and light-based treatments, such as intense pulsed light (IPL), fractional lasers, or Q-switched lasers, may be used to target and lighten pigmented areas of the skin. However, laser treatments should be used with caution during pregnancy and are typically not recommended until after delivery.

- Combination Therapy: Combining multiple treatment modalities, such as topical medications, sun protection, and cosmetic procedures, may provide the most effective results for melasma management.

16.11. Miscarriage

> ➢ *Miscarriage is the spontaneous loss of a pregnancy before the 20th week, often due to genetic abnormalities or maternal health factors.*
>
> ➢ *Symptoms may include vaginal bleeding, abdominal cramps, and passing tissue from the vagina.*
>
> ➢ *Emotional support and medical care are crucial following a miscarriage.*

Symptoms:
- Vaginal bleeding, ranging from light spotting to heavy bleeding
- Abdominal cramping or pain, often similar to menstrual cramps
- Passage of tissue or clots from the vagina
- Back pain or pelvic pressure
- Decreased pregnancy symptoms
- Loss of pregnancy symptoms

Causes and Risk Factors:
- Maternal age: risk increases with advancing maternal age, particularly after age 35
- Previous history of miscarriage
- Genetic or chromosomal abnormalities in the fetus
- Medical conditions: diabetes, thyroid disorders, autoimmune diseases
- Uterine abnormalities or structural issues
- Infections: bacterial vaginosis, sexually transmitted infections
- Lifestyle factors: smoking, alcohol consumption, drug use
- Exposure to environmental toxins or pollutants
- Certain medications or medical treatments: chemotherapy, radiation therapy
- Advanced paternal age
- Obesity or underweight status
- Excessive caffeine consumption

Epidemiology:

Miscarriage is a relatively common pregnancy complication, with an estimated incidence of 10-20% of clinically recognized pregnancies. The risk of miscarriage varies depending on factors such as maternal age, reproductive history, and overall health. Most miscarriages occur in the first trimester (before 12 weeks of gestation), with a smaller proportion occurring in the second trimester.

Diagnosis:
- Physical Examination: assessment of symptoms, vital signs, and pelvic examination to evaluate for signs of miscarriage
- Ultrasound:
    Transabdominal or transvaginal ultrasound can visualize the uterus and fetal development, confirm pregnancy viability, and assess for signs of miscarriage (e.g., absence of fetal heartbeat, empty gestational sac).
- Blood Tests: measurement of quantitative human chorionic gonadotropin (hCG) levels to monitor pregnancy hormone levels and assess for signs of pregnancy loss
- Tissue Analysis: examination of passed tissue or products of conception to confirm the diagnosis and identify any chromosomal abnormalities or other causes of miscarriage

Treatment:
- Expectant Management: allowing the miscarriage to occur naturally without intervention, with close monitoring of symptoms and follow-up care
- Medications: administration of medications such as misoprostol to help induce miscarriage and facilitate the passage of tissue
- Surgical Management: dilatation and curettage (D&C) or suction evacuation to remove remaining tissue from the uterus in cases of incomplete miscarriage or missed miscarriage
- Emotional Support: counseling, support groups, or therapy to help patients cope with the emotional impact of miscarriage and process their grief
- Follow-up Care: monitoring for any complications (e.g., infection, excessive bleeding) and providing appropriate medical care and support as needed

16.12. Cholestasis of Pregnancy

> ➤ *Cholestasis of pregnancy is a liver condition characterized by decreased bile flow, leading to a buildup of bile acids in the blood during pregnancy.*
>
> ➤ *It can cause intense itching, typically on the hands and feet, and may increase the risk of complications for both the mother and the baby, such as preterm birth or stillbirth.*
>
> ➤ *Management involves medication to relieve itching and close monitoring of fetal well-being.*

Symptoms:
- Itching, typically more severe on the palms of the hands and soles of the feet
- Dark urine
- Light-colored stools
- Jaundice
- Fatigue
- Loss of appetite
- Nausea or vomiting
- Upper abdominal pain or discomfort

Causes and Risk Factors:
- Previous history of cholestasis of pregnancy
- Family history of cholestasis of pregnancy
- Multiple pregnancies
- Female gender of the fetus
- Maternal age over 35 years
- Obesity or overweight status
- History of liver or gallbladder disease
- Certain ethnicities (e.g., Scandinavian, Chilean, Swedish)
- In vitro fertilization (IVF) pregnancies

Epidemiology:
- Cholestasis of pregnancy, also known as intrahepatic cholestasis of pregnancy (ICP), is a relatively rare condition occurring in approximately 1-2 pregnancies per 1,000 pregnancies in the United States.

- The prevalence of ICP varies among different populations and is more common in certain ethnic groups, such as those of Scandinavian or Chilean descent. It typically occurs in the third trimester of pregnancy but can develop earlier in some cases.

Diagnosis:
- <u>Clinical Evaluation:</u> assessment of symptoms, medical history, and risk factors for cholestasis of pregnancy
- <u>Blood Tests:</u> measurement of liver function tests (e.g., serum bile acids, alkaline phosphatase, transaminases) to assess liver function and bile acid levels
- <u>Serum Bile Acid Test:</u> elevated serum bile acid levels (>10 μmol/L) are diagnostic for cholestasis of pregnancy
- <u>Fetal Monitoring:</u> Nonstress test (NST) or biophysical profile (BPP) assess fetal well-being and monitor for signs of distress due to the condition.

Treatment:
- <u>Symptomatic Relief:</u> Medications such as antihistamines (e.g., diphenhydramine) or ursodeoxycholic acid (UDCA) alleviate itching and improve liver function.
- <u>Monitoring and Surveillance:</u> regular monitoring of liver function tests and serum bile acid levels to assess disease progression and fetal well-being
- <u>Fetal Surveillance:</u> close monitoring of fetal growth, movement, and well-being through ultrasound and fetal monitoring tests (e.g., NST, BPP)
- <u>Early Delivery:</u> In cases of severe cholestasis or fetal distress, early induction of labor or cesarean delivery may be recommended to prevent complications.

16.13. Postpartum Depression

> *Postpartum depression is a mood disorder that can affect new mothers, typically developing within the first few weeks after childbirth.*
>
> *Symptoms may include sadness, anxiety, and difficulty bonding with the baby, impacting daily functioning.*
>
> *Treatment often involves therapy, support groups, and in some cases, medication.*

Symptoms:
- Persistent feelings of sadness, emptiness, or hopelessness
- Frequent crying or tearfulness
- Loss of interest or pleasure in activities once enjoyed
- Irritability or agitation
- Fatigue or low energy
- Changes in appetite or weight (increased or decreased)
- Sleep disturbances (insomnia or excessive sleep)
- Difficulty concentrating or making decisions
- Feelings of worthlessness or guilt
- Thoughts of self-harm or harming the baby

Causes and Risk Factors:
- Previous history of depression or anxiety
- Personal or family history of postpartum depression or other mood disorders
- Hormonal changes associated with childbirth and breastfeeding
- Stressful life events or lack of social support
- Relationship difficulties or marital discord
- Financial problems or socioeconomic stressors
- Complications during pregnancy or childbirth
- History of trauma or abuse
- Chronic medical conditions or pregnancy complications
- Sleep disturbances or exhaustion from caring for a newborn

Epidemiology:

Postpartum depression affects approximately 10-15% of women following childbirth, making it one of the most common complications of childbirth. The prevalence may be higher in certain populations, such as women with a history of depression, low socioeconomic status, or limited access to healthcare. Postpartum depression can occur within the first few weeks after childbirth or develop gradually over the first year postpartum.

Diagnosis:
- <u>Clinical Evaluation:</u> assessment of symptoms, medical history, and risk factors for postpartum depression

- Screening Tools:

    Use of validated screening questionnaires such as the Edinburgh Postnatal Depression Scale (EPDS) to screen for postpartum depression symptoms during routine postpartum visits.

- Diagnostic Criteria:

    Diagnosis of postpartum depression based on criteria outlined in the Diagnostic and Statistical Manual of Mental Disorders (DSM-5), including the presence of depressive symptoms lasting more than two weeks and causing significant distress or impairment in functioning.

Treatment:

- Psychotherapy:

    Cognitive-behavioral therapy (CBT) or interpersonal therapy (IPT) to address negative thought patterns, improve coping skills, and strengthen social support networks.

- Antidepressant Medications:

    Selective serotonin reuptake inhibitors (SSRIs) or serotonin-norepinephrine reuptake inhibitors (SNRIs) may be prescribed for moderate to severe postpartum depression.

- Supportive Interventions:

    Support groups, peer counseling, or patient counseling provide emotional support, validation, and practical assistance for women experiencing postpartum depression.

- Lifestyle Modifications:

    Adequate rest, healthy nutrition, regular exercise, and stress-reduction techniques (e.g., mindfulness, relaxation exercises) promote overall well-being.

- Family and Social Support:

    Involvement of partners, family members, and friends in caregiving and emotional support help alleviate the burden of postpartum depression and promote recovery.

16.14. Multiple Gestation

> ➤ *Multiple gestation refers to a pregnancy with two or more fetuses, such as twins or triplets, developing simultaneously in the womb.*
> ➤ *It can occur naturally or through assisted reproductive technologies like in vitro fertilization.*
> ➤ *Multiple pregnancies often require closer monitoring for complications such as preterm birth and low birth weight.*

Symptoms:
- Rapidly expanding abdomen
- Excessive weight gain
- Increased fetal movement
- Severe morning sickness (hyperemesis gravidarum)
- Elevated levels of maternal hormones
- Higher levels of discomfort and fatigue compared to singleton pregnancies
- Increased frequency of prenatal visits and ultrasounds

Causes and Risk Factors:
- Advanced maternal age: over 35 years
- Assisted reproductive technology (ART) procedures such as in vitro fertilization (IVF) or ovulation induction
- Previous history of multiple gestation pregnancies
- Family history of twins or multiples
- Ethnicity: Certain ethnic groups have a higher incidence of multiple gestation pregnancies.
- Use of fertility drugs or medications to induce ovulation
- History of multiple miscarriages
- Obesity
- Maternal height: taller women may have a higher likelihood of conceiving twins.
- Parity: Women who have already had multiple pregnancies are at increased risk.

Epidemiology:

The incidence of multiple gestation pregnancies has been increasing in recent years, primarily due to the widespread use of assisted reproductive technologies (ART) and the trend of delaying childbearing. Twins account for the majority of multiple pregnancies, followed by triplets and higher-order multiples. The overall prevalence of twins in the general population is approximately 1 in 30 pregnancies, while the prevalence of triplets or higher-order multiples is much lower.

Diagnosis:

- Ultrasound:

    The definitive method for diagnosing multiple gestation pregnancies, typically performed during the first trimester or early second trimester. Ultrasound can identify multiple gestational sacs, embryos/fetuses, and chorionicity (whether the multiples share a placenta).

- Maternal Serum Alpha-Fetoprotein (MSAFP) Screening:

    Elevated levels of MSAFP may indicate a multiple gestation pregnancy, although this test is less accurate than ultrasound and is typically used in conjunction with other screening tests.

- Physical Examination: Fundal height measurement may be larger than expected for gestational age in multiple gestation pregnancies, although this method is less reliable than ultrasound.

Treatment:

- Prenatal Care: Close monitoring by healthcare providers specializing in high-risk pregnancies, including more frequent prenatal visits, ultrasounds, and laboratory tests.

- Nutritional Counseling:

    Adequate nutrition is crucial for supporting the growth and development of multiple fetuses. Women carrying multiples may need to increase their calorie and nutrient intake.

- Bed Rest: In some cases, The APh may recommend bed rest or reduced activity to minimize the risk of complications such as preterm labor or fetal growth restriction.

- Preterm Birth Prevention:

    Administration of medications such as progesterone or cervical cerclage (stitching the cervix closed) may be used to prevent preterm labor and prolong pregnancy in women carrying multiples.

- Delivery Planning:

    The timing and mode of delivery depend on various factors, including gestational age, fetal presentation, chorionicity, and maternal and fetal health status. Vaginal delivery is often possible for twins, but cesarean delivery may be recommended for higher-order multiples or other complicating factors.

16.15. Gestational Thyroid Disorders

> ➤ *Gestational thyroid disorders involve thyroid dysfunction during pregnancy, including hyperthyroidism or hypothyroidism.*
> ➤ *They can impact maternal and fetal health, leading to complications like preterm birth, preeclampsia, or developmental issues in the baby.*
> ➤ *Treatment may involve medication adjustments and close monitoring to ensure thyroid hormone levels remain within a safe range.*

Symptoms:
- Fatigue
- Weight changes: either weight loss or weight gain
- Palpitations or rapid heartbeat
- Heat intolerance or excessive sweating
- Cold intolerance
- Changes in bowel habits: diarrhea or constipation
- Muscle weakness or tremors
- Mood changes: anxiety, irritability, depression
- Menstrual irregularities
- Goiter: causes swelling of the neck

Risk Factors:
- History of thyroid disorders like hypothyroidism or hyperthyroidism
- Autoimmune diseases: Hashimoto's thyroiditis, Graves' disease
- Family history of thyroid disorders
- Age: risk increases with advancing maternal age
- Previous history of thyroid surgery or radiation therapy to the neck
- History of infertility or miscarriage
- Use of certain medications such as amiodarone or lithium
- Iodine deficiency or excess
- Pregnancy-related factors: multiple gestation, history of preterm birth

- Presence of thyroid antibodies: thyroid peroxidase antibodies, thyroid-stimulating immunoglobulins

Epidemiology:

Gestational thyroid disorders include both hypothyroidism and hyperthyroidism that develop during pregnancy. Hypothyroidism affects approximately 2-3% of pregnant women, while hyperthyroidism is less common, occurring in about 0.2-0.4% of pregnancies. The prevalence of gestational thyroid disorders may vary depending on factors such as iodine intake, maternal age, and underlying medical conditions.

Diagnosis:

- <u>Thyroid Function Tests:</u>
  - Measurement of serum thyroid-stimulating hormone (TSH) levels to assess thyroid function. Abnormal TSH levels may indicate hypothyroidism (elevated TSH) or hyperthyroidism (decreased TSH).
  - Measurement of free thyroxine (FT4) levels to further evaluate thyroid function. Abnormal FT4 levels may confirm the diagnosis of hypothyroidism (low FT4) or hyperthyroidism (high FT4).
- <u>Thyroid Antibody Testing:</u>

  Measurement of thyroid antibodies (e.g., thyroid peroxidase antibodies, thyroid-stimulating immunoglobulins) to assess for autoimmune thyroid disorders such as Hashimoto's thyroiditis or Graves' disease.
- <u>Ultrasound:</u> Thyroid ultrasound may be performed to evaluate the size, shape, and texture of the thyroid gland and identify any nodules or abnormalities.
- <u>Clinical Assessment:</u> evaluation of symptoms, medical history, and risk factors for thyroid disorders during pregnancy

Treatment:

- <u>Hypothyroidism:</u>

  Thyroid hormone replacement therapy with levothyroxine to maintain adequate thyroid hormone levels during pregnancy. Dosage adjustments may be necessary based on thyroid function tests and clinical response.
- <u>Hyperthyroidism:</u>
  - Management may include antithyroid medications such as propylthiouracil (PTU) or methimazole (MMI) to control hyperthyroid symptoms and normalize thyroid function.

- Beta-blocker medications may be used to manage symptoms such as palpitations, tremors, and anxiety.
- **Monitoring:** Regular monitoring of thyroid function tests throughout pregnancy to ensure thyroid hormone levels remain within the normal range and adjust treatment as needed.
- **Multidisciplinary Care:**

    Collaboration with endocrinologists, obstetricians, and other healthcare providers to optimize management and monitor maternal and fetal well-being during pregnancy.

16.16. Endometriosis

> ➤ *Endometriosis is a chronic condition where tissue similar to the lining of the uterus grows outside the uterus, commonly causing pelvic pain and infertility.*
>
> ➤ *Symptoms may include painful menstruation, pain during intercourse, and fatigue.*
>
> ➤ *Treatment options include medication, surgery, and lifestyle changes to manage symptoms and improve fertility.*

Symptoms:
- Pelvic pain: pain before and during menstruation, during intercourse, or during bowel movements or urination
- Heavy menstrual bleeding
- Infertility: Endometriosis can affect fertility by causing scar tissue and adhesions that block fallopian tubes or disrupt the function of reproductive organs.
- Other symptoms may include fatigue, diarrhea, constipation, and bloating.

Causes and Risk Factors:
- Family history of endometriosis
- Menstrual periods lasting longer than 7 days or shorter than 27 days
- Low body mass index (BMI)
- Never giving birth
- Starting menstruation at an early age (before age 11)
- Uterine abnormalities

Epidemiology:

Endometriosis is estimated to affect 10-15% of women of reproductive age worldwide. It is one of the most common gynecological disorders, with a prevalence of approximately 5-10% in women of reproductive age. Endometriosis can occur at any age but is most commonly diagnosed in women in their 30s and 40s.

Diagnosis:

- Pelvic Exam: to feel for abnormalities such as cysts or scars behind the uterus
- Imaging Tests: Ultrasound or MRI may be used to create images of the pelvic area.
- Laparoscopy: surgical procedure to view the inside of the abdomen and pelvis, allowing for direct visualization and biopsy of endometrial tissue

Treatment:

- Pain Medication: Over-the-counter pain relievers such as ibuprofen or prescription medications may help manage pain.
- Hormone Therapy: Birth control pills, hormonal patches, or hormone-containing intrauterine devices (IUDs) can help control the menstrual cycle and reduce symptoms.
- Surgery: Laparoscopic surgery to remove endometrial tissue, scar tissue, or ovarian cysts may be necessary for severe cases or infertility.
- Assisted Reproductive Technologies (ART): In cases of infertility, techniques such as in vitro fertilization (IVF) may be used to help conceive.
- Lifestyle Changes: Regular exercise, stress reduction techniques, and dietary changes may help manage symptoms.

16.17. Uterine Fibroids

> ➢ *Fibroids are noncancerous growths that develop in the uterus, commonly during childbearing years.*
>
> ➢ *They can vary in size and number, causing symptoms such as heavy menstrual bleeding, pelvic pain, and pressure on the bladder or rectum.*
>
> ➢ *Treatment options include medication, minimally invasive procedures, or surgery depending on the severity of symptoms and desire for fertility.*

Symptoms:

- Menorrhagia: heavy menstrual bleeding
- Prolonged menstrual periods or bleeding between periods
- Pelvic pain or pressure
- Frequent urination or difficulty emptying the bladder
- Constipation or difficulty with bowel movements
- Enlargement of the lower abdomen
- Pain during intercourse
- Infertility or recurrent pregnancy loss (in some cases)

Causes and Risk Factors:

- Age: Fibroids are more common in women of reproductive age and tend to shrink after menopause.
- Family history: Having a first-degree relative with fibroids increases the risk.
- Ethnicity: African American women are more likely to develop fibroids and tend to have larger and more symptomatic fibroids than women of other racial/ethnic groups.
- Hormonal factors: Estrogen and progesterone play a role in fibroid growth, and factors that increase hormone levels (such as pregnancy or hormone therapy) may contribute to fibroid development.
- Obesity: Being overweight or obese increases the risk of fibroids.
- Diet: Some studies suggest that a diet high in red meat and low in fruits and vegetables may increase the risk of fibroids.

Epidemiology:

Fibroids are a common gynecological condition, affecting millions of women worldwide. They are estimated to occur in up to 70-80% of women by the age of 50. Fibroids are less common before puberty and tend to regress after menopause. The prevalence of fibroids varies among different racial and ethnic groups, with African American women having the highest prevalence.

Diagnosis:

- Pelvic Exam: to feel for abnormalities or changes in the uterus or ovaries
- Imaging Tests: Transvaginal ultrasound, MRI, or hysterosonography may be used to visualize the size, number, and location of fibroids.
- Hysteroscopy: procedure to examine the inside of the uterus using a thin, lighted tube inserted through the vagina and cervix
- Biopsy: Rarely, a sample of tissue may be taken (usually during hysteroscopy) to confirm the diagnosis if cancer is suspected.

Treatment:

- Watchful Waiting: In many cases, fibroids do not cause symptoms and may not require treatment. Regular monitoring may be recommended to track changes in size or symptoms.
- Medications: Hormonal therapies, such as birth control pills, GnRH agonists, or progestin-releasing intrauterine devices (IUDs), can help control heavy bleeding and reduce fibroid size.
- Minimally Invasive Procedures:

    Uterine artery embolization, myomectomy (surgical removal of fibroids), or focused ultrasound surgery (FUS) may be recommended to treat symptomatic fibroids while preserving the uterus.

- Hysterectomy: In severe cases or when fertility is not a concern, surgical removal of the uterus (hysterectomy) may be recommended to permanently relieve symptoms.

16.18. Pelvic Pain

> ➤ *Pelvic pain refers to discomfort or pain in the lower abdomen, pelvis, or genital area, lasting for more than six months.*
> ➤ *Causes can include menstrual cramps, endometriosis, pelvic inflammatory disease, or urinary tract infections.*
> ➤ *Diagnosis involves a medical history, physical examination, and sometimes imaging tests or laparoscopy for further evaluation and management.*

Symptoms:
- Dull, aching pain in the lower abdomen or pelvis
- Sharp or stabbing pain
- Dyspareunia: pain during sexual intercourse
- Dysmenorrhea: pain during menstruation
- Pain with urination or bowel movements
- Bloating or pressure in the pelvic area
- Irregular menstrual cycles
- Nausea or vomiting

Causes and Risk Factors:
- History of pelvic inflammatory disease (PID) or sexually transmitted infections (STIs)
- Previous pelvic surgery or trauma
- Endometriosis or fibroids
- Chronic constipation or irritable bowel syndrome (IBS)
- History of pelvic inflammatory disease (PID) or sexually transmitted infections (STIs)
- Psychological factors such as stress, anxiety, or depression
- Obesity or sedentary lifestyle

Epidemiology:

Pelvic pain is a common complaint, affecting women of all ages. It is one of the most frequent reasons for gynecological consultations and hospital admissions. The prevalence of chronic pelvic pain in women of reproductive age ranges from 5% to 26%, depending on the population studied and the definition of pelvic pain used.

Diagnosis:
- <u>Medical History and Physical Examination:</u> assessing the location, severity, and duration of pain, as well as associated symptoms, medical history, and risk factors
- <u>Imaging Studies:</u> Transvaginal ultrasound, MRI, or CT scans may be used to visualize pelvic organs and detect abnormalities such as cysts, fibroids, or pelvic masses.
- <u>Laboratory Tests:</u> Blood tests may be performed to assess hormone levels, rule out infections, or evaluate for inflammatory markers.

- Diagnostic Procedures: Laparoscopy or hysteroscopy may be performed to directly visualize pelvic organs and obtain tissue samples for biopsy.

Treatment:
- Conservative Management: Lifestyle modifications such as dietary changes, regular exercise, stress management techniques, and over-the-counter pain relievers may help alleviate symptoms.
- Medications:
    Hormonal therapies (such as birth control pills, GnRH agonists, or progestin-releasing IUDs), nonsteroidal anti-inflammatory drugs (NSAIDs), or muscle relaxants may be prescribed to manage pain and inflammation.
- Physical Therapy: Pelvic floor physical therapy, biofeedback, or relaxation techniques may help relieve pelvic muscle tension and improve symptoms.
- Minimally Invasive Procedures: Procedures such as nerve blocks, trigger point injections, or nerve ablation may be recommended for refractory cases.
- Surgery: In some cases, surgical intervention may be necessary to address underlying causes of pelvic pain, such as endometriosis, fibroids, ovarian cysts, or pelvic adhesions.

16.19. Vaginal Discharge

> *Vaginal discharge is a normal bodily function involving the secretion of fluid and cells from the vagina.*
>
> *It can vary in consistency, color, and odor depending on factors like menstrual cycle, sexual activity, and hormonal changes.*
>
> *While some changes are normal, unusual discharge accompanied by itching, burning, or a foul odor may indicate infection and should be evaluated by a healthcare provider.*

Symptoms:
- Changes in color, consistency, or odor of vaginal discharge
- Itching or irritation in the vaginal area
- Burning sensation during urination
- Pain during sexual intercourse
- Swelling or redness around the vaginal opening

Causes and Risk Factors:
- Hormonal changes: Fluctuations in estrogen levels, such as those occurring during pregnancy, menopause, or the menstrual cycle, can affect vaginal discharge.
- Increased sexual activity, especially with new or multiple partners, can alter vaginal flora and increase the risk of infections.
- Antibiotic use can disrupt the balance of vaginal bacteria, leading to changes in vaginal discharge and an increased risk of yeast infections.
- Poorly controlled diabetes can increase the risk of vaginal yeast infections due to elevated blood sugar levels.
- Immunosuppression: Conditions or medications that weaken the immune system, such as HIV/AIDS or corticosteroid therapy, can predispose individuals to vaginal infections.

Epidemiology:

Vaginal discharge is a common gynecological symptom experienced by women of all ages. While most cases of vaginal discharge are benign and transient, certain infections such as bacterial vaginosis, yeast infections, or sexually transmitted infections (STIs) can cause abnormal vaginal discharge and require medical attention. The prevalence of specific causes of vaginal discharge may vary depending on factors such as age, sexual activity, and geographical location.

Diagnosis:
- Medical History: The APh will inquire about symptoms, sexual activity, menstrual history, contraceptive use, and recent medications
- Physical Examination: A pelvic exam may be performed to assess the appearance of vaginal discharge and check for signs of infection or inflammation.
- Laboratory Tests: Vaginal swabs or cultures may be collected to identify the presence of infectious organisms such as bacteria, yeast, or parasites.
- pH Testing: Testing the acidity (pH) of vaginal discharge can help differentiate between different causes of vaginal infections.

Treatment:
- Antifungal Medications: Antifungal creams, suppositories, or oral medications may be prescribed to treat yeast infections.
- Antibiotics: may be necessary to treat bacterial infections such as bacterial vaginosis or sexually transmitted infections

- **Topical Treatments:** Over-the-counter or prescription topical treatments may help relieve symptoms of itching, irritation, or inflammation.
- **Hormonal Therapy:** Estrogen therapy may be recommended for menopausal women experiencing vaginal dryness or atrophy.
- **Lifestyle Modifications:** Practicing good hygiene, wearing breathable cotton underwear, avoiding douching or scented feminine hygiene products, and practicing safe sex can help prevent vaginal infections and maintain vaginal health.

16.20. Infertility

> - *Infertility is the inability to conceive after one year of unprotected intercourse, affecting around 10-15% of couples.*
> - *Causes can include issues with ovulation, sperm quality, fallopian tube blockages, or underlying health conditions.*
> - *Treatment options may include medication, surgery, assisted reproductive technology, or lifestyle changes depending on the underlying cause.*

Symptoms:
- Inability to conceive after one year of regular, unprotected intercourse
- Amenorrhea: irregular menstrual cycles or absent periods
- Dysmenorrhea or menorrhagia: painful or heavy menstrual periods
- Hormonal imbalances, such as abnormal levels of estrogen, progesterone, or thyroid hormones
- Physical symptoms such as weight gain, hair growth, or acne (in women with polycystic ovary syndrome)
- Erectile dysfunction or decreased libido (in men)

Causes and Risk Factors:
- Age: Fertility declines with age, especially after age 35 for women and age 40 for men.
- Medical conditions: Conditions such as endometriosis, polycystic ovary syndrome (PCOS), thyroid disorders, diabetes, or sexually transmitted infections (STIs) can affect fertility.

- Lifestyle factors: Smoking, excessive alcohol consumption, drug use, obesity, poor nutrition, and high levels of stress can negatively impact fertility.
- Environmental factors: Exposure to environmental toxins, pollutants, radiation, or chemicals can affect reproductive health.
- Genetic factors: Certain genetic conditions or chromosomal abnormalities may be associated with infertility.
- Reproductive history: Previous pelvic surgeries, infections, or complications during pregnancy or childbirth may affect fertility.

Epidemiology:

Infertility is a common problem worldwide, affecting an estimated 10-15% of couples of reproductive age. The prevalence of infertility may vary depending on factors such as age, geographical location, socioeconomic status, and access to healthcare services. In many cases, infertility is a multifactorial condition involving both male and female factors, and the underlying causes may be complex and varied.

Diagnosis:

- Medical History: The APh will review the individual and couple's medical history, including reproductive history, previous pregnancies, menstrual cycles, and lifestyle factors.
- Physical Examination: A physical examination may be performed to assess for signs of hormonal imbalances, anatomical abnormalities, or reproductive health issues.
- Laboratory Tests: Blood tests may be conducted to evaluate hormone levels, thyroid function, ovarian reserve, or other factors affecting fertility.
- Imaging Studies: Ultrasound, hysterosalpingography (HSG), or pelvic MRI may be used to assess the anatomy of the reproductive organs and identify any structural abnormalities.
- Semen Analysis: to evaluate sperm count, motility, morphology, and other parameters of sperm quality in men

Treatment:

- Lifestyle Modifications: Regular exercise, balanced nutrition, weight management, smoking cessation, and reducing alcohol or caffeine intake can help improve fertility.
- Medications: Fertility medications may be prescribed to regulate ovulation, stimulate egg production, or treat underlying hormonal imbalances.

- Assisted Reproductive Technologies (ART):

    Techniques such as in vitro fertilization (IVF), intrauterine insemination (IUI), or intracytoplasmic sperm injection (ICSI) may be recommended for couples with infertility due to male factor infertility, tubal factor infertility, or unexplained infertility.

- Surgery: Laparoscopy, hysteroscopy, or varicocele repair may be performed to correct structural abnormalities, remove blockages, or treat conditions such as endometriosis or fibroids.

- Counseling and Support: Counseling, support groups, or therapy may be beneficial for individuals or couples experiencing infertility-related stress, anxiety, or depression.

16.21. Irregular Menstruation

> ➤ *Irregular menstruation refers to variations in the length, duration, or intensity of menstrual cycles.*
>
> ➤ *Causes can include hormonal imbalances, stress, diet, exercise, or underlying health conditions such as polycystic ovary syndrome (PCOS) or thyroid disorders.*
>
> ➤ *Treatment depends on the underlying cause and may include lifestyle modifications, hormone therapy, or medication.*

Symptoms:

- Variations in menstrual cycle length (shorter or longer than usual)
- Inconsistent menstrual periods (skipped periods or frequent spotting)
- Menorrhagia: heavy or prolonged menstrual bleeding
- Hypomenorrhea: light or scanty menstrual bleeding
- Dysmenorrhea: painful menstrual periods
- Changes in menstrual flow or color of menstrual blood

Causes and Risk Factors:

- Hormonal imbalances: Fluctuations in estrogen, progesterone, thyroid hormones, or other hormones can disrupt the menstrual cycle.
- Age: Adolescents may experience irregular menstrual cycles as they establish regular ovulation patterns after menarche. Perimenopausal women may also experience irregular periods as they approach menopause.

- Polycystic ovary syndrome (PCOS): PCOS is a hormonal disorder characterized by irregular menstrual cycles, ovarian cysts, and androgen excess.
- Thyroid disorders: Hypothyroidism or hyperthyroidism can affect menstrual regularity by altering hormone levels.
- Obesity or underweight: Extreme changes in body weight or body mass index (BMI) can disrupt hormone balance and menstrual cycles.
- Stress: Psychological stress, physical stress (such as excessive exercise or chronic illness), or lifestyle stressors can affect the hypothalamic-pituitary-ovarian axis and menstrual regularity.

Epidemiology:

Irregular menstrual cycles are common among women of reproductive age, with estimates suggesting that up to 30% of women experience irregular periods at some point in their lives. The prevalence of irregular menstrual cycles may vary depending on factors such as age, hormonal status, geographical location, and access to healthcare services. Certain conditions such as PCOS, thyroid disorders, or hormonal imbalances may be associated with a higher risk of irregular periods.

Diagnosis:

- Medical History: The APh will inquire about menstrual history, including the length, duration, and pattern of menstrual periods, as well as associated symptoms, medical conditions, medications, and lifestyle factors.
- Physical Examination: to assess for signs of hormonal imbalances, thyroid disorders, or reproductive health issues
- Laboratory Tests: Blood tests may be conducted to evaluate hormone levels, thyroid function, or other factors affecting menstrual regularity.
- Imaging studies: Ultrasound may be used to assess the ovaries, uterus, and pelvic organs for structural abnormalities or signs of polycystic ovary syndrome (PCOS).

Treatment:

- Lifestyle Modifications: Regular exercise, balanced nutrition, stress management, and adequate sleep can help regulate hormonal balance and improve menstrual regularity.
- Hormonal Therapy: Birth control pills, patches, or hormonal intrauterine devices (IUDs), may be prescribed to regulate menstrual cycles and relieve symptoms of irregular periods.

- **Medications:** Nonsteroidal anti-inflammatory drugs (NSAIDs) or tranexamic acid may be used to manage heavy menstrual bleeding or dysmenorrhea.
- **Treatment of Underlying Conditions:** Treating PCOS, thyroid disorders, or hormonal imbalances may help restore regularity.
- **Fertility Preservation:** In some cases, ovulation induction or assisted reproductive technologies (ART) may be recommended for women with irregular periods who desire pregnancy.

16.22. Ovarian Cysts

> *Ovarian cysts are fluid-filled sacs that form on the ovaries, often as a normal part of the menstrual cycle.*
>
> *They can range in size from small to large and may cause symptoms such as pelvic pain, bloating, or irregular menstruation.*
>
> *While many cysts resolve on their own, others may require monitoring or treatment, especially if they cause symptoms or complications.*

Symptoms:
- Pelvic pain or discomfort, ranging from dull and aching to sharp and severe
- Bloating or abdominal fullness
- Pressure or heaviness in the pelvic area
- Changes in menstrual cycles, including irregular periods or spotting between periods
- Dyspareunia: pain during sexual intercourse
- Difficulty emptying the bladder or frequent urination
- Nausea or vomiting: in cases of cyst rupture or torsion
- Infertility or difficulty conceiving (in some cases)

Causes and Risk Factors:
- Age: Ovarian cysts are more common in women of reproductive age, with peak incidence occurring during the childbearing years.
- Hormonal fluctuations, such as those associated with the menstrual cycle, pregnancy, or hormone therapy, may contribute to ovarian cyst development.

- Polycystic ovary syndrome (PCOS) is a hormonal disorder characterized by multiple ovarian cysts, irregular menstrual cycles, and androgen excess.
- Endometriosis, a condition in which tissue similar to the lining of the uterus grows outside the uterus, may lead to the formation of ovarian cysts (endometriomas).
- Pregnancy: Ovarian cysts, known as corpus luteum cysts, may develop during pregnancy and typically resolve on their own without intervention.
- Previous history: Women who have previously had ovarian cysts may be at increased risk of developing new cysts in the future.

Epidemiology:

Ovarian cysts are a common gynecological condition, with most women developing at least one ovarian cyst during their lifetime. The prevalence of ovarian cysts may vary depending on factors such as age, reproductive status, and underlying health conditions. While many ovarian cysts are asymptomatic and go undetected, others may cause symptoms or complications requiring medical evaluation and treatment.

Diagnosis:

- Pelvic Examination: The APh may perform a pelvic exam to feel for abnormalities such as ovarian enlargement or tenderness.
- Imaging Tests: Transvaginal ultrasound, pelvic MRI, or CT scans may be used to visualize the ovaries and identify the presence, size, and characteristics of ovarian cysts.
- Blood Tests: to measure levels of certain hormones (such as CA-125) or tumor markers that may be associated with ovarian cysts or ovarian cancer
- Laparoscopy: In some cases, a surgical procedure called laparoscopy may be performed to directly visualize the ovaries and remove or biopsy ovarian cysts.

Treatment:

- Watchful Waiting:

    Many ovarian cysts, particularly small, asymptomatic cysts, may resolve on their own without treatment. Regular monitoring with imaging tests may be recommended to track changes in cyst size or appearance.

- Pain Management: Over-the-counter pain relievers such as ibuprofen or acetaminophen may help alleviate pelvic pain or discomfort associated with ovarian cysts.

- Hormonal Therapy:

    Hormonal contraceptives (such as birth control pills), GnRH agonists, or progestin-releasing intrauterine devices (IUDs) may be prescribed to regulate menstrual cycles, prevent new cyst formation, or shrink existing cysts.

- Surgical Removal:

    If an ovarian cyst is large, persistent, causing severe symptoms, or suspected to be cancerous, surgical removal (cystectomy) may be recommended. In some cases, a hysterectomy (removal of the uterus and ovaries) may be necessary.

- Fertility Preservation: In women of reproductive age with ovarian cysts who desire fertility, efforts may be made to preserve ovarian function and fertility during surgical procedures.

16.23. Abnormal Uterine Bleeding

> - *Abnormal uterine bleeding refers to irregularities in menstrual bleeding, including heavy or prolonged periods, bleeding between periods, or postmenopausal bleeding.*
> - *Causes can include hormonal imbalances, uterine fibroids, polyps, or underlying medical conditions.*
> - *Diagnosis involves a medical history, physical examination, and sometimes imaging or laboratory tests to determine the underlying cause and guide treatment.*

Symptoms:

- Heavy menstrual bleeding: bleeding that lasts longer than usual or involves passing large blood clots
- Irregular menstrual cycles: variations in the length, duration, or pattern of menstrual periods, including spotting between periods or prolonged bleeding episodes
- Bleeding after menopause: Any vaginal bleeding that occurs after menopause should be evaluated promptly as it may indicate underlying health concerns.
- Bleeding after sexual intercourse
- Intermenstrual bleeding: bleeding that occurs between menstrual periods

- Pelvic pain or discomfort: Pain or cramping in the lower abdomen or pelvis may accompany abnormal uterine bleeding in some cases.

Causes and Risk Factors:

- Hormonal imbalances: Fluctuations in estrogen and progesterone levels, such as those associated with puberty, perimenopause, or hormonal contraceptive use, may increase the risk of abnormal uterine bleeding.
- Structural abnormalities: Conditions such as uterine fibroids, polyps, adenomyosis, or endometrial hyperplasia may disrupt the normal menstrual cycle and lead to abnormal uterine bleeding.
- Endocrine disorders: Thyroid disorders, polycystic ovary syndrome (PCOS), or disorders of the adrenal glands may affect hormone levels and menstrual regularity.
- Blood clotting disorders: Conditions such as von Willebrand disease or thrombocytopenia may increase the risk of heavy menstrual bleeding.
- Reproductive tract infections or inflammation: Infections or inflammatory conditions affecting the uterus or cervix may cause abnormal uterine bleeding.
- Medications: Certain medications, such as anticoagulants, hormonal contraceptives, or hormone replacement therapy, may cause changes in menstrual bleeding patterns.
- Cancer or precancerous conditions: Conditions such as endometrial hyperplasia or endometrial cancer may cause abnormal uterine bleeding, particularly in postmenopausal women.

Epidemiology:

Abnormal uterine bleeding is a common gynecological complaint, affecting women of all ages. The prevalence of AUB may vary depending on factors such as age, reproductive status, underlying health conditions, and access to healthcare services. While many cases of abnormal uterine bleeding are benign and transient, some may be associated with underlying medical conditions requiring medical evaluation and treatment.

Diagnosis:

- Medical History:

    The APh will inquire about menstrual history, including the length, duration, and pattern of menstrual periods, as well as associated symptoms, medical conditions, medications, and lifestyle factors.

- Physical Examination:

    A pelvic exam may be performed to assess for signs of structural abnormalities, such as uterine fibroids or polyps, and to evaluate the cervix and vagina for signs of infection or inflammation.

- Laboratory Tests: to measure levels of thyroid hormones or reproductive hormones or to assess for signs of anemia.
- Imaging Studies: Transvaginal ultrasound, pelvic MRI, or hysteroscopy may be used to visualize the uterus and ovaries and identify structural abnormalities or lesions affecting the uterine lining.
- Endometrial Biopsy: A biopsy may be performed for further evaluation under a microscope, particularly if cancer or precancerous conditions are suspected.

Treatment:

- Hormonal Therapy:

    Hormonal contraceptives (such as birth control pills), progestin therapy, or hormone replacement therapy may be prescribed to regulate menstrual cycles, reduce bleeding, or treat underlying hormonal imbalances.

- Nonsteroidal Anti-Inflammatory Drugs (NSAIDs): Ibuprofen or naproxen may help reduce menstrual bleeding and relieve associated pain or cramping.
- Tranexamic Acid: medication that helps reduce menstrual bleeding by promoting blood clotting
- Uterine Procedures:

    Procedures such as endometrial ablation, uterine artery embolization, or surgical removal of uterine fibroids or polyps may be recommended to treat structural abnormalities or reduce menstrual bleeding.

- Hysterectomy:

    In severe cases or when conservative treatments are ineffective, surgical removal of the uterus (hysterectomy) may be recommended to alleviate symptoms and prevent recurrence of abnormal uterine bleeding.

16.24. Dysmenorrhea

> ➤ *Dysmenorrhea is a common menstrual disorder characterized by painful cramps in the lower abdomen before or during menstruation.*
>
> ➤ *Primary dysmenorrhea is typically caused by hormonal changes, while secondary dysmenorrhea may result from underlying conditions like endometriosis or fibroids.*
>
> ➤ *Management options include pain medication, hormonal birth control, and lifestyle changes to alleviate symptoms.*

Symptoms:

- Pelvic pain or cramping: typically located in the lower abdomen but may radiate to the lower back or thighs
- Pain intensity: ranges from mild to severe and may interfere with daily activities
- Nausea or vomiting
- Diarrhea or constipation
- Headaches or dizziness
- Fatigue or weakness
- Emotional symptoms: mood swings, irritability, or anxiety

Causes and Risk Factors:

- Age: Dysmenorrhea is most common in adolescents and young women, with symptoms often improving with age or after childbirth.
- Family history: Having a family history of dysmenorrhea may increase the risk of experiencing painful menstrual cramps.
- Early menarche: Starting menstruation at a younger age may be associated with a higher risk of dysmenorrhea.
- Heavy menstrual bleeding: Women with heavy periods may be more likely to experience dysmenorrhea.
- Smoking: Smoking has been associated with increased menstrual pain severity.
- Psychological factors: Stress, anxiety, or depression may exacerbate symptoms of dysmenorrhea.

Epidemiology:

Dysmenorrhea is a prevalent gynecological complaint affecting a significant proportion of women during their reproductive years. Primary dysmenorrhea is estimated to affect up to 50-90% of menstruating women, while secondary dysmenorrhea may occur in approximately 5-20% of cases. The prevalence of dysmenorrhea may vary depending on factors such as age, geographical location, cultural beliefs, and access to healthcare services.

Diagnosis:

- Medical History:

    The APh will inquire about menstrual history, including the onset, duration, severity, and pattern of menstrual cramps, as well as associated symptoms, medical conditions, medications, and lifestyle factors.

- Physical Examination: A pelvic exam may be performed to assess for signs of underlying pelvic pathology, such as endometriosis, fibroids, or pelvic inflammatory disease (PID).

- Imaging Studies: Ultrasound or MRI may be used to visualize the pelvic organs and identify structural abnormalities.

- Diagnostic Tests: In cases of suspected secondary dysmenorrhea, additional diagnostic tests such as laparoscopy or hysteroscopy may be recommended to evaluate the pelvic organs directly.

Treatment:

- Pain Management: Over-the-counter pain relievers such as nonsteroidal anti-inflammatory drugs (NSAIDs) or acetaminophen may help alleviate menstrual cramps and reduce pain severity.

- Hormonal Therapy: Hormonal contraceptives (such as birth control pills, patches, or hormonal intrauterine devices) may be prescribed to regulate menstrual cycles, reduce pain, and prevent ovulation.

- Nonpharmacological Interventions:

    Heat therapy (such as heating pads or warm baths), relaxation techniques (such as deep breathing or meditation), acupuncture, or physical exercise may help relieve menstrual cramps and improve symptoms.

- Dietary Modifications: Consuming a balanced diet rich in fruits, vegetables, whole grains, and omega-3 fatty acids may help reduce inflammation and alleviate menstrual pain.

- Surgical Interventions:

    In cases of severe or refractory dysmenorrhea secondary to underlying pelvic pathology (such as endometriosis or fibroids), surgical procedures such as laparoscopy or hysterectomy may be recommended to remove or treat the underlying cause.

16.25. Polycystic Ovary Syndrome

> ➢ *Polycystic ovary syndrome (PCOS) is a hormonal disorder common among women of reproductive age, characterized by irregular menstrual periods, excess androgen levels, and polycystic ovaries on ultrasound.*
>
> ➢ *Symptoms may include acne, hirsutism, and infertility, and it's often associated with insulin resistance and obesity.*
>
> ➢ *Treatment focuses on managing symptoms, regulating menstrual cycles, and addressing underlying metabolic concerns through medication, lifestyle changes, and fertility treatments as needed.*

Symptoms:

- Irregular menstrual cycles: Women with PCOS may experience irregular periods or missed periods due to ovulatory dysfunction.
- Excess androgen levels: Elevated levels of androgens such as testosterone may cause symptoms such as hirsutism, acne, or male-pattern baldness.
- Polycystic ovaries: Enlarged ovaries with multiple small cysts may be detected on ultrasound examination.
- Insulin resistance: PCOS is associated with insulin resistance, which may lead to symptoms such as weight gain, abdominal obesity, or difficulty losing weight.
- Infertility: Ovulatory dysfunction and irregular menstrual cycles may contribute to infertility or difficulty conceiving.
- Metabolic disturbances: PCOS is associated with an increased risk of metabolic conditions such as type 2 diabetes, dyslipidemia, or cardiovascular disease.
- Psychological symptoms: Women with PCOS may experience symptoms such as depression, anxiety, or decreased quality of life.

Risk Factors:

- Family history: Having a family history of PCOS or related metabolic conditions may increase the risk of developing PCOS.
- Hormonal imbalances: Elevated levels of androgens or insulin resistance may contribute to the development of PCOS.
- Obesity: Excess body weight or obesity is associated with an increased risk of PCOS and may exacerbate symptoms.

- Ethnicity: Certain ethnic groups, such as South Asian or African American women, may have a higher prevalence of PCOS.
- Age: PCOS can occur at any age, but symptoms often become more apparent during adolescence or early adulthood.
- Sedentary lifestyle: Lack of physical activity or sedentary behavior may increase the risk of PCOS and metabolic disturbances.

Epidemiology:

PCOS is one of the most common endocrine disorders affecting women of reproductive age, with estimates suggesting a prevalence of 5-10% worldwide. The prevalence of PCOS may vary depending on factors such as age, ethnicity, geographical location, and diagnostic criteria used. PCOS is a complex condition with heterogeneous clinical manifestations, and the exact prevalence may be difficult to determine due to variations in diagnostic criteria and population characteristics.

Diagnosis:
- Medical History: The APh will inquire about menstrual history, symptoms, family history, medical conditions, medications, and lifestyle factors.
- Physical Examination: A pelvic exam may be performed to assess for signs of androgen excess and to evaluate the ovaries for enlargement or cysts.
- Laboratory Tests:

    Blood tests may be conducted to measure levels of hormones such as testosterone, luteinizing hormone (LH), follicle-stimulating hormone (FSH), and insulin, as well as markers of metabolic health such as glucose and lipid levels.
- Imaging Studies: Transvaginal ultrasound may be used to visualize the ovaries and identify the presence of polycystic ovaries.

Treatment:
- Lifestyle Modifications: Regular exercise, balanced nutrition, weight management, and stress reduction may help improve symptoms and reduce the risk of complications associated with PCOS.
- Hormonal Therapy: Hormonal contraceptives may be prescribed to regulate menstrual cycles, reduce androgen levels, and improve symptoms such as hirsutism or acne.
- Insulin-Sensitizing Medications: Medications such as metformin may be prescribed to improve insulin sensitivity and reduce the risk of metabolic complications associated with PCOS.

- Ovulation Induction: Fertility medications such as clomiphene citrate or letrozole may be prescribed to induce ovulation and improve fertility in women with PCOS who are trying to conceive.
- Anti-Androgen Medications: Medications such as spironolactone may be used to reduce symptoms of androgen excess, such as hirsutism or acne.
- Surgical Interventions: Ovarian drilling or ovarian wedge resection may be considered to induce ovulation in women with PCOS who do not respond to other treatments.

16.26. Sexual Discomfort

> ➢ *Sexual discomfort encompasses physical or psychological discomfort during sexual activity, including pain, discomfort, or emotional distress.*
>
> ➢ *Causes can range from medical conditions like vaginal infections or endometriosis to psychological factors such as relationship issues or past trauma.*
>
> ➢ *Treatment involves addressing underlying causes, communication with partners, and sometimes therapy or medical interventions for symptom relief.*

Symptoms:
- Pain or discomfort during sexual intercourse
- Burning, stinging, or itching sensations in the genital area
- Vaginal dryness or inadequate lubrication
- Muscle tension or spasms in the pelvic floor muscles
- Anxiety, fear, or apprehension related to sexual activity
- Avoidance of sexual activity or loss of interest in sex
- Difficulty achieving orgasm or premature ejaculation

Causes and Risk Factors:
- Physical factors: Underlying medical conditions such as genital infections, pelvic inflammatory disease (PID), endometriosis, vaginal atrophy, or pelvic floor disorders may increase the risk of sexual discomfort.
- Psychological factors: Mental health conditions such as anxiety, depression, post-traumatic stress disorder (PTSD), or a history of sexual trauma may contribute to sexual discomfort.

- Relationship issues: Relationship conflicts, communication problems, lack of emotional intimacy, or sexual dissatisfaction may impact sexual function and contribute to discomfort.
- Hormonal changes: Hormonal fluctuations associated with menopause, pregnancy, breastfeeding, or hormonal contraceptive use may affect vaginal lubrication and increase the risk of sexual discomfort.
- Cultural influences: Cultural beliefs, taboos, or social norms surrounding sexuality and sexual expression may influence sexual attitudes, behaviors, and comfort levels.
- Medications: Certain medications such as antidepressants, antipsychotics, hormone therapy, or chemotherapy drugs may affect sexual function and contribute to discomfort.

Epidemiology:

Sexual discomfort is a common issue affecting individuals of all ages and genders, but it is often underreported and may vary depending on factors such as age, gender, sexual orientation, cultural background, and relationship status. Estimates suggest that up to 20-30% of women and a smaller percentage of men experience some form of sexual discomfort or pain during their lifetime.

Diagnosis:
- Medical History: The APh will inquire about sexual history, symptoms, medical conditions, medications, relationship status, and psychosocial factors.
- Physical Examination: A pelvic exam may be performed to assess for signs of genital infections, pelvic floor muscle tension, or other physical conditions contributing to sexual discomfort.
- Psychological Assessment: A mental health evaluation may be conducted to assess for symptoms of anxiety, depression, PTSD, or other mental health conditions impacting sexual function.
- Laboratory Tests: Vaginal swabs, blood tests, or imaging studies may be conducted to evaluate for underlying medical conditions such as infections, hormonal imbalances, or structural abnormalities.

Treatment:

Treatment of underlying medical conditions such as infections, endometriosis, vaginal atrophy, or pelvic floor disorders may help alleviate sexual discomfort.

- Counseling or Therapy:

    Cognitive-behavioral therapy (CBT), sex therapy, couples therapy, or psychotherapy may be beneficial for addressing psychological factors, relationship issues, or trauma-related symptoms contributing to sexual discomfort.

- Hormonal Therapy: Estrogen therapy or testosterone replacement therapy may be prescribed to address hormonal imbalances affecting sexual function and vaginal lubrication.

- Pelvic Floor Therapy: Pelvic floor physical therapy or relaxation techniques may help reduce muscle tension or spasms in the pelvic floor muscles and improve sexual comfort.

- Lubricants and Moisturizers: Over-the-counter vaginal lubricants or moisturizers may help reduce friction and improve vaginal dryness during sexual activity.

- Lifestyle Modifications: Stress management, regular exercise, adequate sleep, and balanced nutrition may improve overall sexual health and reduce discomfort.

- Medication Adjustments: Adjusting or discontinuing medications that may affect sexual function or arousal may help alleviate sexual discomfort.

- Surgical Interventions: In cases of structural abnormalities or refractory sexual discomfort, surgical procedures such as vaginal dilation, hymenectomy, or corrective surgery may be considered.

16.27. Menopause

> ➤ *Menopause marks the end of a woman's menstrual cycles, typically occurring around age 50, when ovaries stop producing eggs and estrogen levels decline.*
>
> ➤ *Symptoms may include hot flashes, mood changes, and vaginal dryness, impacting quality of life.*
>
> ➤ *Management often involves hormone therapy, lifestyle changes, and medications to alleviate symptoms and reduce long-term health risks.*

Symptoms:

- Irregular menstrual cycles: Menstrual periods may become irregular in the years leading up to menopause before ceasing entirely.
- Hot flashes: sudden feelings of warmth, flushing, or sweating, often accompanied by rapid heartbeat and chills

- Night sweats: episodes of excessive sweating during sleep, often disrupting sleep quality
- Vaginal dryness: reduced vaginal lubrication and elasticity, leading to discomfort or pain during sexual intercourse
- Sleep disturbances: insomnia, difficulty falling asleep or staying asleep, or waking up frequently during the night
- Mood changes: Mood swings, irritability, anxiety, or depression may occur during menopause due to hormonal fluctuations and psychosocial factors.
- Fatigue or decreased energy levels
- Memory problems or difficulty concentrating
- Joint pain or stiffness
- Changes in sexual desire or sexual function
- Urinary symptoms: Increased frequency of urination, urinary urgency, or urinary incontinence may occur due to changes in bladder function and pelvic floor muscles.

Causes and Risk Factors:
- Age: Advancing age is the primary risk factor for menopause, with the average age of onset typically between 45 and 55 years.
- Family history: A family history of early menopause may increase the risk of experiencing menopause at a younger age.
- Reproductive factors: Factors such as nulliparity, early menarche, or late menopause may influence the timing of menopause.
- Surgical factors: Surgical removal of the ovaries or hysterectomy may induce menopause at an earlier age.
- Lifestyle factors: Smoking, excessive alcohol consumption, poor nutrition, sedentary lifestyle, or high levels of stress may affect hormonal balance and increase the risk of menopausal symptoms.
- Medical conditions: Autoimmune diseases, thyroid disorders, or cancer treatments may affect ovarian function and influence the timing or experience of menopause.

Epidemiology:

Menopause is a universal and inevitable transition that affects women as they age. The average age of natural menopause in most populations is around 51 years, but the timing of menopause may vary widely among individuals. Ethnic and cultural factors, socioeconomic status, and access to healthcare services may also influence the experience of menopause and its associated symptoms.

Diagnosis:
- Clinical History: The APh will inquire about menstrual history, symptoms, medical conditions, medications, reproductive history, and lifestyle factors.
- Physical Examination: A pelvic exam may be performed to assess for signs of vaginal atrophy, pelvic organ prolapse, or other gynecological conditions.
- Laboratory Tests: Blood tests may be conducted to measure levels of hormones such as follicle-stimulating hormone (FSH), luteinizing hormone (LH), estrogen, and thyroid hormones to confirm menopausal status.
- Imaging Studies: Pelvic ultrasound or bone mineral density (BMD) scans may be performed to assess for signs of osteoporosis or other age-related changes.

Treatment:
- Hormone Therapy:

    Hormone replacement therapy (HRT) may be prescribed to relieve menopausal symptoms such as hot flashes, vaginal dryness, or night sweats. HRT may include estrogen therapy alone or combined estrogen-progestin therapy, depending on factors such as the presence of a uterus and individual health risks.

- Nonhormonal Therapies:

    Nonhormonal treatments such as selective serotonin reuptake inhibitors (SSRIs), serotonin-norepinephrine reuptake inhibitors (SNRIs), gabapentin, or clonidine may be prescribed to manage symptoms such as hot flashes, mood changes, or sleep disturbances.

- Vaginal Estrogen Therapy: Topical estrogen products such as creams, tablets, or rings may be used to alleviate symptoms of vaginal dryness, itching, or pain during intercourse.
- Lifestyle Modifications: Regular exercise, balanced nutrition, stress management, adequate sleep, and smoking cessation may help reduce the severity of menopausal symptoms.
- Complementary and Alternative Therapies:

    Acupuncture, yoga, meditation, or herbal supplements may provide symptom relief for some women, although evidence supporting their efficacy is limited.

- Osteoporosis Prevention:

Calcium and vitamin D supplementation, weight-bearing exercise, and bone-strengthening medications may be recommended to reduce the risk of osteoporosis and fractures associated with menopause.

16.28. Vaginitis

> ➢ *Vaginitis is inflammation of the vagina often caused by infections, such as bacterial vaginosis, yeast infections, or trichomoniasis.*
> ➢ *Symptoms include vaginal itching, discharge, and irritation.*
> ➢ *Treatment varies based on the underlying cause and may involve antibiotics, antifungal medications, or other medications to relieve symptoms.*

Symptoms:

- Vaginal discharge: Changes in vaginal discharge color, consistency, odor, or amount may occur depending on the underlying cause of vaginitis.
- Vaginal itching or irritation: itching or burning sensations in the vaginal area, often accompanied by redness or swelling
- Pain or discomfort: pain during urination or sexual intercourse
- Vaginal odor: unusual or foul-smelling vaginal odor, particularly with certain types of infections
- Redness or inflammation: The vaginal tissues may appear red, swollen, or irritated on visual inspection.

Causes and Risk Factors:

- Poor hygiene: Improper genital hygiene practices, such as using harsh soaps or douching, may disrupt the natural balance of vaginal flora and increase the risk of vaginitis.
- Sexual intercourse, particularly with multiple partners or new partners, may increase the risk of sexually transmitted infections (STIs) that can cause vaginitis.
- Hormonal fluctuations associated with pregnancy, menopause, or the use of hormonal contraceptives may predispose women to vaginal infections or inflammation.
- Antibiotics can disrupt the normal balance of vaginal bacteria (vaginal microbiota) and increase the risk of developing vaginitis.

- Uncontrolled diabetes or high blood sugar levels may increase the risk of vaginal yeast infections (candidiasis) due to changes in vaginal pH and sugar content.
- Immune suppression: Conditions or medications that weaken the immune system, such as HIV/AIDS, chemotherapy, or immunosuppressive drugs, may predispose individuals to vaginal infections.
- Allergies or sensitivities: Allergic reactions to certain products such as perfumes, soaps, laundry detergents, or latex condoms may cause vaginal irritation or inflammation.

Epidemiology:

Vaginitis is a common condition affecting women of all ages and ethnicities worldwide. The prevalence of vaginitis may vary depending on factors such as geographical location, socioeconomic status, sexual behaviors, and access to healthcare services. Certain types of vaginitis, such as bacterial vaginosis and candidiasis, are among the most common vaginal infections encountered in clinical practice.

Diagnosis:
- <u>Medical History:</u> The APh will inquire about symptoms, medical history, sexual history, hygiene practices, recent antibiotic use, and other relevant factors.
- <u>Physical Examination:</u> A pelvic exam may be performed to assess for signs of vaginal inflammation, discharge, or other abnormalities.
- <u>Laboratory Tests:</u> Samples of vaginal discharge may be collected for laboratory testing to identify the underlying cause of vaginitis. Tests may include:
  - Wet mount microscopy: microscopic examination of vaginal discharge for the presence of yeast cells, bacterial cells, or other microorganisms
  - pH testing: measurement of vaginal pH level to assess acidity or alkalinity, which can help differentiate between different types of vaginitis
  - Vaginal cultures: culturing of vaginal swabs to identify specific pathogens, such as Candida species or bacterial strains
  - STI testing: screening for STIs such as chlamydia, gonorrhea, trichomoniasis, or herpes simplex virus (HSV), if indicated based on clinical suspicion or risk factors

Treatment:

- Antifungal Medications: Antifungal creams, suppositories, or oral medications may be prescribed to treat yeast infections (candidiasis).
- Antibiotics: Antibiotic therapy may be recommended to treat bacterial vaginosis or other bacterial infections causing vaginitis.
- Antiviral Medications: Antiviral drugs may be prescribed to treat viral infections such as herpes simplex virus (HSV) or human papillomavirus (HPV) if present.
- Antiparasitic Medications: Medications such as metronidazole or tinidazole may be used to treat parasitic infections such as trichomoniasis.
- Hormonal Therapy: Estrogen therapy or vaginal moisturizers may be recommended to relieve symptoms of vaginal dryness or atrophy associated with menopause.
- Symptom Management: Over-the-counter remedies such as vaginal lubricants, antihistamines, or corticosteroid creams may help alleviate symptoms such as itching or irritation.
- Avoidance of Irritants: Avoiding potential irritants such as scented products, douches, or harsh soaps may help prevent recurrent episodes of vaginitis.

16.29. Amenorrhea

> ➤ *Amenorrhea refers to the absence of menstrual periods in women of reproductive age, either primary (never having a period by age 15) or secondary (periods stopping for more than three months in women who have previously menstruated).*
>
> ➤ *Causes can include hormonal imbalances, pregnancy, stress, or underlying medical conditions such as polycystic ovary syndrome or thyroid disorders.*
>
> ➤ *Treatment involves addressing the underlying cause, which may include lifestyle changes, medication, or hormonal therapy.*

Symptoms:

- Absence of menstrual periods: The primary symptom of amenorrhea is the absence of menstrual bleeding for an extended period.
- Changes in secondary sexual characteristics: In primary amenorrhea, delayed onset of secondary sexual characteristics such as breast development or pubic hair growth may be observed.

- Symptoms related to underlying conditions: Depending on the cause of amenorrhea, individuals may experience additional symptoms such as hot flashes, vaginal dryness, hair loss, weight changes, or changes in libido.

Causes and Risk Factors:
- Hormonal imbalances: Conditions such as polycystic ovary syndrome (PCOS), thyroid disorders, or hyperprolactinemia may disrupt normal menstrual function and increase the risk of amenorrhea.
- Anatomical abnormalities: Structural abnormalities of the reproductive organs, such as congenital defects or scarring from surgery or infections, may interfere with menstruation.
- Excessive exercise: Intense physical training, excessive exercise, or rigorous athletic training regimens may lead to hypothalamic dysfunction and amenorrhea, a condition known as exercise-induced amenorrhea.
- Eating disorders: Anorexia nervosa or bulimia nervosa can disrupt hormonal balance and lead to amenorrhea.
- Stress: Chronic stress or psychological factors such as depression, anxiety, or emotional trauma may affect the hypothalamic-pituitary-ovarian axis and contribute to amenorrhea.
- Medications: Hormonal contraceptives, antipsychotics, chemotherapy drugs, or medications that affect thyroid function may cause menstrual irregularities or amenorrhea.

Epidemiology:

The prevalence of amenorrhea varies depending on factors such as age, geographical location, cultural practices, and access to healthcare services. Primary amenorrhea is relatively uncommon, with estimates suggesting a prevalence of less than 1% in the general population. Secondary amenorrhea is more prevalent, particularly among women of reproductive age, and may affect up to 5-10% of menstruating women at some point in their lives.

Diagnosis:
- <u>Medical History:</u> The APh will inquire about menstrual history, symptoms, medical conditions, medications, reproductive history, lifestyle factors, and potential underlying causes of amenorrhea.
- <u>Physical Examination:</u> A pelvic exam may be performed to assess for signs of anatomical abnormalities, ovarian function, or other gynecological conditions.

- Blood Tests: to measure levels of hormones such as follicle-stimulating hormone (FSH), luteinizing hormone (LH), estrogen, progesterone, thyroid hormones, prolactin, and other markers of hormonal function
- Imaging Studies: Pelvic ultrasound or magnetic resonance imaging (MRI) may be performed to evaluate the reproductive organs and assess for structural abnormalities or ovarian pathology.

Treatment:
- Hormonal Therapy: Hormone replacement therapy (HRT) or oral contraceptives containing estrogen and progestin may be prescribed to regulate menstrual cycles and restore hormonal balance.
- Medications: Dopamine agonists (for hyperprolactinemia), thyroid hormone replacement (for thyroid disorders), or metformin (for PCOS) may be prescribed to treat underlying hormonal imbalances.
- Surgical Interventions: Laparoscopic surgery (for ovarian cysts or endometriosis), hysteroscopy (for intrauterine adhesions), or ovarian drilling (for PCOS) may be recommended in certain cases.
- Lifestyle Modifications: Reducing stress, adopting a balanced diet, maintaining a healthy weight, and moderating exercise intensity may help improve menstrual regularity.
- Psychological support: Counseling, psychotherapy, or support groups may be beneficial for individuals with underlying psychological factors contributing to amenorrhea, such as eating disorders or stress-related conditions.

References
- American College of Obstetricians and Gynecologists. (2019). ACOG Practice Bulletin No. 200: Early pregnancy loss. Obstetrics & Gynecology, 133(5), e308-e324.
- Barnhart, K. T., Sammel, M. D., & et al. (2006). Risk factors for ectopic pregnancy in women with symptomatic first-trimester pregnancies. Fertility and Sterility, 86(1), 36-43.
- Pennick, V. E., & Young, G. (2007). Interventions for preventing and treating pelvic and back pain in pregnancy. Cochrane Database of Systematic Reviews, (2), CD001139.
- Niebyl, J. R. (2010). Clinical practice. Nausea and vomiting in pregnancy. New England Journal of Medicine, 363(16), 1544-1550.
- American Diabetes Association. (2020). 14. Management of Diabetes in Pregnancy: Standards of Medical Care in Diabetes—2020. Diabetes Care, 43(Supplement 1), S183-S192.

- American College of Obstetricians and Gynecologists. (2019). ACOG Practice Bulletin No. 202: Gestational hypertension and preeclampsia. Obstetrics & Gynecology, 133(1), e1-e25.
- Milman, N., & Taylor, C. L. (2016). Iron status in pregnant women and women of reproductive age in Europe. The American Journal of Clinical Nutrition, 103(2), 367S-368S.
- Maheswari, U., & Grover, S. (2016). Pruritus in pregnancy. In Pruritus (pp. 253-264). Springer, Berlin, Heidelberg.
- Osman, H., Rubeiz, N., & Tamim, H. (2007). Risk factors for the development of striae gravidarum. American Journal of Obstetrics and Gynecology, 196(1), 62-e1.
- Ortonne, J. P., & Bissett, D. L. (2008). Latest insights into skin hyperpigmentation. Journal of Investigative Dermatology Symposium Proceedings, 13(1), 10-14.
- Regan, L., Rai, R., & et al. (2000). Risk of miscarriage in women with vaginal bleeding in early pregnancy: A systematic review and meta-analysis. The Lancet, 356(9237), 1853-1857.
- Glantz, A., & Marschall, H. U. (2006). Lammert F. Intrahepatic cholestasis of pregnancy: a randomized controlled trial comparing dexamethasone and ursodeoxycholic acid. Hepatology, 42(6), 1399-1405.
- O'Hara, M. W., & McCabe, J. E. (2013). Postpartum depression: Current status and future directions. Annual Review of Clinical Psychology, 9, 379-407.
- Martin, J. A., Hamilton, B. E., & et al. (2019). Births: Final data for 2018. National Vital Statistics Reports, 68(13), 1-47.
- Casey, B. M., & Leveno, K. J. (2006). Thyroid disease in pregnancy. Obstetrics & Gynecology, 108(5), 1283-1292.

Part III:

Ancillary Services: Labs, Biostatistics, Wound Care, Surgical Care, and Imaging

Chapter 17: Blood Labs and EKG Interpretations

The APh should compare the test results to reference ranges while considering patient demographics, medical history, symptoms, and combining clinical exams to assess potential health conditions or abnormalities.

The APh may use this data to assess diseases, monitor treatment effectiveness, and guide patient management strategies.

17.1. Complete Blood Count

> ➢ *A Complete Blood Count (CBC) is a blood test that provides information about the types and numbers of blood cells in the body, including red blood cells, white blood cells, and platelets.*
>
> ➢ *It helps diagnose conditions such as anemia, infection, other blood disorders, and also monitors overall health and response to treatment.*
>
> ➢ *This test measures parameters like hemoglobin, white blood cell count, and platelet count, providing valuable insights into the patient's health status.*

Test	Description	Normal Range
Hemoglobin (Hb)	Amount of oxygen-carrying protein in the blood	• Adult male: 13.8 - 17.2 g/dL • Adult female: 12.1 - 15.1 g/dL
Hematocrit (Hct)	Percentage of blood volume occupied by red blood cells	• Adult male: 40.7% - 50.3% • Adult female: 36.1% - 44.3%
Red Blood Cell (RBC)	Number of red blood cells per volume of blood	• Adult male: 4.7 - 6.1 cells/mcL • Adult female: 4.2 - 5.4 cells/mcL
Mean Corpuscular Volume (MCV)	Average volume of red blood cells	80 - 100 fL
Mean Corpuscular Hemoglobin (MCH)	Average amount of hemoglobin per red blood cell	27 - 33 pg
Mean Corpuscular Hemoglobin Concentration (MCHC)	Concentration of hemoglobin in red blood cells	32% - 36%
Red Cell Distribution Width (RDW)	Variation in red blood cell size	11.5% - 14.5 %
White Blood Cell Count (WBC)	Number of white blood cells per volume of blood	4,500 - 11,000 cells/mcL
Platelet Count	Number of platelets per volume of blood	150,000 - 400,000 cells/mcL

Interpretation:

- Abnormalities in the CBC may indicate various conditions such as anemia, infection, inflammation, or bleeding disorders.
- High or low values should be interpreted in clinical context, other lab findings and patient history to determine the underlying cause and appropriate management.

- Hemoglobin (Hb), Hematocrit (Hct), White Blood Cell Count (WBC), Platelet Count: Assess for anemia, infection, inflammation, and thrombocytopenia or thrombocytosis.

17.2. Comprehensive Metabolic Panel

> ➢ *The Comprehensive Metabolic Panel (CMP) is a blood test that assesses various aspects of a person's metabolism and organ function.*
> ➢ *It includes measurements of glucose, electrolytes, kidney function, liver function, and protein levels.*
> ➢ *The CMP helps diagnose conditions such as diabetes, kidney disease, and liver disorders, and monitors overall health and response to treatment.*

Test		Description	Normal Range
Glucose		Blood sugar levels	70 - 100 mg/dL (when fasting)
Blood Urea Nitrogen (BUN)		Amount of nitrogen in blood coming from urea	7 - 20 mg/dL
Creatinine		Amount of creatinine in blood to measure kidney function	• Male: 0.6 - 1.3 mg/dL • Female: 0.5 - 1.1 mg/dL
Electro-lytes	Sodium (Na)	Maintains proper balance of water and minerals, an important role in nerve and muscle function	80 - 100 fL
	Potassium (K)	Important for nerve function and muscle contractions	2.5 - 5.0 mEq/L
	Chloride (Cl)	Maintains fluid balance	98 - 106 mEg/L
	Carbon Dioxide (CO2)	Reflects the body's acid-base balance	22- 29 mEq/L
Total Protein		Amount of protein in the blood	6.0 - 8.3 g/dL
Albumin		A type of protein made by the liver to help maintain blood volume and pressure	3.5 - 5.0 g/dL
Total Bilirubin		Amount of bilirubin in the blood. Elevated level indicates liver or bile duct dysfunction	0.1 - 1.2 mg/dL
Alkaline Phosphatase (ALP)		An enzyme found in various tissues, mainly in liver and bones. Elevated level indicates liver or bone disease	44 - 147 IU/L
Alanine Aminotransferase		Enzymes found in the liver. Elevated level indicates	• ALT: 7 - 56 IU/L

(ALT) and Aspartate Aminotransferase (AST)	liver damage	• AST: 10 - 40 IU/L

Interpretation:
- Abnormalities in the CMP may indicate various conditions such as kidney or liver disease, electrolyte imbalances, or acid-base disorders.
- High or low values should be interpreted in clinical context, other lab findings and patient history to determine the underlying cause and appropriate management.

17.3. Urinalysis

> ➤ Urinalysis (UA) is a common diagnostic test that examines the physical, chemical, and microscopic properties of urine.
> ➤ It assesses hydration status, kidney function, and detects conditions like urinary tract infections, kidney stones, or diabetes.
> ➤ The test involves analyzing urine for color, clarity, pH, protein, glucose, blood cells, and bacteria under a microscope.

Physical Appearance Observation:
- Color: Normal urine color ranges from pale yellow to amber. Abnormal colors may indicate various conditions such as dehydration, liver disease, or urinary tract infections.
- Clarity: Normal urine is clear. Cloudy urine may indicate the presence of bacteria, pus, or other substances.

Chemical Examination:

Examination	Description	Interpretation
pH	Measures the acidity or alkalinity of urine	• Normal range: 4.6 to 8.0 • Abnormal specific gravity may indicate dehydration, kidney dysfunction, or diabetes
		• Normal range: 1.005 to 1.030

Specific Gravity	Measures urine concentration	• Abnormal specific gravity may indicate dehydration, kidney dysfunction, or diabetes
Protein	Detects the presence of protein in urine	Abnormal levels may indicate kidney disease such as diabetic kidney disease, multiple myeloma, or problems in pregnancy
Glucose	Detects the presence of glucose in urine	Abnormal levels may indicate diabetes or kidney dysfunction
Ketones	Detects the presence of ketones in urine	Abnormal levels may indicate diabetic ketoacidosis, starvation, or certain metabolic disorders
Blood	Detects the presence of red blood cells in urine	Abnormal levels may indicate urinary tract infections or malignancy, kidney stones, kidney cysts or other kidney conditions
Nitrites	Detects the presence of bacteria that convert nitrate to nitrite in urine	Abnormal levels may indicate urinary tract infections

Microscopic Examination:

- Red Blood Cells (RBCs): Normal range: **0-2 RBCs per high-power field (HPF).** Elevated levels may indicate kidney disease, urinary tract infections, or other conditions.
- White Blood Cells (WBCs): Normal range: **0-5 WBCs per HPF.** Elevated levels may indicate urinary tract infections or inflammation.
- Bacteria: The presence of bacteria in urine may indicate urinary tract infections.
- Crystals: The presence of crystals in urine may indicate kidney stones or metabolic disorders.

Interpretation:

- Abnormalities in urinalysis results may indicate various urinary tract disorders, kidney dysfunction, metabolic disorders, or systemic diseases.
- Results should be interpreted in conjunction with other clinical findings and patient history to determine the underlying cause and appropriate management.

17.4. Lipid Panel

> ➤ A lipid panel is a blood test that measures levels of cholesterol and triglycerides, essential for assessing cardiovascular health and risk factors.
>
> ➤ It typically includes measurements of total cholesterol, HDL cholesterol (good cholesterol), LDL cholesterol (bad cholesterol), and triglycerides.
>
> ➤ The results can guide the APh in managing cholesterol levels to reduce the risk of heart disease and stroke.

Type	Description	Range
Total Cholesterol	Desirable	<200 mg/dL
	Borderline high	200-239 mg/dL
	High	240 mg/dL and above
Low-density Lipoprotein (LDL) Cholesterol	Optimal	<100 mg/dL
	Near optimal/above optimal	100-129 mg/dL
	Borderline high	130-159 mg/dL
	High	160-189 mg/dL
	Very high	190 mg/dL and above
High-density Lipoprotein (HDL) Cholesterol	Low (increased risk)	• <40 mg/dL (men) • <50 mg/dL (women)
	Good	• 40-59 mg/dL (men) • 50-59 mg/dL (women)
	High (protective)	60 mg/dL and above
Triglycerides	Normal	<150 mg/dL

	Borderline high	150-199 mg/dL
	High	200-499 mg/dL
	Very high	500 mg/dL and above
Non-HDL Cholesterol	Goal	30 mg/dL higher than the LDL cholesterol level

Interpretation:

- High levels of total cholesterol, LDL cholesterol, and triglycerides, as well as low levels of HDL cholesterol, are associated with an increased risk of cardiovascular disease.
- Elevated LDL cholesterol is particularly concerning as it can lead to the buildup of plaque in the arteries, increasing the risk of heart disease and stroke.
- Low HDL cholesterol is also a risk factor for cardiovascular disease, as HDL helps remove LDL cholesterol from the bloodstream.
- Triglyceride levels may be influenced by factors such as diet, physical activity, and alcohol consumption. Elevated triglyceride levels are associated with an increased risk of heart disease, especially when combined with other lipid abnormalities.

In addition to lipid levels, other factors such as age, gender, blood pressure, smoking status, diabetes, and family history of cardiovascular disease should be considered when assessing overall cardiovascular risk.

17.5. Thyroid Panel

> ➤ *A thyroid panel is a blood test that assesses thyroid function by measuring levels of thyroid hormones and thyroid-stimulating hormone (TSH).*
>
> ➤ *It helps diagnose thyroid disorders such as hypothyroidism, hyperthyroidism, and autoimmune thyroid diseases.*
>
> ➤ *The panel typically includes measurements of TSH, free thyroxine (T4), and sometimes triiodothyronine (T3) levels.*

Type	Description	Range
Thyroid-Stimulating Hormone (TSH)	Normal range	Typically between 0.4 to 4.0 mIU/L
	Elevated TSH (hypothyroidism)	• TSH levels above the upper limit of the normal range suggest an underactive thyroid (hypothyroidism) • Mildly elevated TSH levels (between 4.0 and 10.0 mIU/L) with normal levels of thyroxine (T4) may indicate subclinical hypothyroidism, especially if accompanied by symptoms (mild) and risk factors
	Decreased TSH (Hyperthyroidism)	• TSH levels below the lower limit of the normal range suggest an overactive thyroid (hyperthyroidism). • Low TSH levels are typically seen in conditions such as Graves' disease or toxic nodular goiter
Free Thyroxine (FT4)	Normal range	Typically between 0.8 to 1.8 ng/dL or 10 to 23 pmol/L
	Elevated FT4	High levels of FT4 may indicate hyperthyroidism
	Decreased FT4	Low levels of FT4 may indicate hypothyroidism
Triiodothyronine (T3)	Normal range	• Typically between 80 to 200 ng/dL or 1.2 to 3.1 nmol/L • T3 levels are less commonly measured in routine thyroid panels but may be evaluated in specific clinical contexts

Interpretation:

- Elevated TSH with normal or low FT4 levels suggests primary hypothyroidism, where the thyroid gland fails to produce enough thyroid hormones.
- Decreased TSH with elevated FT4 levels suggests primary hyperthyroidism, where the thyroid gland produces too much thyroid hormone.

- Subclinical hypothyroidism refers to mildly elevated TSH levels with normal FT4 levels. It is often temporary but may progress to overt hypothyroidism over time.
- Subclinical hyperthyroidism refers to mildly decreased TSH levels with normal FT4 levels. It may progress to overt hyperthyroidism or resolve spontaneously.
- Thyroid antibody tests (such as anti-thyroid peroxidase antibodies or anti-thyroglobulin antibodies) may be performed to evaluate for autoimmune thyroid diseases such as Hashimoto's thyroiditis or Graves' disease.

17.6. ANA Level

> ➤ *ANA (antinuclear antibody) testing is used to detect the presence of antibodies that target the body's own cell nuclei.*
>
> ➤ *Elevated ANA levels can indicate an autoimmune condition, but they can also be present in healthy patients or patients with non-autoimmune conditions.*

Normal ANA levels

In healthy patients, ANA levels are typically low or undetectable. A negative ANA test result usually indicates that no significant autoimmune activity is present.

Elevated ANA levels

ANA levels are considered elevated when they are above a certain threshold, typically measured in titers (e.g., 1:80, 1:160, 1:320).

- Low-level elevations (e.g., 1:80): may be seen in healthy patients, especially older adults, and may not necessarily indicate autoimmune disease.
- Higher elevations (e.g., 1:160 or greater): are more likely to be associated with autoimmune conditions, but further evaluation is needed to determine the specific cause.

Interpretation in the context of symptoms and other tests

- ANA testing is not diagnostic of a specific autoimmune disease but rather indicates the presence of autoantibodies that may be associated with various conditions.
- The interpretation of ANA levels should be considered in the context of the patient's clinical presentation, medical history, and other laboratory findings.

- Additional tests, such as specific autoantibody tests (e.g., anti-dsDNA, anti-Smith antibodies) and clinical evaluation, are often needed to confirm a diagnosis of autoimmune disease.

Associated conditions
- Elevated ANA levels may be seen in a variety of autoimmune and non-autoimmune conditions, including systemic lupus erythematosus (SLE), Sjögren's syndrome, rheumatoid arthritis, scleroderma, autoimmune hepatitis, and others.
- ANA testing may also be positive in patients with infections, certain medications, cancer, or other non-autoimmune conditions.
- **Positive ANA and anti-histone antibodies** are classically associated with drug-induced lupus erythematosus (procainamide, hydralazine, etanercept, isoniazid...)

Follow-up and further evaluation
- If ANA levels are elevated, especially at moderate to high titers, further evaluation by a healthcare provider, typically a rheumatologist, is recommended.
- Additional tests and examinations may be performed to determine the underlying cause of the elevated ANA levels and to guide appropriate management and treatment.

The APhs should be aware that ANA testing alone is not sufficient for diagnosing autoimmune diseases. A thorough clinical evaluation, including medical history, physical examination, and additional laboratory tests, is necessary for accurate diagnosis and appropriate management.

The APh will interpret ANA test results in the context of a patient's overall health and recommend further evaluation or treatment if needed.

17.7. ESR/CRP Level

> ➢ *ESR (Erythrocyte Sedimentation Rate) and CRP (C-reactive Protein) are markers of inflammation commonly measured in blood tests.*

ESR (Erythrocyte Sedimentation Rate)

ESR measures the rate at which red blood cells settle in a tube of blood over time. It is a nonspecific marker of inflammation.
- Normal ESR: Values vary based on age and gender but are typically below 20 mm/hr for men and below 30 mm/hr for women.
- Elevated ESR: Elevated values indicate increased inflammation in the body but do not specify the cause.

- Possible reasons for elevated ESR include infections, autoimmune diseases (such as rheumatoid arthritis or lupus), certain cancers, and other inflammatory conditions.

CRP (C-Reactive Protein)

CRP is a protein produced by the liver in response to inflammation. It is a more specific marker of acute inflammation compared to ESR.

- Normal CRP are typically below 10 mg/L, although the reference range may vary slightly between laboratories.
- Elevated CRP indicates acute inflammation in the body. CRP can rise dramatically in response to infections, tissue injury, autoimmune diseases, and other inflammatory conditions.

CRP levels can also be used to monitor response to treatment in certain conditions.

- A decrease in CRP levels over time may indicate improvement or resolution of inflammation.
- hs-CRP (high-sensitivity CRP) usually elevated in patients with myocardial infarction; high levels of hs-CRP in otherwise healthy people is linked to an increased risk of future heart attack, stroke, sudden cardiac death and/or peripheral artery disease.

Interpretation:

- Elevated ESR and CRP levels indicate the presence of inflammation in the body but do not provide specific information about the underlying cause.
- Further evaluation, including a thorough medical history, physical examination, and additional diagnostic tests, is often needed to determine the cause of inflammation.
- It's essential to interpret ESR and CRP levels in conjunction with other clinical findings and tests to guide diagnosis and treatment decisions accurately.

17.8. Lupus Panel

> A lupus panel, also known as an autoimmune panel or connective tissue disease panel, is a blood test used to help diagnose systemic lupus erythematosus (SLE) and other autoimmune connective tissue diseases.

Antinuclear Antibody (ANA, as explained above)

ANA is a marker of autoimmune activity.

- A positive ANA test suggests the presence of autoantibodies targeting the cell nuclei.
- ANA is not specific to lupus and can be positive in other autoimmune diseases and even in healthy patients.
- ANA testing is typically done using indirect immunofluorescence, and results are reported as titers (e.g., 1:80, 1:160, 1:320).

Anti-double-stranded DNA (anti-dsDNA) Antibodies

Anti-dsDNA antibodies specifically target double-stranded DNA and are more specific to lupus.

- Elevated levels of anti-dsDNA antibodies are strongly associated with active lupus and lupus nephritis (kidney involvement).

Anti-Sm Antibodies

Anti-Sm antibodies target a specific nuclear protein called Smith (Sm) antigen. It has low sensitivity but high specificity for SLE.

- Anti-Sm antibodies are found in about 20-30% of patients with lupus, more commonly in African Americans and Asians than Causcasians.

Anti-Ro (SSA) and Anti-La (SSB) Antibodies

Anti-Ro and anti-La antibodies target the Ro and La proteins, respectively.

- These antibodies are associated with conditions such as Sjögren's syndrome and neonatal lupus (when passed from mother to fetus).

Anti-RNP Antibodies

Anti-RNP antibodies target the ribonucleoprotein (RNP) complex.

- Elevated levels of anti-RNP antibodies are associated with mixed connective tissue disease (MCTD) but can also be found in lupus and other autoimmune conditions.

Complement Levels (C3 and C4)

Complement proteins (C3 and C4) are part of the immune system and may be consumed in the presence of immune complex formation in lupus.

- Low levels of complement proteins may indicate lupus activity, especially if accompanied by other clinical manifestations.

Interpretation:

- A positive ANA test is often the first step in diagnosing lupus, but it is not sufficient on its own for a lupus diagnosis.
- The presence of anti-dsDNA antibodies, anti-Sm antibodies, or other lupus-specific antibodies supports the diagnosis of lupus, especially when accompanied by compatible clinical features.

- Complement levels may help assess disease activity, with low levels indicating complement consumption in active lupus.
- Interpretation of a lupus panel should consider the overall clinical picture, including symptoms, physical examination findings, and other laboratory tests.

Follow-Up:
- A positive lupus panel may prompt further evaluation, including assessment for organ involvement (e.g., kidney, skin, joints) and monitoring disease activity over time.
- Additional tests or consultations with specialists (e.g., rheumatologists, nephrologists) may be needed to confirm the diagnosis and guide treatment decisions.

17.9. Rheumatoid Arthritis Panel

> ➤ RF (Rheumatoid Factor) and anti-CCP (anti-Cyclic Citrullinated Peptide) antibodies are blood tests commonly used in the diagnosis and management of rheumatoid arthritis (RA) and other autoimmune rheumatic diseases.

Rheumatoid Factor (RF)

RF is an autoantibody that targets the Fc portion of immunoglobulin G (IgG) antibodies.

- Elevated RF levels can be found in various autoimmune diseases, but they are most commonly associated with rheumatoid arthritis.
- RF positivity is found in a significant proportion of patients with RA, particularly those with seropositive RA.
- RF can also be positive in other conditions such as Sjögren's syndrome, systemic lupus erythematosus, and hepatitis C infection.

Anti-Cyclic Citrullinated Peptide (anti-CCP) Antibodies

Anti-CCP antibodies target citrullinated peptides, which are present in inflamed joints of patients with rheumatoid arthritis.

- Anti-CCP antibodies are highly specific to rheumatoid arthritis and are present in a significant proportion of patients with RA, especially those with early or aggressive disease.
- Anti-CCP positivity is associated with more severe disease and joint damage in RA.

Interpretation
- A positive RF or anti-CCP antibody test, especially in the presence of compatible clinical features, supports the diagnosis of rheumatoid arthritis.
- The presence of both RF and anti-CCP antibodies further increases the likelihood of rheumatoid arthritis, especially in patients with early or undifferentiated arthritis.
- However, it's important to note that RF and anti-CCP antibodies can also be present in other autoimmune and non-autoimmune conditions, and their presence alone is not diagnostic of rheumatoid arthritis.
- Interpretation of RF and anti-CCP antibody results should be done in the context of the overall clinical picture, including symptoms, physical examination findings, imaging studies, and other laboratory tests.

Follow-Up

A positive RF or anti-CCP antibody test may prompt further evaluation, including imaging studies (e.g., X-rays, ultrasound, MRI) and consultation with a rheumatologist.
- Additional tests or procedures may be needed to confirm the diagnosis, assess disease activity, and guide treatment decisions.

17.10. Cancer Markers

> ➤ *Cancer markers, also known as tumor markers, are substances produced by cancer cells or by the body in response to cancer.*
> ➤ *These markers can be detected in blood, urine, or tissue samples and are used for various purposes in cancer diagnosis, prognosis, monitoring, and treatment.*

Prostate-Specific Antigen (PSA)
- Used for screening and monitoring prostate cancer.
- Elevated PSA levels can indicate prostate cancer, but they can also be caused by non-cancerous conditions such as benign prostatic hyperplasia (BPH) or prostatitis.

CA 125
- Associated with ovarian cancer.

- Elevated CA 125 levels may indicate ovarian cancer, but they can also be elevated in other conditions such as endometriosis, pelvic inflammatory disease (PID), or uterine fibroids.

Carcinoembryonic Antigen (CEA)
- Associated with colorectal cancer and other gastrointestinal cancers.
- Elevated CEA levels can indicate colorectal cancer, but they can also be elevated in other cancers (e.g., pancreatic, lung) and non-cancerous conditions such as inflammatory bowel disease (IBD) or smoking.

Alpha-Fetoprotein (AFP)
- Associated with liver cancer (hepatocellular carcinoma) and certain types of germ cell tumors.
- Elevated AFP levels may indicate liver cancer, but they can also be elevated in other liver diseases (e.g., hepatitis, cirrhosis) and certain non-cancerous conditions.

CA 19-9
- Associated with pancreatic cancer and other gastrointestinal cancers.
- Elevated CA 19-9 levels may indicate pancreatic cancer, but they can also be elevated in other gastrointestinal cancers and non-cancerous conditions such as pancreatitis or biliary obstruction.

CA 15-3 and CA 27.29
- Associated with breast cancer.
- Elevated CA 15-3 and CA 27.29 levels may indicate breast cancer, particularly in advanced or metastatic disease, but they can also be elevated in other conditions.

CA 72-4
- Associated with gastrointestinal cancers, including stomach (gastric) cancer.
- Elevated CA 72-4 levels may indicate stomach cancer, but they can also be elevated in other gastrointestinal cancers and non-cancerous conditions.

HER2/neu (Human Epidermal Growth Factor Receptor 2)
- Associated with breast cancer and some other cancers.
- HER2/neu testing is used to determine the HER2 status of breast cancer tumors, which helps guide treatment decisions such as targeted therapy with drugs like trastuzumab (Herceptin).

AFP-L3%
- A subtype of alpha-fetoprotein associated with liver cancer (hepatocellular carcinoma).
- AFP-L3% testing can help differentiate between hepatocellular carcinoma and other liver conditions.

Ki-67
- A marker of cellular proliferation associated with various cancers.
- Ki-67 testing is used to assess tumor aggressiveness and predict response to treatment in certain cancers, including breast cancer and neuroendocrine tumors.

17.11. Vitamin D Level

> ➤ *Vitamin D is a fat-soluble vitamin crucial for calcium absorption in the gut, promoting bone health and playing a vital role in immune function, inflammation reduction, and muscle strength.*
>
> ➤ *Vitamin D is obtained through skin exposure to sunlight, certain foods (like fatty fish, fortified dairy products, and egg yolks), and dietary supplements.*
>
> ➤ *Insufficient vitamin D levels can lead to bone disorders such as rickets in children and osteoporosis in adults.*

25(OH)D Levels	Range	Description
Severe Deficiency	<10 ng/mL (25 nmol/L)	Symptoms of vitamin D deficiency may include muscle weakness, bone pain, fatigue, and an increased risk of fractures and osteoporosis
Deficiency	10-20 ng/mL (25-50 nmol/L)	
Insufficiency	21-29 ng/mL (50-74 nmol/L)	Some experts consider levels below 30 ng/mL (75 nmol/L) as insufficient for optimal health, as higher levels may provide additional benefits beyond bone health
Adequacy	30-100 ng/mL (75-250 nmol/L)	Levels above 30 ng/mL (75 nmol/L) are generally considered adequate for maintaining bone health and overall health, although optimal levels for other health outcomes are still debated

Optimal Range	40-60 ng/mL (100-150 nmol/L)	Patient requirements for vitamin D may vary based on factors such as age, ethnicity, geographic location, sun exposure, diet, and medical conditions
Toxicity	>150 ng/mL (375 nmol/L)	Vitamin D toxicity is rare but can occur with very high doses of supplementation, leading to elevated blood calcium levels (hypercalcemia) and symptoms such as nausea, vomiting, weakness, and kidney stones

Interpretation:

- Interpretation of vitamin D levels should consider the patient's clinical context, including symptoms, risk factors for deficiency or insufficiency, and medical history.
- Testing may be indicated for patients with symptoms suggestive of vitamin D deficiency, those at higher risk (e.g., older adults, patients with limited sun exposure, certain medical conditions), or as part of routine health screening.
- The APP may recommend supplementation or lifestyle modifications (such as increased sun exposure and dietary changes) based on vitamin D levels and patient factors
- Regular monitoring of vitamin D levels may be recommended for patients at risk of deficiency or insufficiency or those undergoing supplementation to ensure optimal levels and prevent potential adverse effects.

17.12. Vitamin B12 Level

> ➤ Vitamin B12, also known as cobalamin, is essential for red blood cell formation, brain function, and DNA synthesis.
>
> ➤ It's naturally found in animal products, such as meat, fish, poultry, eggs, and dairy, with supplementation recommended for vegans or people with absorption issues.
>
> ➤ Deficiency in vitamin B12 can lead to anemia, neurological disorders, and cognitive impairments.

Normal Range:

- The normal range for serum vitamin B12 levels typically falls between 200 and 900 pg/mL or between 150 and 670 pmol/L.

However, the reference range may vary slightly between laboratories.

Deficiency:
- Vitamin B12 deficiency is typically defined as a serum B12 level below 200 pg/mL (148 pmol/L).
- Symptoms of vitamin B12 deficiency may include fatigue, weakness, numbness or tingling in the hands and feet, difficulty walking, memory problems, and mood changes.
- Severe deficiency can lead to pernicious anemia, neurological complications, and other health problems if left untreated.

Borderline Deficiency:
- Serum B12 levels between 200 and 300 pg/mL (148-222 pmol/L) may be considered borderline deficient and may warrant further evaluation, especially if accompanied by symptoms or risk factors.

Elevated Levels:
- Elevated vitamin B12 levels are less common but may occur in certain medical conditions such as liver disease, kidney failure, and myeloproliferative disorders.
- High levels of vitamin B12 are generally considered non-toxic, as excess B12 is usually excreted in the urine.

Interpretation:
- Interpretation of vitamin B12 levels should consider the patient's clinical context, including symptoms, risk factors for deficiency, medical history, and other laboratory tests.
- Testing for vitamin B12 deficiency may be indicated in patients with symptoms suggestive of deficiency (such as fatigue, anemia, neuropathy), those with conditions associated with malabsorption or impaired absorption of B12 (such as pernicious anemia, gastrointestinal disorders, or certain medications), or as part of routine health screening in older adults.
- Medications inhibit B12 absorption: metformin, colchicine, proton pump inhibitors, etc.
- Additional tests, such as methylmalonic acid (MMA) and homocysteine levels, may be used to further evaluate suspected vitamin B12 deficiency and differentiate between true deficiency and functional deficiency.
- Treatment for vitamin B12 deficiency typically involves oral or intramuscular supplementation with vitamin B12, depending on the underlying cause and severity of the deficiency.

17.13. Hemoglobin A1c and Blood Sugar Level

> *Hemoglobin A1c (HbA1c) measures the average blood sugar level over the past three months, reflecting the percentage of hemoglobin coated with sugar.*

Hemoglobin A1c (HbA1c) Interpretation

- Normal range: Less than 5.7%
- Prediabetes: 5.7% to 6.4%
- Diabetes: 6.5% or higher

Blood Sugar (Glucose) Interpretation

Fasting Plasma Glucose (FPG):

- Normal fasting glucose: Less than 100 mg/dL
- Prediabetes (impaired fasting glucose): 100 to 125 mg/dL
- Diabetes: 126 mg/dL or higher on two separate occasions

Oral Glucose Tolerance Test (OGTT):

- Normal glucose tolerance: Less than 140 mg/dL two hours after the glucose load
- Prediabetes: 140 to 199 mg/dL two hours after the glucose load
- Diabetes: 200 mg/dL or higher two hours after the glucose load

Random Plasma Glucose:

- Diabetes: 200 mg/dL or higher with classic symptoms of hyperglycemia
- Note: Random glucose levels may not be reliable for diagnosing prediabetes

Interpretation in Conjunction

- Elevated HbA1c levels, along with elevated fasting or postprandial glucose levels, indicate poor glycemic control and may suggest the need for treatment intensification or lifestyle modifications.
- HbA1c levels provide a long-term measure of glycemic control, while blood sugar measurements (FPG, OGTT, random glucose) offer a snapshot of glucose levels at specific times.
- Consistency between HbA1c and blood sugar measurements supports the reliability of the assessment of glycemic control.

Clinical Decision-Making
- The APP should use both HbA1c and blood sugar measurements to diagnose diabetes, assess glycemic control, and adjust treatment plans.
- Treatment goals are often based on both HbA1c targets and blood sugar measurements to reduce the risk of diabetes-related complications.
- Regular monitoring of HbA1c and blood sugar levels is essential for patients with diabetes to evaluate treatment efficacy and adjust management strategies as needed.

Patient Variability
- It's essential to consider patient variability and factors that may affect HbA1c and blood sugar measurements, such as age, ethnicity, comorbidities (kidney failure, liver disease, or severe anemia), medications, and adherence to treatment and monitoring regimens.

17.14. Uric Acid Level

> ➤ *Uric acid is a waste product formed from the breakdown of purines, substances found in various foods and drinks and naturally occurring in the body.*
>
> ➤ *Normally excreted in urine, elevated levels of uric acid can lead to gout, a form of arthritis characterized by painful joint inflammation, and can also be associated with kidney stones and renal failure.*
>
> ➤ *Management of high uric acid levels includes dietary changes, hydration, and medications to reduce production or increase excretion of uric acid.*

Normal Range
- The normal range for serum uric acid levels is typically:
    - For men: 3.4 to 7.0 mg/dL (200 to 420 µmol/L)
    - For women: 2.4 to 6.0 mg/dL (140 to 360 µmol/L)
- However, the reference range may vary slightly between laboratories.

Elevated Levels
- Elevated uric acid levels, known as hyperuricemia, may indicate increased production or decreased excretion of uric acid.

- Hyperuricemia can be caused by various factors, including dietary intake (high-purine foods), obesity, certain medications (e.g., thiazide diuretics), chronic kidney disease, metabolic syndrome, and genetic factors.
- Persistent hyperuricemia may increase the risk of developing gout, a type of arthritis caused by the deposition of urate crystals in the joints, as well as kidney stones and other health problems.

Low Levels

- Low uric acid levels are less common and may be seen in rare genetic disorders, certain medications (e.g., allopurinol), or conditions associated with increased excretion of uric acid (e.g., Fanconi syndrome).

Interpretation:

- Interpretation of uric acid levels should consider the patient's clinical context, including symptoms, medical history, and other laboratory tests.
- Uric acid testing may be indicated in patients with symptoms suggestive of gout (e.g., sudden joint pain, swelling, redness), kidney stones, or other conditions associated with hyperuricemia.
- Elevated uric acid levels may prompt further evaluation to identify the underlying cause and assess the risk of developing gout or other complications.
- Treatment for hyperuricemia and gout may involve lifestyle modifications (e.g., dietary changes, weight loss), medications to reduce uric acid levels (e.g., allopurinol, febuxostat), and management of comorbidities such as hypertension and kidney disease.

17.15. Protein and Urine Electrophoresis

> ➤ *Protein and urine electrophoresis are laboratory techniques used to separate and identify different proteins in the blood and urine, respectively, based on their size and charge.*
>
> ➤ *These tests are valuable in diagnosing and monitoring disorders such as multiple myeloma, chronic inflammatory conditions, and kidney diseases, by detecting abnormal levels and patterns of proteins.*
>
> ➤ *The results can help address specific protein abnormalities, guiding treatment decisions and monitoring disease progression or response to therapy.*

Total Protein in Urine

- Elevated total protein levels in urine, known as proteinuria, may indicate kidney damage or dysfunction, inflammation, infection, or systemic diseases affecting the kidneys.
- Proteinuria can be quantified as:
  - Trace or 1+ (mild proteinuria): 30 to 150 mg/dL
  - 2+ (moderate proteinuria): 150 to 300 mg/dL
  - 3+ (marked proteinuria): 300 to 1000 mg/dL
  - 4+ (severe proteinuria): >1000 mg/dL

Urinary Protein Electrophoresis

- Urinary protein electrophoresis separates and identifies different protein fractions in the urine, including albumin, globulins, and other proteins.
- The pattern of protein bands observed on the electrophoresis gel can provide insights into the underlying cause of proteinuria.
- Common patterns include increased albumin, increased alpha-2 globulins, and the presence of monoclonal bands.

Interpretation:

- Interpretation of protein and urine electrophoresis results should consider the patient's clinical context, including symptoms, medical history, and other laboratory tests.
- Proteinuria may be transient or persistent and can be caused by various conditions such as glomerular diseases (e.g., nephrotic syndrome, glomerulonephritis), tubular disorders, urinary tract infections, diabetes mellitus, hypertension, and systemic diseases (e.g., systemic lupus erythematosus, multiple myeloma).
- The pattern of protein bands observed on urine electrophoresis can help differentiate between different types of proteinuria and guide further diagnostic evaluation and management.

Follow-Up and Management:

- Elevated total protein levels and abnormal protein patterns on urine electrophoresis may warrant further evaluation, including additional laboratory tests (e.g., serum protein electrophoresis, urine immunofixation), imaging studies, and kidney biopsy.
- Treatment for proteinuria depends on the underlying cause and may involve medications to control blood pressure, reduce inflammation, or treat underlying systemic diseases.

- Regular monitoring of proteinuria and urinary protein patterns may be necessary to assess treatment efficacy, disease progression, and kidney function.

17.16. Iron Panel

> ➢ An iron panel evaluates iron levels in the body, including tests for serum iron, total iron-binding capacity (TIBC), transferrin saturation, and ferritin.
>
> ➢ It helps diagnose conditions like iron deficiency anemia or iron overload. Interpretation considers low or high levels of these markers, indicating potential iron-related disorders in the context of clinical findings.

Test	Normal Range	Interpretation
Serum Iron	• 60-170 µg/dL (men) • 50-150 µg/dL (women)	Measures the amount of iron in the blood • Low levels may indicate iron deficiency • High levels may suggest iron overload
Total Iron-Binding Capacity (TIBC)	240-450 µg/dL	Measures all proteins available to bind with iron, including transferrin • High levels often indicate iron deficiency, as the body produces more transferrin to try to capture more iron • Low levels may suggest iron overload or chronic illness
Transferrin Saturation	20-50%	Calculated by dividing serum iron by TIBC and multiplying by 100 • Low percentages (<20%) suggest iron deficiency • High percentages (>50%) indicate iron overload

Ferritin	• 20-500 ng/mL (men) • 20-200 ng/mL (women)	Reflects the amount of iron stored in the body • Low levels indicate iron deficiency • High levels may suggest iron overload or an acute phase reactant (indicative of inflammation)

Interpretation

- Iron Deficiency Anemia: Characterized by low serum iron, high TIBC, low transferrin saturation, and low ferritin.
- Anemia of Chronic Disease: May show normal or slightly low serum iron, low TIBC, normal or low transferrin saturation, and normal or high ferritin.
- Iron Overload (Hemochromatosis): Indicated by high serum iron, low TIBC, high transferrin saturation, and high ferritin.

17.17. Sex Hormones Panel

> ➤ *A sex hormone panel evaluates hormones related to reproductive health, including estradiol, testosterone, follicle-stimulating hormone (FSH), luteinizing hormone (LH), and progesterone, to diagnose conditions like infertility, polycystic ovary syndrome (PCOS), and menopause.*
>
> ➤ *Normal ranges vary by sex, age, and, for women, the menstrual cycle phase.*
>
> ➤ *Interpretation should consider hormonal values and clinical symptoms to guide treatment strategies.*

Sex Hormones	Gender	Range	Interpretation
Estradiol (E2)	Women	Levels vary significantly with the menstrual cycle: • Follicular phase: 30-120 pg/mL • Ovulatory peak: 130-370 pg/mL • Luteal phase: 70-250 pg/mL • Postmenopausal: <10-20 pg/mL	• High levels can indicate ovarian tumors or hyperstimulation • Low levels may suggest menopause or hypogonadism
	Men	10-50 pg/mL	High levels could be due to estrogen therapy, liver disease, or obesity
Testosterone	Women	15-70 ng/dL	High levels could suggest conditions like polycystic ovary syndrome (PCOS) or an adrenal or ovarian tumor
	Men	Normal range is typically 300-1,000 ng/dL (vary slightly depending on the lab)	Low levels may indicate hypogonadism
Follicle-Stimu-lating Hormone (FSH)	Women	Varied by cycle phase: • Follicular phase : 5-20 IU/L • Mid-cycle peak: ~20-30 IU/L • Luteal phase: 1-10 IU/L • Postmenopausal: 30-120 IU/L	High levels can indicate menopause or diminished ovarian reserve

	Men	1-15 IU/L	• High levels may suggest testicular failure • Low levels could indicate problems with the pituitary gland or hypothalamus
Luteinizing Hormone (LH)	Women	Varied by cycle phase: • Follicular phase: 1-10 IU/L • Mid-cycle peak: ~10-60 IU/L • Luteal phase: 1-15 IU/L • Postmenopausal: 15-60 IU/L	• High LH levels are typical around ovulation and in conditions like PCOS • Low levels in both sexes could suggest hypopituitarism
	Men	1-15 IU/L	High levels may indicate primary testicular failure
Progesterone	Women	Varied by cycle phase: • Follicular phase: <1 ng/mL • Mid-luteal phase: 5-20 ng/mL • Pregnant: >11 ng/mL, varies greatly with gestational age • Postmenopausal: <0.2 ng/mL	• Progesterone levels are used to confirm ovulation and assess placental and ovarian function during pregnancy • Low levels can indicate lack of ovulation or ectopic pregnancy
	Men	10-57 nmol/L	• High levels can decrease

	Women	18-144 nmol/L	the availability of testosterone, leading to symptoms of hypogonadism despite normal total testosterone levels
Sex Hormone-Bin-ding Globulin (SHBG)			• Low levels can increase the availability of testosterone, potentially exacerbating conditions sensitive to androgens like PCOS

17.18. Other Hormones

Type	Hormone	Normal Range	Interpretation
Adrenal Hormone	Cortisol	10-20 µg/dL	• High levels may indicate Cushing's syndrome • Low levels suggest Addison's disease or secondary adrenal insufficiency
	ACTH	10-60 pg/mL	Levels are interpreted in conjunction with cortisol levels to assess adrenal and pituitary functions
	Insulin	<25 µIU/mL	High levels may indicate insulin resistance or early type 2 diabetes
Prolactin Hormone	Prolactin	• Women (non-pregnant): 2-29 ng/mL • Men: 2-18 ng/mL	Pregnant Women: Levels can rise significantly, up to 10-209 ng/mL or higher, especially in the third trimester

17.19. Hepatitis Panel

> ➤ A hepatitis panel includes various markers to diagnose and monitor hepatitis A, B, and C infections, indicating acute or chronic infection, immunity, or the need for vaccination.
>
> ➤ Key markers include HBsAg and Anti-HBs for hepatitis B, Anti-HAV IgM/IgG for hepatitis A, and Anti-HCV and HCV RNA for hepatitis C.
>
> ➤ Interpretation depends on a combination of these markers to assess infection status, immunity, and infectivity.

Hepatitis A

- Anti-HAV IgM: Indicates acute hepatitis A infection.
- Anti-HAV IgG: Indicates past infection and immunity to hepatitis A.

Hepatitis B

- HBsAg (Hepatitis B surface antigen): Indicates current hepatitis B infection. Persistent presence for more than six months suggests chronic infection.
- Anti-HBs (Hepatitis B surface antibody): Indicates recovery and immunity to hepatitis B. Can also indicate successful vaccination.
- Anti-HBc IgM (Hepatitis B core antibody, IgM): Indicates recent infection with hepatitis B, generally within the last 6 months.
- Anti-HBc IgG (Hepatitis B core antibody, IgG): Indicates past or ongoing infection with hepatitis B; can be present in those who have recovered or in those with chronic infection.
- HBeAg (Hepatitis B e antigen): Indicates active replication of the virus and high infectivity.
- Anti-HBe (Hepatitis B e antibody): Indicates a lower level of virus replication and reduced infectivity.

Hepatitis C

- Anti-HCV (Hepatitis C antibody): Indicates exposure to the hepatitis C virus. A positive result requires further testing with HCV RNA to determine if the infection is current.
- HCV RNA (Hepatitis C viral RNA): Indicates active hepatitis C infection. Quantitative tests measure the virus's load in the blood, important for treatment decisions and monitoring response.

Hepatitis Interpretation

- Acute Hepatitis: Suggested by positive IgM antibodies for hepatitis A (Anti-HAV IgM) or hepatitis B (Anti-HBc IgM), or by the presence of

HCV RNA for hepatitis C with or without Anti-HCV antibodies depending on the timing of testing post-exposure.

- Chronic Hepatitis: Indicated by the persistence of HBsAg for more than six months in hepatitis B, or by the presence of HCV RNA in hepatitis C without clearance over time.
- Immunity: Demonstrated by positive Anti-HAV IgG for hepatitis A, Anti-HBs for hepatitis B indicating recovery or successful vaccination, and the absence of Anti-HCV in the context of previous exposure without chronic infection development.
- Infectivity: Suggested by positive HBeAg for hepatitis B, indicating high viral replication and higher risk of transmission.

Tips to consider for the APh

- Confirmatory testing is essential for hepatitis C due to the possibility of false positives or past resolved infections.
- Chronic hepatitis B and C infections require careful monitoring for liver function and damage, as well as assessment for antiviral treatment eligibility.
- Vaccination history should be considered, especially for hepatitis B, as it can influence the interpretation of Anti-HBs.

17.20. Sexually Transmitted Disease Panel

> ➤ An STD panel is a comprehensive set of tests designed to screen for various sexually transmitted diseases, including HIV, syphilis, hepatitis B and C, herpes simplex virus, chlamydia, gonorrhea, and human papillomavirus (HPV).
>
> ➤ These tests help detect infections that may be asymptomatic and ensure timely treatment to prevent complications.
>
> ➤ Regular screening is recommended for sexually active individuals, especially those with new or multiple partners, to maintain sexual health and prevent disease transmission.

Disease	Test
HIV (Human Immunodeficiency Virus)	Antibody/antigen combination tests (4th generation tests), followed by confirmatory testing with Western blot or PCR for acute HIV infection

Syphilis	Non-treponemal tests (VDRL, RPR) for screening, followed by treponemal tests (FTA-ABS, TPPA) for confirmation
Hepatitis B	Surface antigen (HBsAg) to detect active infection, surface antibody (Anti-HBs) to assess immunity, and core antibody (Anti-HBc) to identify previous or ongoing infection
Hepatitis C	Anti-HCV antibody test followed by HCV RNA PCR tests for confirmation and to assess viral load
Herpes Simplex Virus	Type-specific serologic tests to detect antibodies to HSV-1 (oral herpes) and HSV-2 (genital herpes). PCR tests can be used for acute infection diagnosis
Chlamydia	Nucleic acid amplification tests (NAAT) from urine samples or swabs from genital areas, the throat, or the rectum
Gonorrhea	NAAT from urine samples or swabs from the urethra, cervix, throat, or rectum to detect Neisseria gonorrhoeae
Human Papillomavirus (HPV)	High-risk HPV testing, often from cervical swab samples, especially for HPV types associated with the risk of cervical cancer

STD Interpretation

- Positive Results: Require confirmatory testing, clinical evaluation, and appropriate treatment. Partner notification and treatment may also be necessary to prevent reinfection and transmission.
- Negative Results: May need to be repeated if testing occurs during the window period of an infection. Regular screening is recommended for sexually active individuals with new or multiple partners.

Prevention and Counseling

- Part of STD testing includes counseling on safe sex practices, the importance of regular screening, and, if necessary, vaccination (e.g., HPV and hepatitis B vaccines).

17.21. Prostate Panel

> ➤ A prostate lab panel typically includes the Prostate-Specific Antigen (PSA) test to screen for prostate cancer, with elevated levels indicating the need for further evaluation.
>
> ➤ Additional tests like Free PSA, Prostate Health Index (PHI), and PCA3 may also be used to assess prostate cancer risk more accurately.
>
> ➤ These tests, combined with physical exams such as the Digital Rectal Exam (DRE), help diagnose and monitor prostate health conditions, guiding treatment decisions.

Prostate-Specific Antigen (PSA)

- Purpose: Measures the level of PSA in the blood, a protein produced by both cancerous and noncancerous tissue in the prostate.
- Normal Range: Generally, a PSA level under 4 ng/mL is considered normal, but this can depend on age and race. Levels between 4-10 ng/mL are considered a gray area, and above 10 ng/mL is considered elevated.
- Interpretation:
    - Elevated PSA levels can indicate prostate cancer, BPH, or prostatitis. However, PSA levels can also be influenced by age, prostate size, and other factors.
    - The rate of PSA changes over time (PSA velocity) can also provide important diagnostic information.

Free PSA

- Purpose: Measures the percentage of PSA that is not bound to proteins in the blood. Used in conjunction with total PSA testing.
- Interpretation: A lower percentage of free PSA (<25%) might indicate a higher risk of prostate cancer in men with slightly elevated total PSA levels.

Digital Rectal Exam (DRE)

- Though not a lab test, the DRE is a physical exam that's often performed as part of prostate health screening.
- The APh feels the prostate through the rectal wall to check for bumps, soft or hard spots, and overall size and shape.

Additional Tests for Prostate Evaluation
- Prostate Health Index (PHI): Combines total PSA, free PSA, and [-2]proPSA levels for a more accurate assessment of prostate cancer risk.
- 4Kscore Test: Measures four prostate-specific biomarkers, providing a risk score for aggressive prostate cancer.
- PCA3 Test: A urine test after DRE that looks for the presence of the PCA3 gene in urine, which is overexpressed in prostate cancer cells.
- Transrectal Ultrasound (TRUS) and MRI: Imaging tests that provide visual images of the prostate, used for diagnosis and biopsy guidance.
- Prostate Biopsy: Recommended if other tests suggest the possibility of cancer. It involves collecting small samples of prostate tissue to look for cancer cells.

PSA Interpretation
- Elevated or borderline PSA levels often lead to further testing to determine the cause, which may include repeat PSA testing, imaging, or biopsy.
- The decision to proceed with more invasive testing like a biopsy should consider the patient's overall health, PSA level, DRE results, and personal preference.

17.22. Basic EKG

> ➢ An EKG interpretation involves a systematic analysis of the waveform to evaluate the heart's electrical activity, structure, and function.
>
> ➢ This process can identify not only arrhythmias but also signs of cardiac ischemia, structural heart disease, electrolyte imbalances, and other conditions.

Rate and Rhythm
- Rate: Calculate the heart rate by counting the number of QRS complexes on the EKG strip (for a 6-second strip, multiply by 10; for other lengths, adjust accordingly).
- Rhythm: Determine if the rhythm is regular or irregular by measuring the intervals between consecutive QRS complexes.

P Wave Analysis
- Presence and Morphology: Confirm that there is a P wave before each QRS complex, indicating normal atrial depolarization. Assess for

variations in shape, which may indicate atrial enlargement or ectopic atrial rhythms.

- P Wave Axis: The normal axis for P waves is between 0° and +75°, reflecting atrial depolarization from the SA node.

PR Interval

- Length: Measure the PR interval from the beginning of the P wave to the start of the QRS complex. The normal range is 0.12 to 0.20 seconds. Variations can indicate conduction delays or pre-excitation syndromes.

QRS Complex

- Duration: A normal QRS duration is up to 0.10 seconds. Longer durations may indicate bundle branch blocks or ventricular conduction abnormalities.
- Morphology: Evaluate for the presence of Q waves, which can indicate previous myocardial infarction, and the overall morphology for signs of hypertrophy or conduction defects.

ST Segment and T Wave

- ST Segment: Analyze for elevation or depression, which may suggest myocardial ischemia, injury, or pericarditis.
- T Wave: Assess amplitude and direction. Inverted or peaked T waves can indicate ischemia, hyperkalemia, or other conditions.

QT Interval

- Measurement: From the start of the QRS complex to the end of the T wave, adjusting for heart rate. A prolonged QT interval increases the risk of torsades de pointes and other arrhythmias.

Axis Determination

- Frontal Plane Axis: Calculate the heart's electrical axis in the frontal plane by analyzing the QRS complex in limb leads. The normal axis is between -30° and +90°. Deviations can indicate underlying cardiac or pulmonary conditions.

Identification of Additional Features

- Look for other features such as premature beats, signs of chamber enlargement, and evidence of previous cardiac events.

References

- Briggs, C., Culp, N., Davis, B., & d'Onofrio, G. (2019). ICSH guidelines for the laboratory diagnosis of nonimmune hereditary red cell membrane disorders. International Journal of Laboratory Hematology, 41(S1), 24-37.

- Cervinski, M. A., Lee, H. K., & Martin, C. S. (2019). Clinical implications of pseudohyponatremia in a patient with hyperglycemia: A case report. BMC Endocrine Disorders, 19(1), 1-5.
- Wu, A. H. B., & Briggs, C. (2017). Assessment of glomerular filtration rate using urine measurements. In Laboratory Tests and Diagnostic Procedures (Vol. 1, pp. 1707-1710). John Wiley & Sons.
- Stone, N. J., Robinson, J. G., & et al. (2014). 2013 ACC/AHA guideline on the treatment of blood cholesterol to reduce atherosclerotic cardiovascular risk in adults: A report of the American College of Cardiology/American Heart Association Task Force on Practice Guidelines. Circulation, 129(25_suppl_2), S1-S45.
- Brent, G. A. (2012). Clinical practice. Graves' disease. New England Journal of Medicine, 358(24), 2594-2605.
- Hanly, J. G., & Pisetsky, D. S. (2010). Diagnosis and management of patients with antinuclear antibody-negative systemic lupus erythematosus. Best Practice & Research Clinical Rheumatology, 24(4), 531-542.
- McLean-Tooke, A., & Spickett, G. P. (2009). Association between antinuclear antibody and thrombosis: A case report and literature review. Rheumatology International, 29(12), 1493-1496.
- Hochberg, M. C. (1997). Updating the American College of Rheumatology revised criteria for the classification of systemic lupus erythematosus. Arthritis & Rheumatism, 40(9), 1725.
- Aletaha, D., Neogi, T., & et al. (2010). 2010 rheumatoid arthritis classification criteria: An American College of Rheumatology/European League Against Rheumatism collaborative initiative. Arthritis & Rheumatism, 62(9), 2569-2581.
- Duffy, M. J. (2013). Tumor markers in clinical practice: A review focusing on common solid cancers. Medical Principles and Practice, 22(1), 4-11.
- Holick, M. F. (2007). Vitamin D deficiency. New England Journal of Medicine, 357(3), 266-281.
- Langan, R. C., & Zawistoski, K. J. (2017). Update on vitamin B12 deficiency. American Family Physician, 89(12), 979-986.
- American Diabetes Association. (2020). 6. Glycemic targets: Standards of medical care in diabetes—2020. Diabetes Care, 43(Supplement 1), S66-S76.
- Richette, P., & Bardin, T. (2010). Gout. The Lancet, 375(9711), 318-328.
- Simerville, J. A., Maxted, W. C., & Pahira, J. J. (2005). Urinalysis: A comprehensive review. American Family Physician, 71(6), 1153-1162.

Chapter 18: Basic Biostatistics for the APh

18.1. Introduction to Biostatistics

> ➢ *Biostatistics, also known as biometry or biometrics, is the application of statistical methods to biological, health, and medical data.*
>
> ➢ *It plays a crucial role in healthcare by providing tools and techniques to analyze, interpret, and draw conclusions from data collected in various biomedical research studies and clinical trials.*

Study Design
- Biostatistics is fundamental in designing research studies and clinical trials to investigate hypotheses, assess outcomes, and evaluate interventions.
- Proper study design ensures the validity and reliability of study findings and minimizes bias and confounding factors.

Data Collection and Management
- Biostatistics helps in planning and executing data collection procedures, including sample size determination, randomization, and data quality control measures.
- It also involves the development of data collection tools, such as questionnaires, surveys, and electronic health records, to capture relevant information accurately.

Descriptive Statistics
- Biostatistical methods are used to summarize and describe the characteristics of populations or samples, including measures of central tendency (e.g., mean, median) and variability (e.g., standard deviation, range).

Inferential Statistics
- Biostatistics enables researchers to make inferences and draw conclusions about populations based on sample data.
- Inferential statistics include hypothesis testing, confidence intervals, regression analysis, and survival analysis, which are used to assess associations, compare groups, and predict outcomes in healthcare research.

Epidemiological Studies

- Biostatistics plays a crucial role in epidemiological research by quantifying the distribution and determinants of diseases within populations.
- Epidemiological studies use statistical methods to calculate measures of disease occurrence (e.g., incidence, prevalence), assess risk factors, and identify trends or outbreaks of diseases.

Clinical Trials

- Biostatistics is essential in designing, analyzing, and interpreting results from clinical trials, which evaluate the safety and efficacy of new drugs, treatments, or medical devices.
- Statistical methods such as randomization, blinding, and intention-to-treat analysis are used to minimize bias and estimate treatment effects accurately.

Evidence-Based Medicine

- Biostatistics provides the foundation for evidence-based medicine (EBM), which integrates clinical expertise, patient values, and the best available scientific evidence to guide clinical decision-making.
- Biostatistical methods are used to critically appraise research studies, synthesize evidence, and conduct meta-analyses to inform clinical practice guidelines and healthcare policies.

Quality Improvement

- Biostatistics facilitates quality improvement initiatives in healthcare by monitoring and analyzing healthcare outcomes, patient satisfaction, and healthcare processes.
- Statistical process control (SPC) methods help identify variations, trends, and areas for improvement in healthcare delivery and patient care.

18.2. Descriptive Statistics

> ➢ *Descriptive statistics are methods used to summarize and describe the characteristics of a dataset.*
>
> ➢ *These statistics provide a concise overview of the data's central tendency, dispersion, and shape, allowing researchers and analysts to understand and interpret the data more effectively.*
>
> ➢ *They are typically the first step in data analysis and are essential for gaining insights into the distribution and patterns within the data.*

Key Measures of Descriptive Statistics:

Measures of Central Tendency:
- Mean: The arithmetic average of a dataset, calculated by summing all values and dividing by the total number of observations.
- Median: The middle value of a dataset when arranged in ascending or descending order. It represents the 50th percentile and is less sensitive to outliers compared to the mean.
- Mode: The value that occurs most frequently in a dataset. A dataset may have one mode (unimodal), two modes (bimodal), or more (multimodal).

Measures of Dispersion:
- Range: The difference between the maximum and minimum values in a dataset, providing a measure of the spread or variability.
- Variance: The average of the squared differences between each value and the mean, indicating the extent of dispersion around the mean.
- Standard Deviation: The square root of the variance, representing the average deviation of data points from the mean. It provides a measure of the spread of data relative to the mean.

Measures of Shape:
- Skewness: A measure of the asymmetry of the distribution, indicating whether the data is skewed to the left (negative skew) or right (positive skew) relative to the mean.

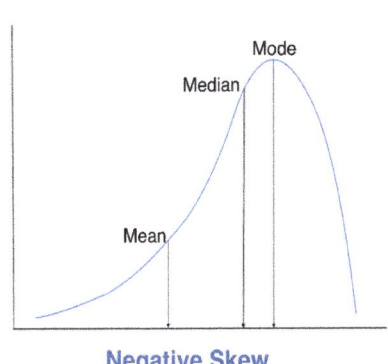
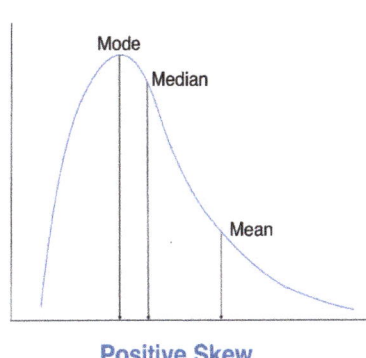

- Kurtosis: A measure of the peakedness or flatness of the distribution, indicating whether the data has heavy tails (leptokurtic) or light tails (platykurtic) compared to a normal distribution.

Percentiles and Quartiles:
- Percentiles: Values that divide a dataset into hundredths, representing the percentage of data points below a certain value. For

example, the 25th percentile (Q1) represents the value below which 25% of the data falls.

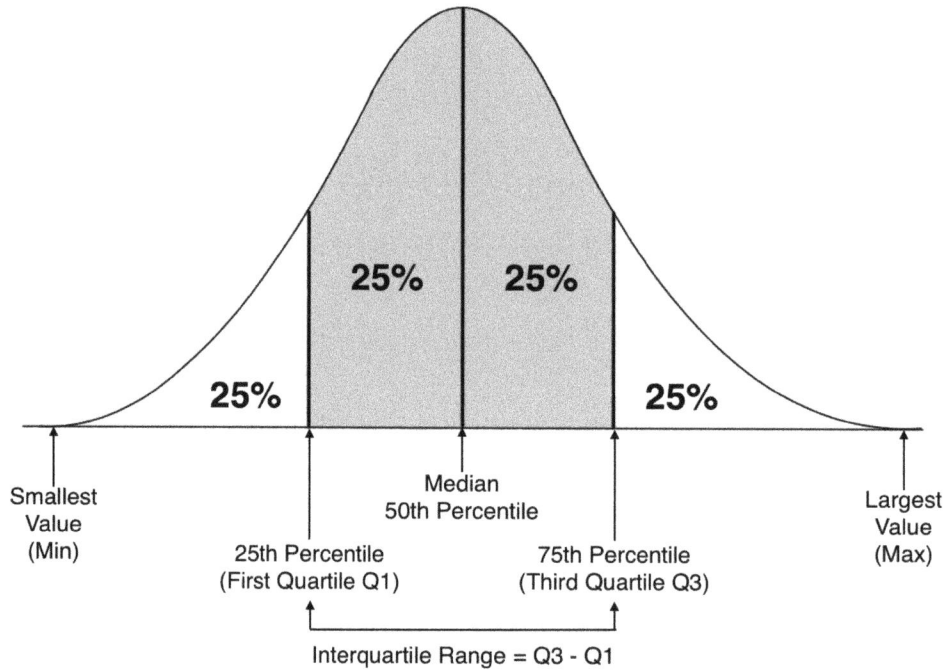

- Quartiles: Values that divide a dataset into quarters, representing the 25th (Q1), 50th (median), and 75th (Q3) percentiles.

Frequency Distributions:

- Histogram: A graphical representation of the frequency distribution of continuous data, with bars representing the frequency of data points within predefined intervals (bins).
- Frequency Table: A tabular summary of the frequency distribution of categorical or discrete data, showing the count or proportion of observations in each category.

Applications of Descriptive Statistics

Data Summarization:

- Descriptive statistics provide a concise summary of the main characteristics of a dataset, including its central tendency, variability, and shape.

Data Visualization:

- Descriptive statistics are often visualized using graphs, charts, and plots to help researchers and analysts visualize the distribution and patterns within the data.

Data Cleaning:
- Descriptive statistics can help identify and address missing values, outliers, or errors in the data, ensuring data quality and reliability for further analysis.

Exploratory Data Analysis (EDA):
- Descriptive statistics are used in EDA to explore relationships, trends, and patterns within the data, guiding subsequent analysis and hypothesis testing.

Comparative Analysis:
- Descriptive statistics enable comparisons between different groups or subsets of data, allowing researchers to identify differences or similarities in their characteristics.

18.3. Inferential Statistics

> ➢ Inferential statistics is a branch of statistics that involves making inferences or predictions about populations based on sample data.
>
> ➢ Unlike descriptive statistics, which summarize and describe the characteristics of a dataset, inferential statistics use probability theory and hypothesis testing to draw conclusions about populations, parameters, or relationships between variables.

Key Concepts in Inferential Statistics

Population and Sample:
- Population: The entire group of interest from which data is collected. Population parameters, such as the population mean or standard deviation, are characteristics of the entire population.
- Sample: A subset of the population selected for study. Inferential statistics use sample data to estimate population parameters and make inferences about the population as a whole.

Sampling Distribution:
- Sampling Distribution: The distribution of a sample statistic (e.g., sample mean or proportion) across all possible samples of a given size from the population. The Central Limit Theorem states that, for large sample sizes, the sampling distribution of the sample mean tends to be normally distributed regardless of the shape of the population distribution.
- Standard Error: The standard deviation of a sampling distribution, representing the variability of sample statistics across different

samples. It quantifies the precision of an estimate and decreases as the sample size increases.

Estimation:

- Point Estimation: Estimating a population parameter based on a single value or point estimate derived from sample data (e.g., sample mean or proportion).
- Interval Estimation: Estimating a range or interval that is likely to contain the true population parameter with a certain level of confidence. Confidence intervals provide a range of values within which the population parameter is expected to lie, based on sample data and a specified confidence level (e.g., 95% confidence interval).

Hypothesis Testing:

- Null Hypothesis (H0): A statement or assumption that there is no significant difference or effect in the population, often denoted as H0. It represents the status quo or default position that researchers aim to test.
- Alternative Hypothesis (Ha): A statement or assertion that contradicts the null hypothesis, suggesting the presence of a significant difference, effect, or relationship in the population.
- Significance Level (α): The probability threshold used to determine whether to reject the null hypothesis. Common significance levels include $\alpha = 0.05$ (5%) or $\alpha = 0.01$ (1%).
- P-value: The probability of obtaining observed sample results (or more extreme) under the assumption that the null hypothesis is true. A low p-value indicates strong evidence against the null hypothesis and supports the rejection of H0.
    - *Type I Error:* Rejecting the null hypothesis when it is actually true, leading to a false positive conclusion. The probability of a Type I error is equal to the significance level (α).
    - *Type II Error:* Failing to reject the null hypothesis when it is actually false, resulting in a false negative conclusion. The probability of a Type II error is denoted as β.

Parametric vs. Nonparametric Tests:

- Parametric Tests: Statistical tests that make assumptions about the distribution of the data (e.g., normality) and the parameters of the population (e.g., mean, variance). Examples include t-tests, ANOVA, and linear regression.
- Nonparametric Tests: Statistical tests that do not rely on specific distributional assumptions and are based on the rankings or order of

data values. Nonparametric tests are often used when data are skewed or non-normally distributed. Examples include the Wilcoxon rank-sum test and the Kruskal-Wallis test.

Applications of Inferential Statistics

Hypothesis Testing:
- Inferential statistics are used to test hypotheses and make decisions based on sample data, such as comparing group means, assessing the significance of treatment effects, or evaluating the strength of associations between variables.

Parameter Estimation:
- Inferential statistics provide methods for estimating population parameters based on sample data, including point estimation (e.g., sample mean) and interval estimation (e.g., confidence intervals).

Prediction and Forecasting:
- Inferential statistics can be used to make predictions or forecasts about future outcomes based on historical data or observed trends, such as predicting sales figures, disease incidence rates, or stock prices.

Generalization:
- Inferential statistics allow researchers to generalize findings from a sample to the larger population, providing insights into population characteristics, trends, and relationships.

Decision Making:
- Inferential statistics provide a basis for decision-making in various fields, including business, healthcare, and policy, by providing evidence, support, and guidance for informed decisions and actions.

18.4. Study Design and Research Methodology

> ➤ *Study design and research methodology are fundamental components of the scientific process, guiding the planning, execution, and analysis of research studies.*
> ➤ *They encompass the selection of appropriate study designs, data collection methods, sampling strategies, and statistical analyses to address research questions and objectives effectively.*

Research Question and Objectives
- Define the specific research question or hypothesis that the study aims to address.

- Clearly articulate the research objectives and goals to guide study design and methodology.

Study Design
- Choose an appropriate study design based on the research question, study objectives, and available resources.
- Common study designs include:
  - Experimental designs (e.g., randomized controlled trials [RCTs], quasi-experimental studies)
  - Observational designs (e.g., cross-sectional, case-control, cohort studies)
  - Qualitative research designs (e.g., interviews, focus groups, ethnography)

Sampling Strategy
- Determine the target population or study population from which participants will be selected.
- Select a sampling method (e.g., random sampling, stratified sampling, convenience sampling) to recruit study participants.
- Calculate sample size requirements to ensure adequate statistical power and precision in estimating study outcomes.

Data Collection Methods
- Choose appropriate data collection instruments and techniques based on the study design and research objectives.
- Examples of data collection methods include:
  - Surveys and questionnaires
  - Interviews (structured, semi-structured, or unstructured)
  - Observational methods (e.g., direct observation, chart review)
  - Biological specimen collection (e.g., blood samples, tissue biopsies)

Variables and Measurements
- Identify key variables of interest and define operational definitions for each variable.
- Determine appropriate measurement scales (e.g., nominal, ordinal, interval, ratio) for data collection.
- Develop valid and reliable measurement instruments to assess study outcomes and covariates.

Data Analysis Plan

- Specify the statistical methods and techniques to be used for data analysis.
- Outline the primary and secondary endpoints, hypotheses to be tested, and potential confounding variables.
- Consider appropriate statistical tests based on the study design and nature of the data (e.g., parametric tests, nonparametric tests, regression analysis).

Ethical Considerations

- Obtain approval from institutional review boards (IRBs) or ethics committees to ensure the protection of human subjects in research.
- Adhere to ethical principles and guidelines (e.g., informed consent, confidentiality, beneficence, nonmaleficence) throughout the research process.

Data Management and Quality Assurance

- Establish data management protocols to ensure the accuracy, completeness, and integrity of collected data.
- Implement quality assurance measures (e.g., data validation, inter-rater reliability checks) to minimize errors and bias in data collection and entry.

Timeline and Budget

- Develop a timeline or project plan outlining key milestones, activities, and deadlines for the study.
- Estimate the budget required for conducting the study, including personnel, equipment, supplies, and administrative costs.

Dissemination and Reporting

- Plan for the dissemination of study findings through peer-reviewed publications, presentations at conferences, or other dissemination channels.
- Prepare a comprehensive research report or manuscript following relevant reporting guidelines (e.g., CONSORT for clinical trials, STROBE for observational studies).

18.5. A Good Clinical Study

> ➤ A good study requires a well-defined and ethically sound protocol, including a clear hypothesis, objectives, and methodology. It must have Institutional Review Board (IRB) approval to ensure the safety and rights of participants are protected.
>
> ➤ A good study should also include a representative sample population to enhance generalizability, rigorous data collection and analysis methods to ensure reliability and validity, and transparent reporting of results, regardless of the outcome.
>
> ➤ Additionally, informed consent from all participants is crucial, along with strict adherence to regulatory standards and guidelines.

Understanding Study Design
- Recognize the study design used in the research, whether it's an observational study, randomized controlled trial (RCT), case-control study, or cohort study.
- Understand the strengths and limitations of each study design and how they may impact the interpretation of study findings.

Statistical Tests and Measures
- Familiarize yourself with the statistical tests and measures used in the study, such as t-tests, chi-square tests, regression analysis, or survival analysis.
- Understand the meaning and implications of statistical measures, including p-values, confidence intervals, effect sizes, and odds ratios.

Clinical Relevance
- Evaluate the clinical relevance of study findings by considering the magnitude of effect, clinical significance, and relevance to patient care.
- Determine whether the observed differences or associations are clinically meaningful and applicable to your patient population.

Confounding Factors and Bias
- Consider potential confounding factors and sources of bias that may influence the interpretation of study results.
- Assess whether the study adequately controlled for confounders and addressed sources of bias to ensure the validity of the findings.

Contextualization and Generalization
- Contextualize study findings within the broader clinical context, considering factors such as patient demographics, comorbidities, treatment adherence, and healthcare settings.
- Determine the extent to which study findings can be generalized to your patient population and clinical practice.

Consistency and Reproducibility
- Evaluate the consistency of study findings with existing evidence from other studies or systematic reviews.
- Consider whether study results are reproducible and whether they have been independently validated in other settings or populations.

Causality vs. Association
- Differentiate between causality and association when interpreting study results. Correlation does not imply causation, so be cautious when inferring causal relationships based on observational data.
- Consider the strength of evidence supporting causal relationships, including temporal sequence, dose-response relationships, and consistency across studies.

Clinical Decision Making
- Use statistical data to inform clinical decision-making, treatment planning, and patient management strategies.
- Consider the balance between benefits and risks when applying study findings to patients, taking into account patient preferences, values, and goals of care.

References
- Kirkwood, B. R., & Sterne, J. A. (2010). Essential medical statistics. John Wiley & Sons.
- Altman, D. G., & Bland, J. M. (1994). Statistics notes: The normal distribution. BMJ, 309(6960), 434.
- Armitage, P., Berry, G., & Matthews, J. N. S. (2008). Statistical methods in medical research. John Wiley & Sons.
- Porta, M. (2014). A dictionary of epidemiology. Oxford University Press.
- Sackett, D. L., Straus, S. E., Richardson, W. S., Rosenberg, W., & Haynes, R. B. (2000). Evidence-based medicine: How to practice and teach EBM. Churchill Livingstone.

Chapter 19: Wound Care Essentials

Reviewed by
Dean Nguyen, MD, RN

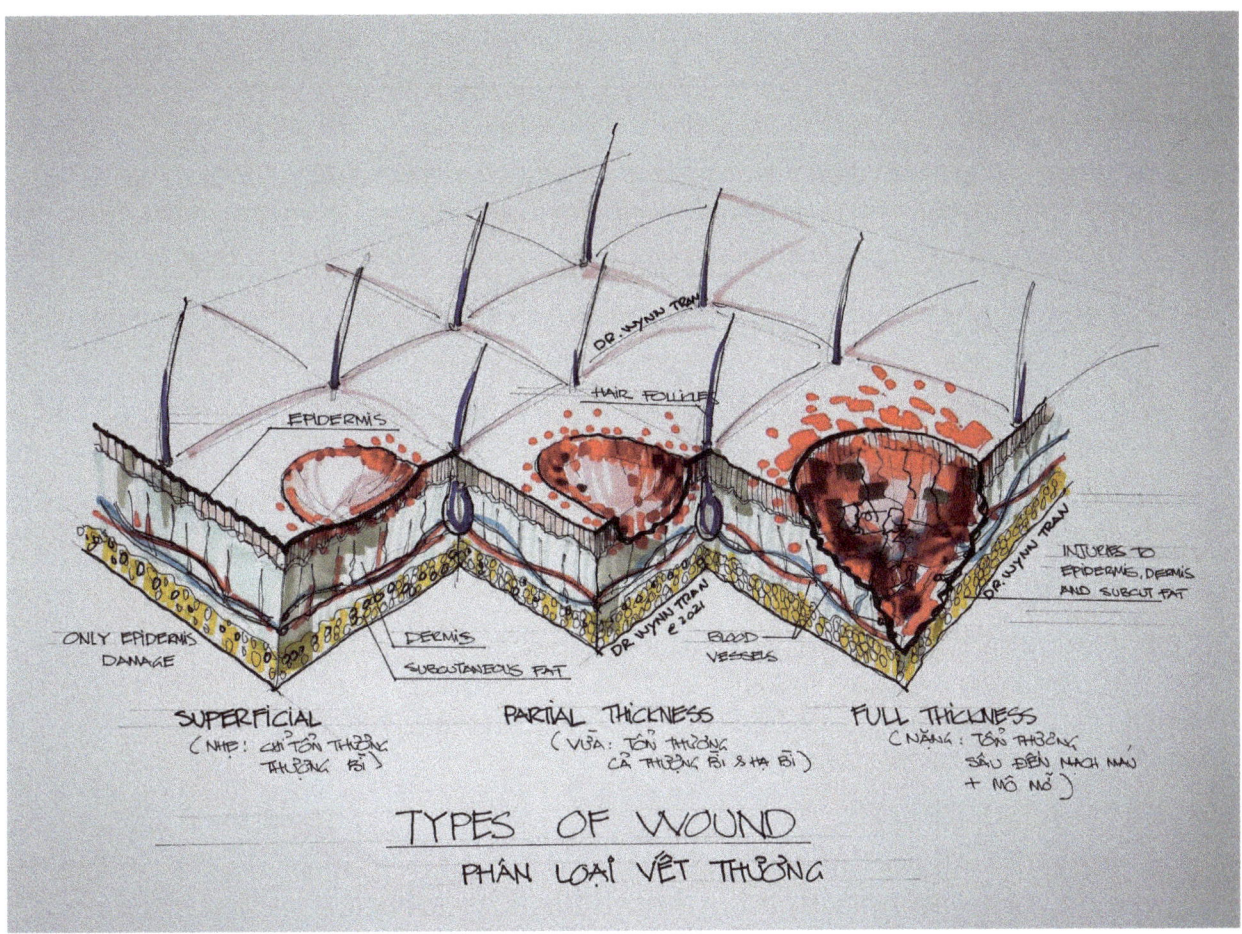

The APh should be familiar with the presentation, diagnosis, and management of these common wounds to provide appropriate care and referral to wound care specialists when necessary.

19.1. Wound Overview

> ➤ Wounds are injuries to the skin or underlying tissues that result from physical trauma, surgery, or underlying medical conditions.
>
> ➤ They can vary in severity, size, and underlying tissue involvement. Understanding the different types and classifications of wounds is essential for the APh to have proper assessment, treatment, and management.

Acute Wounds

Acute wounds are caused by sudden injury or trauma to the skin and typically heal through a series of well-defined stages. Examples include:

- Incisions: Surgical wounds resulting from surgical procedures.
- Lacerations: Jagged or irregular cuts in the skin caused by sharp objects.
- Abrasions: Superficial wounds caused by friction or scraping of the skin.
- Puncture wounds: Penetrating injuries caused by sharp objects puncturing the skin.

Chronic Wounds

Chronic wounds are persistent wounds that fail to progress through the normal stages of wound healing within a reasonable timeframe. They often result from underlying medical conditions, impaired circulation, or prolonged pressure or trauma.

Common types include:

- Pressure ulcers (bedsores): Caused by prolonged pressure on the skin, often in bedridden or immobilized patients.
- Diabetic foot ulcers: Chronic wounds that develop on the feet of patients with diabetes, often due to neuropathy and poor circulation.
- Venous ulcers: Wounds that occur due to venous insufficiency, leading to poor circulation and tissue damage in the lower extremities.

Classification by Depth

Wounds can be classified based on structures (muscle, bone).

Classification by Etiology

Wounds can also be classified based on their underlying causes or etiology:

- Traumatic wounds: Result from physical injury or trauma, such as cuts, abrasions, or burns.

- Surgical wounds: Result from surgical procedures and are classified based on their cleanliness (clean, clean-contaminated, contaminated, dirty).
- Ulcers: Chronic wounds caused by underlying factors such as pressure, ischemia, neuropathy, or infection.

Classification by Healing Process

Wounds can be classified based on their expected healing process and trajectory:

- Healing by primary intention: Wounds with clean, well-approximated edges that heal without significant tissue loss or inflammation, such as surgical incisions.
- Healing by secondary intention: Wounds with irregular edges or tissue loss that require gradual closure through the formation of granulation tissue and epithelialization, such as large abrasions or pressure ulcers.
- Healing by tertiary intention (delayed closure): Wounds initially left open to allow for drainage or resolution of underlying issues before closure, such as contaminated or infected wounds.

Specialized Wound Types

Certain wounds have specific characteristics or etiologies that require specialized management:

- Burn wounds: Caused by thermal, chemical, or electrical injury, requiring specialized assessment and treatment to prevent infection, fluid loss, and tissue damage.
- Necrotizing fasciitis: A rare but serious bacterial infection that affects the skin, subcutaneous tissue, and fascia, leading to rapid tissue necrosis and systemic complications.

Other Classifications

Wounds can also be classified based on additional factors such as:

- Location
- Size
- Infection status. Presence of underlying conditions (e.g., vascular disease, immunosuppression)

19.2. Wound Assessment

> ➤ *Wound assessment involves evaluating factors like size, depth, tissue type, and presence of infection to guide appropriate management strategies.*
>
> ➤ *Principles of wound management focus on promoting healing, preventing infection, minimizing pain, and restoring function through techniques such as debridement, dressing selection, and addressing underlying factors like nutrition and mobility.*

1. **Comprehensive Assessment**
   - Conduct a thorough assessment of the wound, including its location, size, depth, edges, surrounding tissue, and presence of any exudate or necrotic tissue.
   - Evaluate the patient's medical history, comorbidities, medications, nutritional status, and lifestyle factors that may impact wound healing.

2. **Identification of Underlying Factors**
   - Determine the underlying etiology and contributing factors to the wound, such as trauma, pressure, ischemia, infection, or systemic conditions (e.g., diabetes, peripheral vascular disease).
   - Address any modifiable risk factors that may impede wound healing, such as smoking, poor nutrition, immobility, or inadequate wound care.

3. **Wound Classification**
   - Classify the wound based on its type (acute vs. chronic), depth, etiology, and healing trajectory to guide appropriate management strategies.
   - Differentiate between clean, contaminated, or infected wounds to determine the need for antimicrobial therapy and wound debridement.

4. **Wound Debridement**
   - Remove non-viable tissue, debris, and foreign material from the wound bed through mechanical, surgical, enzymatic, or autolytic debridement techniques.
   - Promote the formation of granulation tissue and epithelialization by creating an optimal environment for wound healing.

5. Infection Control
- Assess the wound for signs and symptoms of infection, such as increased pain, erythema, warmth, swelling, purulent drainage, or systemic symptoms (fever, chills).
- Obtain wound cultures if indicated and initiate appropriate antimicrobial therapy based on the results and clinical presentation.

6. Moist Wound Healing
- Maintain a moist wound environment to facilitate cellular proliferation, angiogenesis, and collagen synthesis.
- Use appropriate dressings, such as hydrogels, hydrocolloids, foams, or films, to maintain moisture balance and promote autolytic debridement.

7. Optimal Nutrition and Hydration
- Ensure adequate nutrition and hydration to support wound healing and tissue repair.
- Assess the patient's nutritional status and provide nutritional supplementation or dietary modifications as needed, with a focus on protein, vitamins, and minerals essential for wound healing.

8. Offloading and Pressure Redistribution
- Implement offloading techniques and pressure redistribution devices to relieve pressure and minimize shear forces on pressure ulcers and other wounds.
- Encourage mobility, repositioning, and use of support surfaces (e.g., pressure-relieving mattresses, cushions) to prevent and manage pressure injuries.

9. Pain Management
- Assess and manage pain associated with the wound, using appropriate pharmacological and non-pharmacological interventions.
- Consider the patient's pain tolerance, preferences, and potential adverse effects of analgesic medications in pain management.

19.3. Wound Dressing

> ➤ Wound dressing involves applying a sterile material to a wound to protect it from infection, absorb exudate, maintain a moist environment to promote healing, and provide support and protection to the injured area.
>
> ➤ The choice of dressing depends on the wound type, size, location, and healing stage, ranging from simple adhesive bandages for minor cuts to advanced options like hydrogels, alginate dressings, and silver-impregnated antimicrobial dressings for more complex wounds.

1. **Assessment of the Wound**
   - Begin by assessing the wound, including its size, depth, location, and characteristics (e.g., presence of necrotic tissue, amount of exudate, signs of infection).
   - Consider the patient's overall health status, comorbidities, and preferences when selecting a wound dressing.

2. **Wound Cleansing**
   - Cleanse the wound using a gentle, non-toxic wound cleanser or saline solution to remove debris, bacteria, and excess exudate.
   - Avoid using harsh antiseptics or cytotoxic solutions that may damage healthy tissue.

3. **Selection of Wound Dressing**

Choose a wound dressing based on the characteristics and needs of the wound:

   - Alginate dressings: Suitable for moderate to heavily exuding wounds, providing absorbency and maintaining a moist environment.
   - Hydrocolloid dressings: Ideal for lightly to moderately exuding wounds, promoting autolytic debridement and granulation tissue formation.
   - Foam dressings: Effective for wounds with moderate to heavy exudate, providing absorption, cushioning, and protection.
   - Hydrogel dressings: Recommended for dry or necrotic wounds, hydrating the wound bed and facilitating autolytic debridement.
   - Transparent films: Suitable for superficial wounds or as secondary dressings, providing a barrier against water and bacteria while allowing visualization of the wound.

4. Application Techniques

   a. Wash hands and wear appropriate personal protective equipment (PPE) before applying wound dressings to prevent contamination.

   b. Use aseptic technique when handling wound dressings to minimize the risk of infection.

   c. Cut the dressing to the appropriate size, ensuring that it covers the entire wound bed and extends slightly beyond the wound margins.

   d. Apply the dressing gently to avoid trauma to the wound bed and surrounding tissue.

   e. Secure the dressing in place using medical tape, adhesive strips, or a cohesive bandage, ensuring that it is snug but not too tight to impede circulation.

   f. Consider using additional fixation devices (e.g., adhesive borders, net dressings) for wounds in areas prone to movement or friction.

Monitoring and Replacement

- Regularly monitor the wound and dressing for signs of infection, excessive exudate, or deterioration of the wound bed.
- Change the dressing as needed based on the wound assessment findings, typically every 1-3 days or as recommended by the healthcare provider.
- Document the type of dressing applied, the condition of the wound, and any changes observed during each dressing change.

Patient Education

- Educate the patient and caregivers on the purpose of the wound dressing, proper application technique, and signs of complications to watch for (e.g., increasing pain, redness, swelling, or drainage).
- Provide instructions on wound care, dressing changes, and follow-up appointments to promote optimal wound healing and prevent complications.

19.4. Wound Complications

> ➤ *Complications of wound healing include infection, excessive inflammation, delayed healing, and formation of abnormal scars like keloids or hypertrophic scars.*
>
> ➤ *Appropriate interventions may involve addressing underlying causes, managing infection with antibiotics, promoting a healthy wound environment with appropriate dressings, and considering advanced therapies like negative pressure wound therapy or surgical consult for complex cases.*

Infection
- <u>Signs and Symptoms:</u> Increased pain, redness, swelling, warmth, and purulent discharge from the wound.
- <u>Interventions:</u>
    1. Obtain wound cultures for bacterial identification and sensitivity testing.
    2. Initiate appropriate antimicrobial therapy based on culture results and clinical presentation.
    3. Perform wound debridement to remove infected tissue and promote healing.
    4. Implement infection control measures, such as hand hygiene and aseptic technique during wound care.

Delayed Healing
- <u>Signs and Symptoms:</u> Prolonged wound healing beyond the expected timeframe, failure to progress through the stages of healing.
- <u>Interventions:</u>
    1. Identify and address underlying factors contributing to delayed healing, such as poor nutrition, inadequate blood supply, or systemic diseases.
    2. Optimize wound care interventions, including debridement, dressing selection, and offloading techniques.
    3. Consider adjunctive therapies such as growth factors, hyperbaric oxygen therapy, or advanced wound care modalities.

Excessive Granulation Tissue (Hypergranulation)
- <u>Signs and Symptoms:</u> Overgrowth of granulation tissue above the wound surface, hindering epithelialization and wound closure.

- Interventions:
    1. Trim excess granulation tissue using sterile scissors or electrocautery under local anesthesia.
    2. Apply silver nitrate or topical steroids to reduce hypergranulation and promote wound healing.
    3. Adjust the frequency and type of wound dressings to create a moist wound environment conducive to epithelialization.

Dehiscence
- Signs and Symptoms: Separation of wound edges along the incision line, leading to partial or complete wound opening.
- Interventions:
    1. Provide supportive wound care, including gentle cleansing, debridement of necrotic tissue, and application of appropriate wound dressings.
    2. Implement measures to reduce tension on the wound, such as using sutures, staples, or adhesive strips to approximate wound edges.
    3. Monitor for signs of infection or further wound breakdown and intervene promptly to prevent complications.

Hypertrophic Scarring and Keloids
- Signs and Symptoms: Excessive fibrous tissue formation at the wound site, resulting in raised, thickened scars.
- Interventions:
    1. Initiate early scar management interventions, including silicone gel sheets, pressure therapy, and massage techniques.
    2. Consider corticosteroid injections or laser therapy for hypertrophic scars and keloids to reduce inflammation and promote remodeling of collagen fibers.
    3. Educate patients on scar management strategies and encourage compliance with recommended interventions to optimize outcomes.

Chronic Wound Formation
- Signs and Symptoms: Wounds that fail to progress through the stages of healing and remain open for an extended period.

- Interventions:
    1. Identify and address underlying factors contributing to chronic wound formation, such as vascular insufficiency, pressure, or infection.
    2. Implement a multidisciplinary approach to wound management, involving specialists such as wound care nurses, vascular surgeons, and infectious disease specialists.
    3. Utilize advanced wound care modalities, including negative pressure wound therapy, bioengineered skin substitutes, and electrical stimulation, to promote wound healing and closure.

References

- Falabella, A. F., Kirsner, R. S., & Eaglstein, W. H. (2001). The use of Dermagraft, a cultured human dermis, to treat diabetic foot ulcers. Diabetes Care, 24(2), 290-295.
- Snyder, R. J., Frykberg, R. G., Rogers, L. C., Applewhite, A. J., Bell, D., Bohn, G., ... & Wound Healing Society. (2010). The management of diabetic foot ulcers through optimal off-loading: Building consensus guidelines and practical recommendations to improve outcomes. Journal of the American Podiatric Medical Association, 100(5), 369-378.
- Thomas, S., Loveless, P., & Hay, N. P. (2016). Advanced wound care products: A review of the current evidence. Future Medicine, 8(12), 1013-1025.
- Gottrup, F., Apelqvist, J., Bjarnsholt, T., Cooper, R., Moore, Z., Peters, E., ... & Löndahl, M. (2013). EWMA document: Antimicrobials and non-healing wounds—Evidence, controversies and suggestions. Journal of Wound Care, 22(Sup10), S1-S89.

Chapter 20: Surgical Care Essentials

20.1. Pre-Operative Assessment

> ➢ *For the APh, preoperative assessment involves reviewing patient medical history, current medications, allergies, and lab results to identify potential risks and optimize medication regimens.*
>
> ➢ *Optimization strategies may include adjusting doses, discontinuing medications that increase surgical complications, and initiating prophylactic therapies to minimize perioperative risks such as infection or thrombosis.*
>
> ➢ *Collaboration with the surgical team and PCP ensures comprehensive preoperative care tailored to individual patient needs, optimizing surgical outcomes.*

1. **Comprehensive Medication Review**
   - Conduct a comprehensive review of the patient's medication history, including prescription medications, over-the-counter drugs, herbal supplements, and dietary supplements.
   - Evaluate potential drug interactions, adverse effects, and contraindications that may impact perioperative management.
   - Collaborate with other providers to adjust or modify medications as needed to minimize perioperative risks and optimize medication therapy.

2. **Assessment of Medical History and Comorbidities**
   - Gather and assess the patient's medical history, including past surgical procedures, chronic medical conditions, allergies, and comorbidities.
   - Identify any medical conditions that may affect perioperative management, such as cardiovascular disease, diabetes, hypertension, or respiratory disorders.

3. **Risk Assessment and Stratification**
   - Utilize risk assessment tools, such as the American Society of Anesthesiologists (ASA) Physical Status Classification System or the American College of Surgeons National Surgical Quality Improvement Program (ACS NSQIP) to stratify patients.

4. ASA Physical Status Classification

Classification	Description
ASA I	A healthy patient
ASA II	A patient with mild systemic disease
ASA III	A patient with severe systemic disease but is not incapacitating
ASA IV	A patient with incapacitating systemic disease that is a constant threat to life
ASA V	A moribund patient who is not expected to survive without the operation
ASA VI	A declared brain-dead patient whose organs are being removed for donor purposes

The ACS NSQIP Surgical Risk Calculator Online at
https://riskcalculator.facs.org/RiskCalculator/

- Individualized Risk Assessment: The calculator estimates the chances of various outcomes, such as complications, mortality, and the length of hospital stay, based on a patient's individual risk factors and the type of surgical procedure planned.
- Wide Range of Procedures: It covers a vast array of surgical procedures across multiple specialties, making it a versatile tool for many types of surgeries.
- Evidence-Based: The risk estimates are derived from clinical data collected from hospitals participating in the ACS NSQIP, ensuring that the calculator is grounded in real-world outcomes.

5. Preoperative Medication Management

- Optimize preoperative medications to minimize perioperative complications and ensure optimal perioperative outcomes.
- Provide recommendations for perioperative medication management, including instructions for medication continuation, modification, or discontinuation based on clinical guidelines and best practices.
- Consider the timing of medication administration and potential drug interactions with anesthetic agents.

6. Assessment of Nutritional Status and Fluid Management

- Evaluate the patient's nutritional status and hydration status, as malnutrition and dehydration can increase the risk of perioperative complications and impair wound healing.

- Provide recommendations for preoperative nutritional supplementation or fluid management as needed to optimize perioperative outcomes.
- Consider the patient's fasting status and provide guidance on preoperative fasting guidelines to prevent perioperative complications.

7. **Identification of Anesthetic Considerations**
   - Collaborate with the anesthesia team to identify and address specific anesthetic considerations based on the patient's medical history, medication regimen, and surgical procedure.
   - Discuss potential drug allergies, medication interactions, or adverse reactions to anesthetic agents with the anesthesia provider.
   - Ensure appropriate perioperative monitoring and management of anesthesia-related concerns, such as postoperative nausea and vomiting (PONV) or intraoperative hypotension.

8. **Coordination of Care and Interdisciplinary Collaboration**
   - Collaborate closely with the multidisciplinary healthcare team, including surgeons, anesthesiologists, nurses, and other allied healthcare professionals, to ensure comprehensive preoperative assessment and optimization.
   - Facilitate communication and information sharing between healthcare providers to promote continuity of care and seamless perioperative management.
   - Participate in interdisciplinary rounds, case conferences, and care planning meetings to coordinate perioperative care and address patient-specific needs.

9. **Documentation and Follow-Up**
   - Document preoperative assessments, medication recommendations, and interventions in the patient's medical record in a clear, concise, and timely manner.
   - Ensure accurate and thorough documentation of preoperative medication orders, allergy information, and other pertinent details for perioperative care.
   - Follow up with patients postoperatively to monitor medication adherence, manage postoperative pain, and address any medication-related concerns or complications.

20.2. Anticoagulation for Dental Procedure

> ➢ The American Dental Association (ADA) provides guidance for managing patients on anticoagulation therapy undergoing dental procedures to balance the risk of bleeding with the risk of thromboembolism.

Continuing Anticoagulation Therapy

The ADA suggests that for most dental procedures, including extractions, implant placement, and periodontal surgery, patients can continue their anticoagulant or antiplatelet medication as usual. The risk of thromboembolic events outweighs the risk of post-procedure bleeding, which can usually be managed with local hemostatic measures.

1. Warfarin

Patients on warfarin should have their International Normalized Ratio (INR) checked close to the time of the procedure. Dental treatments can generally proceed safely if the INR is within the therapeutic range, typically 2.0 to 3.5, depending on the indication for anticoagulation.

2. Direct Oral Anticoagulants (DOACs)

For patients taking DOACs (e.g., apixaban, rivaroxaban, dabigatran, and edoxaban), the ADA notes that these medications do not require routine discontinuation for dental procedures. Local hemostatic measures and timing the procedure (considering the half-life and dosing schedule of the medication) can effectively manage bleeding risks.

3. Local Hemostatic Measures

Effective local measures to control bleeding include the use of sutures, pressure packs, local hemostatic agents (such as tranexamic acid mouthwash), and fibrin glue.

4. Communication with Dentist and PCP

It's crucial to communicate with the patient's PCP and dentist, especially for patients with complex medical histories or when performing extensive surgical procedures.

5. Patient Education

Advise patients not to discontinue or alter their anticoagulation medication without consulting their healthcare provider.

Inform patients about signs of excessive bleeding and when to seek immediate care.

20.3. Post-Operative Complications

> - Post-operative complications can vary widely but commonly include infection, bleeding, thromboembolism (such as deep vein thrombosis and pulmonary embolism), and delayed wound healing.
> - These complications can affect recovery time and overall outcomes, necessitating close monitoring and sometimes additional interventions.
> - Risk factors include the type of surgery, patient's age, pre-existing health conditions, and the length of the surgical procedure.

Cause	Key Manifestations	Management
Neurologic		
Delirium Tremens	Altered mental status, hypertension, tachycardia, hallucinations	IV Benzodiazepines
Pulmonary		
Pulmonary Embolism	Acute onset shortness of breath, pleuritis chest pain, hypoxia, tachycardia	CT chest angiogram or lower extremity venous doppler, anticoagulation, early ambulation, inferior vena cava filter if contraindication to anticoagulation
Tension Pneumothorax	<ul><li>Increasing difficulty bag mask ventilation</li><li>Decrease in blood pressure.</li><li>Increase in central venous pressure and jugular vein distention</li></ul>	Needle decompression followed by chest tube
Aspiration Pneumonitis	Vomiting during intubation	NPO prior to procedure, bronchoalveolar lavage
Cardiovascular		

Perioperative Myocardial Infarction	Chest pain, elevated troponin, ST elevation	Percutaneous intervention
Gastrointestinal		
Postoperative Ileus	Abdominal distention, no pain, absent bowel sounds	Observation, treat electrolyte abnormalities such as hypokalemia
Mechanical Bowel Obstruction	Abdominal x-ray with dilated loops and air fluid levels, abdominal pain/distention, tinkling bowel sounds	Decompression with nasogastric tube, bowel rest, +/- surgical intervention for lysis of adhesions
Fistulas	Connection of bowel with bowel, bladder, vagina or skin; fecal material will come out with the connecting organ	Fistulotomy, treat/remove aggravating agents such as foreign bodies, epithelialization, tumors, infection, irradiated tissue, inflammatory bowel disease, or obstruction
Genitourinary		
Postoperative Urinary Retention	Sensation to void, however unable, suprapublic fullness	Early ambulation, bladder scan, indwelling catheter after multiple catheterizations
Renal		
Electrolyte Derangements (sodium, calcium, glucose)	Altered mental status, lethargy, paresthesia (hypocalcemia)	Treat metabolic derangements

20.4. Post-Operative Concerned Symptoms

Concerned Symptoms	Possible Cause
Incisional Pain	Inadequate pain control, wound infection (acute/necrotizing, delayed), wound disruption/dehiscence
Nausea/Vomiting	Reaction to medication (including anesthesia), paralytic ileus
Acute Confusion	Medications, sleep disturbances, dehydration, hemorrhage, sepsis
Tachycardia	Pain, volume depletion, hemorrhage, atrial fibrillation (or other conduction abnormality)
Hypotension	Volume depletion, atrial fibrillation (or other conduction abnormality)
Hypertension	Pain, baseline hypertension (home medications not resumed)
Chest Pain	Myocardial ischemia, reactive airway
Dyspnea	Atelectasis, reactive airway, pneumonia, failure to clear secretions, fluid overload, pulmonary embolism, myocardial ischemia
Leg Swelling	Fluid overload, venous thromboembolism
Low Urine Output	Volume depletion, urinary retention, hemorrhage, urinary tract infection
Fever	Atelectasis, surgical site infection, urinary tract infection, drug reaction

20.5. Post-Operative Monitoring

> ➤ The APh monitors patients postoperatively for complications like pain, infection, thromboembolism, or adverse drug reactions, ensuring timely intervention and optimizing medication therapy.
>
> ➤ Appropriate interventions may include pain management strategies, antibiotic stewardship, anticoagulation therapy, and adjusting medications to prevent or manage complications, collaborating closely with the surgical team and PCP to optimize patient outcomes.

1. **Continuous Monitoring**
   - Implement a system for continuous monitoring of postoperative patients, including vital signs, pain levels, fluid balance, and laboratory values.
   - Utilize electronic health records (EHR) or mobile health applications to track and document postoperative parameters in real-time for timely intervention.

2. **Assessment of Complications**
   - Conduct regular assessments to identify signs and symptoms of postoperative complications, such as surgical site infections, wound dehiscence, deep vein thrombosis (DVT), pulmonary embolism (PE), and adverse drug reactions.
   - Utilize standardized assessment tools and clinical guidelines to systematically evaluate patients for common postoperative complications.

3. **Pain Management**
   - Assess postoperative pain intensity using validated pain scales and patient-reported outcomes.
   - Optimize pain management strategies based on the severity and nature of pain, patient preferences, and response to analgesic therapy.
   - Provide multimodal analgesia and adjunctive therapies to minimize opioid use and reduce the risk of opioid-related adverse effects.

4. **Fluid and Electrolyte Management**
   - Monitor fluid balance, electrolyte levels, and renal function in postoperative patients to prevent dehydration, electrolyte imbalances, and acute kidney injury.

- Provide appropriate intravenous fluids and electrolyte supplementation based on patient patient needs and perioperative fluid losses.

5. **Prevention and Management of Surgical Site Complications**
    - Implement evidence-based strategies to prevent surgical site infections, including perioperative antimicrobial prophylaxis, meticulous surgical technique, and postoperative wound care.
    - Monitor surgical incisions for signs of infection, such as erythema, swelling, warmth, and purulent drainage, and intervene promptly with antimicrobial therapy and wound care as needed.

6. **Prevention and Management of Thromboembolic Events**
    - Assess postoperative patients for risk factors for venous thromboembolism (VTE), such as immobility, obesity, age, and history of VTE.
    - Implement pharmacologic and mechanical thromboprophylaxis measures based on individualized risk assessment and perioperative guidelines.
    - Monitor for signs and symptoms of DVT and PE, such as swelling, pain, redness, dyspnea, and chest pain, and initiate prompt treatment if suspected.

7. **Monitoring and Management of Adverse Drug Reactions**
    - Monitor postoperative patients for adverse drug reactions, drug interactions, and medication errors that may occur during the perioperative period.
    - Conduct medication reconciliation and review medication orders to ensure appropriateness, accuracy, and adherence to evidence-based guidelines.
    - Provide education to patients and caregivers about common adverse effects of postoperative medications and strategies to manage them effectively.

8. **Coordination of Care and Interdisciplinary Collaboration**
    - Collaborate closely with the interdisciplinary healthcare team, including surgeons, anesthesiologists, nurses, and other allied healthcare professionals, to coordinate postoperative care and address patient-specific needs.
    - Facilitate communication and information sharing between healthcare providers to ensure continuity of care and timely intervention for postoperative complications.

9. Patient Education and Support

- Provide postoperative education to patients and caregivers regarding signs and symptoms of common postoperative complications, self-care measures, and follow-up appointments.
- Offer support and guidance to patients throughout the postoperative recovery process, addressing any concerns or questions they may have about their care.

10. Documentation and Quality Improvement

- Document postoperative monitoring parameters, assessments, interventions, and outcomes in a systematic and comprehensive manner using standardized documentation tools and protocols.
- Participate in quality improvement initiatives, adverse event reporting, and medication safety reviews to identify opportunities for enhancing postoperative care and reducing the risk of complications.

20.6. Post-Operative Pain Management

> ➤ *Post-surgical pain management strategies involve a multimodal approach combining analgesic medications, regional anesthesia techniques, and non-pharmacological interventions to optimize pain relief while minimizing side effects.*
>
> ➤ *The APh should consider patient factors, type of surgery, and pain severity, aiming to enhance recovery, improve comfort, and reduce opioid consumption.*
>
> ➤ *Close monitoring, titration of medications, and early intervention for breakthrough pain are key elements in achieving effective pain control in the postoperative period.*

1. Multimodal Analgesia

- Recommend a multimodal approach to pain management combining different classes of analgesic agents with complementary mechanisms of action.
- Utilize non-opioid analgesics such as acetaminophen, nonsteroidal anti-inflammatory drugs (NSAIDs), and COX-2 inhibitors as first-line agents for mild to moderate pain.
- Consider adjuvant analgesics such as gabapentinoids, tricyclic antidepressants, and topical agents for neuropathic pain or as adjunctive therapy to enhance pain relief and reduce opioid requirements.

2. Opioid Analgesics

- Use opioid analgesics judiciously and in accordance with evidence-based guidelines to manage moderate to severe pain not adequately controlled with non-opioid analgesics alone.
- Prescribe opioids at the lowest effective dose and for the shortest duration necessary to achieve adequate pain control while minimizing the risk of opioid-related adverse effects and complications.
- Educate patients about the potential risks of opioid therapy, including respiratory depression, sedation, constipation, tolerance, dependence, and opioid use disorder.

3. Patient-Controlled Analgesia (PCA)

- Consider PCA as an option for patient-controlled delivery of opioid analgesics, allowing patients to self-administer bolus doses within preset limits to manage their pain effectively.
- Provide thorough education and instructions to patients and caregivers on the proper use of PCA devices, including dosing parameters, lockout intervals, and potential adverse effects.

4. Regional Anesthesia Techniques

- Recommend regional anesthesia techniques such as epidural analgesia, peripheral nerve blocks, and local infiltration anesthesia to provide targeted pain relief and minimize systemic opioid exposure.
- Collaborate with the anesthesia team to optimize the selection and administration of regional anesthesia techniques based on the surgical procedure, patient factors, and perioperative goals.

5. Enhanced Recovery After Surgery (ERAS) Protocols

- Advocate for the implementation of ERAS protocols incorporating evidence-based perioperative interventions to optimize pain management, reduce opioid consumption, and accelerate recovery following surgery.
- Encourage early mobilization, nutrition optimization, and multimodal analgesia within the framework of ERAS pathways to enhance postoperative outcomes and minimize complications.

6. Nonpharmacological Pain Management Modalities

- Promote the use of nonpharmacological pain management modalities such as cognitive-behavioral therapy, relaxation techniques, distraction therapy, acupuncture, and physical therapy to complement pharmacologic interventions and enhance pain relief.

- Provide education and resources to patients on self-management strategies and coping mechanisms to empower them in managing their pain effectively.

7. Individualized Pain Management Plans

- Tailor pain management to the patient's needs, preferences, and goals, considering factors such as age, comorbidities, surgical complexity, and prior analgesic response.
- Monitor and reassess pain intensity, functional status, and treatment response regularly to adjust pain management strategies as needed throughout the post-surgical period.

8. Education and Counseling

- Offer comprehensive education and counseling to patients and caregivers on the importance of pain management, expected postoperative pain levels, analgesic options, potential side effects, and strategies for optimizing pain relief.
- Encourage open communication and shared decision-making between patients, caregivers, and The APh to address concerns, manage expectations, and promote collaborative pain management efforts.

20.7. Post-Operative Nutrition and Rehabilitation

> ➤ *Post-surgery, nutritional support focuses on optimizing protein intake, vitamins, and minerals to facilitate wound healing and prevent malnutrition-related complications.*
>
> ➤ *Rehabilitation includes early mobilization, physical therapy, and occupational therapy to restore function, strength, and independence, enhancing overall recovery and quality of life.*

1. Nutritional Support

- Early Assessment: Conduct a thorough assessment of the patient's nutritional status, including weight history, dietary habits, and any existing nutritional deficiencies.
- individualized Plan: Develop a personalized nutrition plan based on the patient's specific needs, considering factors such as age, medical history, type of surgery, and postoperative complications.
- Balanced Diet: Encourage a balanced diet rich in essential nutrients, including protein, vitamins, minerals, and fiber, to support healing and recovery.

- Supplementation: Consider nutritional supplements or specialized formulas to address any deficiencies and promote optimal healing. Vitamin C, zinc, and omega-3 fatty acids may be particularly beneficial for wound healing.

2. **Hydration Management**
   - Fluid Intake: Ensure adequate hydration by encouraging the patient to drink plenty of fluids, such as water, herbal teas, and broth.
   - Electrolyte Balance: Monitor electrolyte levels and provide electrolyte-rich beverages or oral rehydration solutions to maintain proper electrolyte balance.

3. **Physical Rehabilitation:**
   - Early Mobilization: Encourage early mobilization and gradual increases in physical activity to prevent muscle weakness, joint stiffness, and complications such as deep vein thrombosis (DVT).
   - Physical Therapy: Refer patients to physical therapists for tailored rehabilitation programs focusing on strength, flexibility, balance, and functional mobility.
   - Range of Motion Exercises: Teach patients a range of motion exercises to improve joint flexibility and prevent contractures, especially for orthopedic and neurosurgical procedures..

4. **Psychological Support**
   - Emotional Well-being: Address the patient's emotional well-being and provide psychological support to help cope with the stress, anxiety, and depression that may arise during the recovery process.
   - Support Groups: Connect patients with support groups, counseling services, or peer mentors who can offer encouragement, guidance, and empathy.

5. **Wound Care**
   - Wound Assessment: Monitor surgical incisions for signs of infection, inflammation, or delayed healing, and promptly report any concerns to the healthcare provider.
   - Dressing Changes: Perform wound dressing changes according to the surgeon's instructions, using sterile technique and appropriate wound care products.

20.8. Post-Operative Medication Management

> ➤ *Postoperative medication management involves ensuring appropriate pain control, preventing infections, managing chronic conditions, and minimizing adverse drug interactions.*
>
> ➤ *The APh should consider patient factors, surgical procedures, and potential complications to optimize outcomes and promote recovery. Close monitoring, patient education, and collaboration among surgical team, PCP, and specialist providers are essential for safe and effective postoperative medication management.*

1. **Analgesics Medications**
   - <u>Opioid Analgesics:</u> Prescribe opioid analgesics judiciously for pain management, considering the severity of pain, patient's tolerance, and risk of adverse effects such as respiratory depression and opioid dependence.
   - <u>Non-Opioid Analgesics:</u> Utilize non-opioid analgesics such as acetaminophen, nonsteroidal anti-inflammatory drugs (NSAIDs), and COX-2 inhibitors as first-line agents for mild to moderate pain.

2. **Antiemetics Medications**
   - Prescribe antiemetic medications to prevent and manage postoperative nausea and vomiting (PONV), especially in patients at high risk due to factors such as anesthesia type, surgical procedure, and patient susceptibility.
   - Consider the use of serotonin receptor antagonists (e.g., ondansetron), dopamine receptor antagonists (e.g., metoclopramide), and antihistamines (e.g., dimenhydrinate) for prophylaxis and treatment of PONV.

3. **Prophylactic Antibiotics Medications**
   - Administer prophylactic antibiotics before surgery as recommended by evidence-based guidelines to reduce the risk of surgical site infections (SSIs) and other postoperative infections.
   - Select antibiotics based on the type of surgery, local antimicrobial resistance patterns, and patient-specific factors, and adhere to appropriate dosing and duration recommendations.

4. **Anticoagulants and Thromboprophylaxis Medications**
   - Initiate pharmacologic thromboprophylaxis with anticoagulant medications, such as low molecular weight heparin (LMWH), unfractionated heparin (UFH), or direct oral anticoagulants (DOACs),

to prevent venous thromboembolism (VTE) in high-risk surgical patients.
- Individualized thromboprophylaxis regimens based on patient-specific risk factors, surgical procedure, bleeding risk, and contraindications to anticoagulant therapy.

5. Gastrointestinal Prophylaxis Medications
- Consider prophylactic medications such as proton pump inhibitors (PPIs) or histamine-2 receptor antagonists (H2RAs) to prevent stress-related mucosal damage and gastrointestinal bleeding in critically ill or high-risk surgical patients.
- Evaluate the need for gastrointestinal prophylaxis based on patient factors, duration of mechanical ventilation, and risk of stress ulcers.

6. Anticoagulation Reversal Agents
- Familiarize yourself with the appropriate use of anticoagulation reversal agents, such as protamine sulfate for heparin reversal and vitamin K or prothrombin complex concentrates (PCCs) for warfarin reversal, in the event of bleeding complications or urgent surgery.

7. Diabetes Management
- Optimize glycemic control in diabetic patients during the perioperative period to minimize the risk of hyperglycemia-related complications such as wound infection and delayed wound healing.
- Adjust diabetes medications, insulin regimens, and glucose monitoring protocols based on perioperative fasting status, insulin sensitivity, and anticipated changes in nutritional intake.

8. Antihypertensive Agents
- Continue or resume antihypertensive medications in the postoperative period to maintain blood pressure control and prevent hypertensive crises, especially in patients with preexisting hypertension or cardiovascular disease.
- Monitor blood pressure closely and adjust antihypertensive therapy as needed based on hemodynamic stability, fluid status, and patient response to treatment.

9. Psychotropic Medications
- Review and optimize psychotropic medication regimens for patients with preexisting psychiatric conditions, ensuring continuity of care and adherence to treatment protocols during the perioperative period.
- Consider adjustments to psychotropic medications based on factors such as drug interactions, sedation risk, and perioperative stressors.

10. Patient Education and Counseling

- The APh should provide a comprehensive education to patients and caregivers on medication management principles, including medication names, doses, frequencies, indications, adverse effects, and instructions for administration.
- Emphasize the importance of medication adherence, follow-up appointments, and communication with The APh regarding any concerns or changes in symptoms.

References

- Fleisher, L. A., Fleischmann, K. E., Auerbach, A. D., Barnason, S. A., Beckman, J. A., Bozkurt, B., ... & Young, B. (2014). 2014 ACC/AHA guideline on perioperative cardiovascular evaluation and management of patients undergoing noncardiac surgery: a report of the American College of Cardiology/American Heart Association Task Force on practice guidelines. Journal of the American College of Cardiology, 64(22), e77-e137.
- Grocott, M. P. W., Pearse, R. M., & Mythen, M. G. (2017). Perioperative medicine: the value proposition for anesthesia?: a UK perspective on delivering value from anesthesiology. Anesthesiology, 126(2), 182-186.
- Chou, R., Gordon, D. B., de Leon-Casasola, O. A., Rosenberg, J. M., Bickler, S., Brennan, T., ... & Wu, C. L. (2016). Management of postoperative pain: a clinical practice guideline from the American Pain Society, the American Society of Regional Anesthesia and Pain Medicine, and the American Society of Anesthesiologists' Committee on Regional Anesthesia, Executive Committee, and Administrative Council. The journal of pain, 17(2), 131-157.
- McClave, S. A., Taylor, B. E., Martindale, R. G., Warren, M. M., Johnson, D. R., Braunschweig, C., ... & Compher, C. (2016). Guidelines for the provision and assessment of nutrition support therapy in the adult critically ill patient: Society of Critical Care Medicine (SCCM) and American Society for Parenteral and Enteral Nutrition (ASPEN). JPEN Journal of parenteral and enteral nutrition, 40(2), 159-211.
- Vetter, T. R., & Jones, K. A. (2018). Perioperative medication management: fundamentals for the anesthesia provider. Anesthesia & Analgesia, 126(5), 1478-1490.

Chapter 21: Post-Hospitalization Care

21.1. Transition of Care

> ➢ *Transition of care from hospital to home involves coordinating discharge planning, medication reconciliation, and patient education to ensure a smooth and safe transition. The APh should provide clear instructions, arranging follow-up appointments, and connecting patients with community resources for ongoing support.*
>
> ➢ *Effective communication among hospitalists, discharge RN and case manager, patients, and caregivers is essential to prevent complications, readmissions, and promote successful recovery at home.*

1. Medication Reconciliation
- Conduct a thorough medication reconciliation process to ensure accurate and up-to-date medication lists, including prescription medications, over-the-counter products, supplements, and herbal remedies.
- Verify medication names, dosages, frequencies, routes of administration, and indications with the patient, caregivers, and other healthcare providers to prevent medication errors and adverse drug events.

2. Discharge Planning
- Initiate discharge planning early in the hospitalization process, involving interdisciplinary care team members, including physicians, pharmacists, nurses, social workers, and case managers.
- Collaborate with patients, caregivers, and community resources to develop individualized discharge plans addressing post-discharge needs, such as medication management, follow-up appointments, home care services, and rehabilitation programs.

3. Patient Education
- Provide comprehensive education to patients and caregivers on post-discharge care instructions, including medication regimens, dosing schedules, potential side effects, and instructions for monitoring and self-management.

- Use patient-friendly materials, visual aids, and teach-back techniques to enhance patient understanding and adherence to discharge instructions.

4. Medication Counseling

- Conduct medication counseling sessions with patients and caregivers to review pre-hospitalization and post-hospitalization medications, including purpose, dosage, administration, side effects, drug interactions, and precautions.
- Address any concerns or questions raised by patients regarding their medications and provide clarification or additional information as needed.

5. Follow-up Care

- Schedule follow-up appointments with primary care providers, specialists, and other healthcare professionals to ensure continuity of care and ongoing monitoring of the patient's health status.
- Communicate discharge summaries, medication lists, and relevant clinical information to the receiving healthcare providers to facilitate seamless transitions and coordinated care.

6. Home Health Services

- Arrange home health services, if necessary, to provide additional support and assistance with activities of daily living, wound care, medication administration, physical therapy, and other healthcare needs.
- Coordinate with home health agencies, visiting nurses, and other community resources to ensure timely initiation and appropriate provision of services.

7. Remote Monitoring and Telehealth

- Implement remote monitoring technologies and telehealth solutions to remotely monitor patients' vital signs, medication adherence, and clinical status post-discharge.
- Conduct virtual follow-up visits, medication reviews, and patient assessments to enhance access to care, improve patient engagement, and identify potential issues early.

8. Patient Empowerment and Engagement

- Empower patients and caregivers to take an active role in their care management by providing tools, resources, and support for self-monitoring, self-care, and decision-making.
- Foster open communication, shared decision-making, and collaborative goal-setting between patients, caregivers, and

healthcare providers to promote patient-centered care and improve health outcomes.

9. **Continuous Quality Improvement**
   - Participate in quality improvement initiatives, performance metrics tracking, and post-discharge outcome assessments to evaluate the effectiveness of transition of care processes and identify areas for improvement.
   - Implement evidence-based interventions, best practices, and standardized protocols to enhance the quality, safety, and efficiency of transitions of care across care settings.

21.2. Post-Discharge Monitoring

> ➤ *Monitoring for post-discharge complications and readmissions involves implementing early warning systems, conducting follow-up assessments, and utilizing telehealth to detect and address issues promptly.*
>
> ➤ *The APh should understand the key aspects including tracking symptoms, medication adherence, and vital signs, while providing education and support to empower patients in self-management.*
>
> ➤ *Collaborative efforts among healthcare providers, patients, and caregivers aim to minimize complications and prevent unnecessary readmissions.*

1. **Early Warning Signs and Symptoms**
   - Educate patients and caregivers on common signs and symptoms of post-discharge complications, such as fever, pain, shortness of breath, swelling, redness, and changes in mental status.
   - Encourage patients to promptly report any new or worsening symptoms to their healthcare provider or seek medical attention if they experience concerns or difficulties at home.

2. **Scheduled Follow-Up Appointments**
   - Schedule timely follow-up appointments with primary care providers, the APh, specialists, or other healthcare professionals within the first week post-discharge to assess the patient's recovery progress, monitor for complications, and address any ongoing healthcare needs.
   - Ensure that patients are aware of their follow-up appointments, understand the importance of attending them, and have the

necessary resources to access transportation or arrange for support as needed.

3. **Remote Monitoring Technologies**
   - Implement remote monitoring technologies, such as wearable devices, mobile health applications, and telehealth platforms, to remotely track patients' vital signs, symptoms, medication adherence, and functional status post-discharge.
   - Use telehealth visits or virtual check-ins to conduct remote assessments, medication reviews, and patient education sessions, facilitating ongoing communication and support between healthcare providers and patients.

4. **Medication Reconciliation and Adherence**
   - Conduct medication reconciliation processes to ensure that patients understand their prescribed medications, including dosages, frequencies, and instructions for use, and have access to necessary medications post-discharge.
   - Monitor medication adherence and address any barriers or challenges to medication management, such as medication side effects, financial constraints, or difficulty obtaining refills.

5. **Transitional Care Coordination**
   - If possible, identify a designated care coordinator or case manager to oversee the transition of care process, coordinate post-discharge follow-up care, and monitor the patient's progress and outcomes.
   - Facilitate communication and collaboration among healthcare providers, patients, and caregivers to address any issues or concerns that arise during the post-discharge period and ensure continuity of care.

6. **Patient Education and Empowerment**
   - Provide comprehensive education to patients and caregivers on self-care strategies, symptom management techniques, and red flag warning signs indicating the need for medical attention post-discharge.
   - Empower patients to take an active role in their recovery and advocate for their healthcare needs by encouraging open communication, shared decision-making, and engagement in self-monitoring activities.

7. Early Intervention and Support Services
- Implement proactive interventions and support services to address identified risk factors, mitigate potential complications, and prevent hospital readmissions post-discharge.
- Collaborate with community resources, home health agencies, and social services to provide additional assistance with activities of daily living, rehabilitation, transportation, and psychosocial support as needed.

21.3. Patient Education on Self-care and Symptom Recognition

> ➢ *The APh could play an important role in a patient's self-care involving teaching about wound care, medication management, and recognizing signs of complications post-surgery or post-hospitalization.*
>
> ➢ *Emphasis is placed on empowering patients to identify and report symptoms like fever, pain, or wound changes promptly, fostering active participation in their recovery process.*

1. Discharge Instructions
- Provide clear and concise discharge instructions outlining medication regimens, follow-up appointments, activity restrictions, dietary guidelines, and self-care instructions.
- Use plain language and avoid medical jargon to enhance patient comprehension and adherence to post-discharge recommendations.

2. Medication Management
- Review the patient's medication list, including names, dosages, frequencies, and potential side effects.
- Emphasize the importance of medication adherence, proper administration techniques, and strategies for managing medication-related symptoms or adverse effects.

3. Wound Care
- Demonstrate proper wound care techniques, including dressing changes, wound inspection, and signs of infection.
- Educate patients on the importance of keeping the wound clean, dry, and protected, and when to seek medical attention for wound-related concerns.

4. Activity and Mobility
- Provide guidance on gradually resuming activities of daily living, exercise, and mobility following discharge.

- Encourage patients to follow prescribed activity levels, avoid strenuous activities or heavy lifting, and listen to their body's signals to prevent overexertion or injury.

5. **Nutrition and Fluid Intake**
    - Discuss dietary recommendations, including appropriate food choices, portion sizes, and hydration.
    - Highlight the importance of maintaining a balanced diet rich in nutrients, fiber, and fluids to support healing and prevent dehydration.

6. **Signs and Symptoms of Complications**
    - Educate patients on common signs and symptoms of post-discharge complications, such as fever, pain, shortness of breath, swelling, redness, and changes in mental status.
    - Provide specific guidance on when to contact their healthcare provider or seek emergency medical attention if they experience concerning symptoms.

7. **Monitoring Vital Signs**
    - Instruct patients on how to monitor and record vital signs, such as temperature, blood pressure, heart rate, and respiratory rate, at home.
    - Review normal ranges for vital signs and provide guidance on when to seek medical evaluation based on abnormal readings.

8. **Follow-up Care**
    - Stress the importance of attending scheduled follow-up appointments with primary care providers, specialists, or other healthcare professionals.
    - Ensure that patients understand how to arrange transportation, schedule appointments, and obtain necessary referrals or authorizations for follow-up care.

9. **Contact Information**
    - Provide contact information for The APh, including phone numbers, office hours, after-hours support, and instructions for contacting emergency services.
    - Encourage patients to keep a list of emergency contacts and important medical information readily accessible in case of an emergency.

21.4. Coordination with Other Healthcare Providers

> ➤ *Effective coordination with other healthcare providers is essential for ensuring seamless transitions of care and comprehensive post-hospitalization management.*
>
> ➤ *The Advanced Pharmacist Practitioner can facilitate communication and collaboration among interdisciplinary care teams to optimize patient outcomes.*

1. **Interdisciplinary Communication**
   - Establish open lines of communication with primary care providers, specialists, nurses, pharmacists, therapists, social workers, and other healthcare professionals involved in the patient's care.
   - Use secure messaging platforms, electronic health records (EHRs), and telecommunication technologies to share relevant clinical information, coordinate care plans, and address patient needs.

2. **Care Coordination Meetings**
   - Schedule regular care coordination meetings or case conferences involving key stakeholders to discuss patient progress, care plans, treatment goals, and discharge planning.
   - Use multidisciplinary rounds, huddles, or virtual meetings to facilitate real-time communication, problem-solving, and decision-making among team members.

3. **Discharge Planning and Transition Management**
   - Collaborate with case managers, social workers, and discharge planners to develop individualized discharge plans addressing post-hospitalization needs, such as medication management, follow-up appointments, home care services, and rehabilitation programs.
   - Ensure that discharge instructions are communicated clearly to patients and caregivers, with a focus on continuity of care and transition management.

4. **Medication Reconciliation and Management**
   - Coordinate with pharmacists and medication reconciliation specialists to review and reconcile medication lists, resolve discrepancies, and optimize medication regimens post-hospitalization.
   - Facilitate access to medications, prescription refills, and specialty pharmacy services, and provide patient education on medication adherence, side effects, and self-administration techniques.

5. **Home Health and Community Resources**
   - Collaborate with home health agencies, visiting nurses, durable medical equipment (DME) suppliers, and community resources to arrange post-discharge support services, such as home health visits, physical therapy, occupational therapy, and medical equipment rentals.
   - Provide referrals to social services, support groups, and community organizations to address psychosocial needs, transportation barriers, financial assistance, and other social determinants of health.

6. **Remote Monitoring and Telehealth**
   - Leverage remote monitoring technologies and telehealth platforms to monitor patients' vital signs, symptoms, and functional status post-hospitalization.
   - Conduct virtual follow-up visits, medication reviews, and patient assessments to assess recovery progress, address concerns, and provide ongoing support and education remotely.

7. **Specialty Consultations and Referrals**
   - Facilitate timely referrals to specialty care providers, such as cardiologists, pulmonologists, endocrinologists, and wound care specialists, for further evaluation and management of complex medical conditions or surgical complications.
   - Coordinate follow-up appointments, diagnostic tests, and procedures to expedite access to specialty care services and optimize patient outcomes.

8. **Patient-Centered Care Planning**
   - Engage patients and caregivers in care planning discussions, involving them as active participants in decision-making, goal-setting, and treatment planning.
   - Solicit patient feedback, preferences, and priorities to tailor care plans to patient needs, preferences, and cultural beliefs, promoting patient-centered care and shared decision-making.

9. **Continuous Communication and Follow-Up**
   - Maintain ongoing communication with patients, caregivers, and The APh to monitor patient progress, address emerging issues, and adjust care plans as needed.
   - Conduct post-discharge phone calls, telehealth visits, or home visits to assess patient satisfaction, evaluate adherence to care plans, and identify opportunities for improvement in care coordination and transitions of care.

10. Quality Improvement Initiatives

- Participate in quality improvement initiatives, performance metrics tracking, and outcome assessments to evaluate the effectiveness of care coordination efforts and identify areas for enhancement.
- Implement evidence-based practices, standardized protocols, and best practices to optimize care transitions, reduce readmissions, and improve overall quality of care post-hospitalization.

References

- Hansen, L. O., Young, R. S., Hinami, K., Leung, A., & Williams, M. V. (2011). Interventions to reduce 30-day rehospitalization: a systematic review. Annals of internal medicine, 155(8), 520-528.
- Kansagara, D., Englander, H., Salanitro, A., Kagen, D., Theobald, C., Freeman, M., ... & Cheadle, A. (2011). Risk prediction models for hospital readmission: a systematic review. JAMA, 306(15), 1688-1698.
- Coleman, E. A., Parry, C., Chalmers, S., & Min, S. J. (2006). The care transitions intervention: results of a randomized controlled trial. Archives of internal medicine, 166(17), 1822-1828.
- Rennke, S., & Ranji, S. R. (2019). Transitional care strategies from hospital to home: a review for the neurohospitalist. Neurohospitalist, 9(2), 63-72.

Chapter 22: Imaging Modalities

22.1. X-ray (Radiography)

> ➤ X-ray, or radiography, utilizes ionizing radiation to produce images of internal structures such as bones, organs, and tissues.
> ➤ It is commonly used to diagnose fractures, infections, and abnormalities in various medical specialties, offering a quick and relatively low-cost imaging modality.
> ➤ Despite its widespread use, precautions are taken to limit radiation exposure, especially in vulnerable populations.

Indications

1. Bone Fractures:

   X-rays are commonly used to diagnose fractures (broken bones) and assess the extent of the injury. They can help determine the location, severity, and alignment of the fracture.

2. Joint Injuries:

   X-rays are used to evaluate joint injuries, such as dislocations or sprains. They can help identify any misalignment or abnormalities in the joint structure.

3. Pulmonary Conditions:

   X-rays of the chest are used to diagnose and monitor conditions affecting the lungs and surrounding structures, such as pneumonia, lung cancer, tuberculosis, and pleural effusion.

4. Cardiac Conditions:

   Chest X-rays can also provide information about the size, shape, and position of the heart, as well as the presence of fluid or congestion in the lungs (cardiomegaly, pulmonary edema).

5. Abdominal Conditions:

   X-rays of the abdomen can help diagnose conditions such as bowel obstruction, kidney stones, abdominal masses, and foreign objects.

6. Orthopedic Conditions:

   X-rays are used to assess orthopedic conditions, such as degenerative joint disease (osteoarthritis), osteoporosis, scoliosis, and bone infections.

7. Dental Conditions:

   Dental X-rays are used to evaluate oral health, detect tooth decay (cavities), assess the jawbone, and plan dental procedures such as root canals or extractions.

8. Soft Tissue Injuries:

   While X-rays primarily visualize bones, they can also detect soft tissue injuries such as muscle strains, ligament tears, and joint effusions when combined with appropriate techniques (e.g., stress views, and use of contrast agents).

9. X-ray with contrast:

   Contrast-enhanced X-rays are used in visualizing blood vessels (angiography), evaluating the gastrointestinal tract (barium studies), assessing the urinary system (intravenous urography), diagnosing joint issues (arthrography), and imaging spinal cord conditions (myelography).

10. Specialized X-rays:

    DEXA (Dual-Energy X-ray Absorptiometry) is used to measure bone density. Mammogram is used in breast cancer screening.

Interpretation

1. Fractures:

   Fractures appear as discontinuities or breaks in the continuity of the bone on X-ray images. The radiologist or healthcare provider assesses the location, orientation, displacement, and alignment of the fracture to determine the appropriate management.

2. Alignment and Congruence:

   X-rays are used to assess the alignment and congruence of joints and bones. Misalignments, subluxations, or dislocations can be identified, aiding in the diagnosis and treatment planning.

3. Soft Tissue Abnormalities:

   While X-rays primarily visualize bones, they can also provide indirect evidence of soft tissue abnormalities such as swelling, joint effusions, or soft tissue calcifications.

4. Density and Opacity:

   X-ray images display variations in tissue density and opacity, with denser structures appearing whiter (e.g., bones) and less dense structures appearing darker (e.g., air-filled spaces, soft tissues). The radiologist evaluates these variations to identify abnormalities or pathologies.

5. <u>Comparative Analysis:</u>

   When interpreting X-rays, the radiologist often compares current images with previous studies (if available) to assess for any changes over time, such as progression of disease, healing of fractures, or response to treatment.

6. <u>Clinical Correlation:</u>

   X-ray interpretation should always be correlated with the patient's clinical history, symptoms, physical examination findings, and other diagnostic tests to arrive at an accurate diagnosis and treatment plan.

22.2. Computed Tomography

> ➤ *Computed Tomography (CT) combines X-rays and computer processing to generate detailed cross-sectional images of the body.*
>
> ➤ *It provides high-resolution views of internal organs, bones, and tissues, aiding in diagnosis of conditions such as tumors, fractures, and vascular abnormalities.*
>
> ➤ *Despite its diagnostic value, CT scans involve higher radiation doses compared to X-rays and may require contrast agents for enhanced imaging.*

Indications

1. <u>Trauma:</u>

   CT scans are frequently used in emergency settings to evaluate traumatic injuries, such as head trauma, spinal injuries, chest trauma, abdominal trauma, and skeletal fractures.

2. <u>Abdominal and Pelvic Conditions:</u>

   CT scans are valuable for diagnosing and evaluating conditions affecting the abdomen and pelvis, including abdominal pain, gastrointestinal bleeding, appendicitis, kidney stones, liver and spleen injuries, and pelvic masses.

3. <u>Chest Conditions:</u>

   CT scans of the chest are used to assess various pulmonary and mediastinal conditions, such as pneumonia, lung cancer, pulmonary embolism, pleural effusion, pneumothorax, and mediastinal masses.

4. Neurological Conditions:

   CT scans of the brain and spine are used to diagnose and evaluate neurological conditions, including stroke, intracranial hemorrhage, brain tumors, hydrocephalus, spinal cord injuries, and degenerative spine disorders.

5. Orthopedic Conditions:

   CT scans are utilized in orthopedic imaging to assess complex fractures, joint injuries, degenerative joint disease (osteoarthritis), spinal disorders, and pre-operative planning for orthopedic surgeries.

6. Vascular Imaging:

   CT angiography (CTA) is a specialized CT technique used to visualize blood vessels and diagnose vascular conditions such as arterial stenosis, aneurysms, dissections, and peripheral vascular disease.

7. Oncological Imaging:

   CT scans are essential for staging, monitoring, and follow-up of various cancers, including lung cancer, liver cancer, pancreatic cancer, colorectal cancer, lymphoma, and metastatic disease.

8. Interventional Procedures:

   CT guidance is used for image-guided interventions and procedures, including biopsies, drainage procedures, needle aspirations, and catheter placements.

Interpretation

1. Anatomy and Morphology:

   CT images provide detailed cross-sectional views of the body, allowing radiologists to assess the size, shape, and location of organs, tissues, and structures. Abnormalities such as masses, lesions, fluid collections, and anatomical variations can be identified.

2. Density and Contrast Enhancement:

   CT images display variations in tissue density, with denser structures appearing brighter (hyperdense) and less dense structures appearing darker (hypodense). Contrast enhancement with intravenous contrast agents highlights blood vessels, organs, and abnormalities.

3. Lesion Characterization:

   Radiologists analyze the characteristics of lesions, including size, shape, margins, internal composition, enhancement patterns, and surrounding tissue involvement, to determine the nature of the lesion (e.g., benign vs. malignant).

4. Location and Extension:

   CT imaging provides information about the location, extent, and spread of diseases, helping to determine the stage of cancer, assess organ involvement, and plan surgical or radiation therapy.

5. Comparative Analysis:

   Radiologists may compare current CT images with previous studies (if available) to assess for any changes over time, such as disease progression, treatment response, or recurrence.

6. Clinical Correlation:

   Interpretation of CT findings should be correlated with the patient's clinical history, symptoms, physical examination findings, and other diagnostic tests to arrive at an accurate diagnosis and treatment plan.

22.3. Magnetic Resonance Imaging

> - *MRI uses a strong magnetic field and radio waves to generate detailed images of the body's internal structures.*
> - *It is particularly useful for imaging soft tissues such as the brain, spinal cord, muscles, and organs.*
> - *MRI is commonly used to diagnose neurological disorders, joint injuries, tumors, and cardiovascular conditions.*

Indications

1. Neurological disorders:

   MRI is commonly used to evaluate various neurological conditions, including brain tumors, strokes, multiple sclerosis, dementia, epilepsy, and intracranial hemorrhage.

2. Spinal disorders:

   MRI can assess spinal cord compression, disc herniation, spinal tumors, spinal stenosis, and other degenerative spinal conditions.

3. Musculoskeletal disorders:

   MRI is valuable for diagnosing musculoskeletal conditions such as ligament or tendon injuries, joint abnormalities, arthritis, bone tumors, and sports-related injuries.

4. Vascular abnormalities:

   MRI angiography (MRA) can visualize blood vessels and detect vascular abnormalities such as aneurysms, arterial stenosis, or vascular malformations.

5. Abdominal and pelvic conditions:

   MRI is used to evaluate abdominal and pelvic organs for conditions such as liver tumors, pancreatic abnormalities, gastrointestinal disorders, pelvic masses, and gynecological conditions.

6. Breast imaging:

   MRI is utilized for breast cancer screening in high-risk patients and for evaluating breast abnormalities detected on mammography or ultrasound.

7. Cardiovascular imaging:

   MRI can assess cardiac structure and function, detect myocardial infarction, evaluate congenital heart defects, and visualize blood flow in the heart and great vessels.

8. Oncological imaging:

   MRI plays a crucial role in cancer staging, monitoring treatment response, and detecting metastatic disease in various organs.

9. Soft tissue evaluation:

   MRI provides excellent soft tissue contrast, making it useful for assessing soft tissue injuries, infections, inflammatory conditions, and tumors throughout the body.

10. Pediatric imaging:

    MRI is commonly used in pediatric patients for evaluating congenital anomalies, developmental disorders, and neurological conditions.

Interpretation

1. Image quality assessment:

   Radiologists evaluate the quality of MRI images to ensure adequate visualization of anatomical structures and pathology.

2. Anatomical assessment:

   Radiologists identify and characterize normal anatomical structures and any abnormalities present in the scanned region.

3. Lesion detection and characterization:

   Radiologists identify and characterize lesions such as tumors, cysts, hemorrhages, or inflammatory foci based on their size, shape, location, signal intensity, and enhancement characteristics.

4. Tissue characterization:

   MRI provides multi-parametric imaging capabilities, allowing radiologists to assess tissue characteristics such as water content, fat content, vascularity, and tissue composition.

5. Differential diagnosis:

   Radiologists consider various differential diagnoses based on imaging findings, clinical history, and other diagnostic information to provide accurate diagnoses.

6. Reporting:

   Radiologists generate detailed reports summarizing their findings, including a description of abnormalities, their location and extent, and relevant clinical implications. Reports may also include recommendations for further imaging or interventions as necessary.

22.4. Ultrasound

> - *Ultrasound imaging uses high-frequency sound waves to produce real-time images of the body's internal organs and structures.*
> - *It is commonly used to visualize the abdomen, pelvis, heart, blood vessels, and developing fetus during pregnancy.*
> - *Ultrasound is non-invasive and does not use ionizing radiation.*

Indications

1. Abdominal imaging:

   Ultrasound is commonly used to evaluate abdominal organs such as the liver, gallbladder, pancreas, kidneys, spleen, and abdominal aorta for conditions such as liver disease, gallstones, pancreatic tumors, renal cysts, and abdominal masses.

2. Pelvic imaging:

   Ultrasound is utilized to assess the uterus, ovaries, and bladder in both males and females for conditions such as ovarian cysts, uterine fibroids, pelvic inflammatory disease (PID), and urinary tract abnormalities.

3. Obstetric imaging:

   Ultrasound plays a crucial role in prenatal care for assessing fetal growth, development, and anatomy, as well as detecting abnormalities such as congenital anomalies, placental abnormalities, and multiple pregnancies.

4. <u>Vascular imaging</u>:

   Doppler ultrasound is used to evaluate blood flow in arteries and veins throughout the body, including the carotid arteries, peripheral arteries, and deep venous system, for conditions such as arterial stenosis, venous thrombosis, and vascular malformations.

5. <u>Musculoskeletal imaging</u>:

   Ultrasound is employed to assess soft tissue structures, muscles, tendons, ligaments, and joints for conditions such as tendonitis, bursitis, muscle tears, joint effusions, and rheumatologic diseases.

6. <u>Breast imaging</u>:

   Ultrasound is used as an adjunct to mammography for evaluating breast abnormalities, characterizing breast masses, and guiding breast biopsies.

7. <u>Thyroid imaging</u>:

   Ultrasound is commonly performed to evaluate thyroid nodules, thyroid size, and thyroid gland vascularity, and to guide fine-needle aspiration (FNA) biopsy of thyroid nodules.

8. <u>Cardiac imaging</u>:

   Echocardiography, a specialized form of ultrasound, is utilized to assess cardiac structure and function, detect valvular abnormalities, evaluate heart chambers, and assess for pericardial effusion.

9. <u>Pediatric imaging</u>:

   Ultrasound is frequently used in pediatric patients for assessing congenital anomalies, evaluating abdominal pain, and detecting urinary tract abnormalities.

10. <u>Emergency and trauma imaging</u>: Ultrasound is used in emergency settings to assess for free fluid in the abdomen or pelvis, detect abdominal aortic aneurysms, evaluate for appendicitis, and perform focused assessment with sonography in trauma (FAST) scans.

Interpretation

1. <u>Image quality assessment</u>:

   Sonographers and radiologists evaluate the quality of ultrasound images, including resolution, clarity, and artifacts, to ensure diagnostic accuracy.

2. <u>Anatomical assessment</u>:

   Sonographers and radiologists identify and characterize normal anatomical structures and any abnormalities present in the scanned region, including size, shape, echogenicity, and mobility.

3. <u>Lesion detection and characterization</u>:

   Sonographers and radiologists identify and characterize lesions such as cysts, tumors, fluid collections, or masses based on their appearance, location, vascularity, and associated findings.

4. <u>Doppler evaluation</u>:

   Doppler ultrasound is used to assess blood flow patterns, velocities, and directionality in arteries and veins, aiding in the diagnosis of vascular conditions such as stenosis, thrombosis, or arterial-venous malformations.

5. <u>Functional assessment</u>:

   Ultrasound can provide functional information such as cardiac ejection fraction, bladder function, or fetal cardiac activity, enhancing diagnostic capabilities.

6. <u>Real-time guidance</u>:

   Ultrasound can guide interventional procedures such as biopsies, aspirations, injections, or catheter placements in real-time, ensuring accuracy and safety.

7. <u>Reporting</u>:

   Sonographers and radiologists generate detailed reports summarizing their findings, including a description of abnormalities, their location and extent, and relevant clinical implications. Reports may also include recommendations for further imaging or interventions as necessary.

Ultrasound-Guided Procedures

Ultrasound-guided procedures utilize real-time ultrasound imaging to precisely guide needles or catheters for diagnostic and therapeutic interventions.

Common procedures include biopsies, aspirations and drainages, central venous access, nerve blocks, and musculoskeletal interventions. These techniques offer improved accuracy, reduced risk of complications, and increased patient comfort compared to blind techniques.

- Biopsy: Obtaining tissue samples for diagnostic evaluation, such as core needle biopsy or fine-needle aspiration biopsy of the breast, thyroid, liver, prostate, or lymph nodes.

- Aspiration and Drainage: Draining fluid collections (e.g., abscesses, cysts, seromas) or aspirating joint fluid (arthrocentesis) for diagnostic or therapeutic purposes.

- Central Venous Access: Placing central venous catheters (e.g., subclavian, jugular, or femoral veins) for administering medications, fluids, or blood products, or for hemodialysis access.
- Peripheral Nerve Blocks: Delivering local anesthetic agents to block nerve impulses and provide pain relief for various surgical procedures or chronic pain management.
- Paracentesis and Thoracentesis: Removing fluid from the abdominal or pleural cavities, respectively, to relieve symptoms and obtain diagnostic samples.
- Musculoskeletal Interventions: Guiding injections into joints, bursae, tendons, or ligaments for pain management, diagnostic purposes, or therapeutic treatment of conditions like osteoarthritis or tendonitis.
- Thyroid Nodule Ablation: Using radiofrequency or ethanol ablation guided by ultrasound to treat benign thyroid nodules, reducing their size or symptoms.
- Peripheral Vascular Interventions: Guiding procedures such as vascular access for angiography or angioplasty, thrombin injection for pseudoaneurysm, or arterial and venous interventions for peripheral vascular disease.
- Obstetric and Gynecological Procedures: Including amniocentesis, fetal blood sampling, embryo transfer, and aspiration of ovarian cysts or ectopic pregnancies.

22.5. Positron Emission Tomography

> *Positron Emission Tomography (PET) scans use a radioactive tracer injected into the body to detect metabolic activity and physiological processes.*
> *They are often used in combination with CT or MRI to diagnose cancer, evaluate heart function, and assess brain disorders.*

Indications:
- Cancer detection and staging: PET scans are commonly used in oncology to detect primary tumors, assess metastatic spread, and determine the stage of cancer.
- Response assessment: PET scans can monitor the response to cancer treatment, including chemotherapy, radiation therapy, or immunotherapy.
- Evaluation of tumor recurrence: PET scans can help identify recurrent or residual disease after cancer treatment.

- Cardiac imaging: PET scans are used to assess myocardial perfusion, myocardial viability, and myocardial metabolism in patients with coronary artery disease or cardiomyopathy.
- Neurological disorders: PET scans can detect abnormalities in brain metabolism and neuronal function, aiding in the diagnosis and management of neurodegenerative diseases, epilepsy, and brain tumors.
- Infectious diseases: PET scans can localize and characterize infectious foci, such as abscesses, osteomyelitis, or inflammatory conditions.
- Evaluation of inflammatory conditions: PET scans can assess the extent and activity of inflammatory processes in various organs, including the lungs, joints, and blood vessels.
- Evaluation of dementia: PET scans can detect changes in brain metabolism associated with Alzheimer's disease and other forms of dementia.

Interpretation:
- Visual interpretation: Radiologists assess the distribution and intensity of radiotracer uptake in different tissues or organs. Increased uptake may indicate the presence of disease or abnormal metabolic activity.
- Semi-quantitative analysis: Standardized uptake values (SUVs) are calculated to quantify the amount of radiotracer uptake in specific regions of interest. Higher SUVs may suggest increased metabolic activity or disease burden.
- Comparison with anatomical imaging: PET scans are often interpreted in conjunction with computed tomography (CT) or magnetic resonance imaging (MRI) to correlate metabolic findings with anatomical structures and provide comprehensive diagnostic information.
- Clinical correlation: PET scan findings are interpreted in the context of clinical history, physical examination, laboratory tests, and other imaging studies to arrive at a definitive diagnosis and guide patient management.
- Follow-up imaging: Serial PET scans may be performed to monitor disease progression, response to treatment, or recurrence over time.

22.6. Fluoroscopy

> ➤ *Fluoroscopy is a real-time imaging technique that uses X-rays to visualize moving structures within the body, such as the digestive tract, blood vessels, and joints.*
>
> ➤ *It is commonly used during procedures such as angiography, gastrointestinal studies, and orthopedic surgeries.*

Indications:

- Diagnostic imaging: Fluoroscopy is used to visualize internal structures and organs in real-time, allowing for dynamic assessment of anatomical function and pathology.
- Guidance for interventional procedures: Fluoroscopy provides live imaging guidance during minimally invasive procedures, such as catheter placements, angiography, orthopedic interventions, and gastrointestinal studies.
- Orthopedic evaluations: Fluoroscopy is commonly used to assess joint mobility, alignment, and function during orthopedic examinations and procedures, including joint injections, arthrograms, and fracture reductions.
- Gastrointestinal studies: Fluoroscopy is utilized in procedures such as barium swallow studies, upper gastrointestinal series, barium enemas, and small bowel follow-throughs to evaluate the anatomy and function of the digestive tract.
- Pulmonary studies: Fluoroscopy may be used to assess lung function and ventilation during procedures such as bronchoscopy, bronchography, and diaphragmatic fluoroscopy.
- Urological procedures: Fluoroscopy is employed in imaging studies of the urinary tract, including voiding cystourethrography, retrograde pyelograms, and ureteral stent placements.
- Cardiac imaging: Fluoroscopy is utilized in cardiac catheterization procedures, electrophysiology studies, and coronary angiography to visualize the heart and blood vessels.
- Vascular interventions: Fluoroscopy guides endovascular procedures such as angioplasty, stent placements, embolization, and thrombectomy in the treatment of vascular diseases.

Interpretation:

- Real-time visualization: Fluoroscopy provides continuous, live imaging of the area of interest, allowing radiologists and interventionalists to observe anatomical structures and dynamic physiological processes.

- Anatomical assessment: Radiologists interpret fluoroscopic images to evaluate the size, shape, position, and movement of organs, tissues, and anatomical landmarks.

- Pathological findings: Abnormalities such as masses, obstructions, strictures, perforations, fractures, or dislocations may be identified on fluoroscopic images and interpreted in the context of clinical history and patient symptoms.

- Guidance for interventions: During interventional procedures, fluoroscopic images guide the placement of catheters, needles, guidewires, and other instruments, ensuring precise localization and optimal treatment delivery.

- Dynamic assessment: Fluoroscopy captures motion and functional changes in real-time, allowing for the evaluation of physiological processes such as swallowing, peristalsis, cardiac function, joint mobility, and respiratory motion.

- Documentation: Fluoroscopic images may be recorded or captured digitally for documentation, archiving, and subsequent review by healthcare providers, patients, or for medicolegal purposes.

- Communication: Radiologists communicate their findings to referring physicians, surgeons, or other members of the healthcare team, providing diagnostic insights and guidance for patient management and treatment planning.

22.7. Interventional Radiology

> *Interventional radiology (IR) uses various imaging modalities, such as X-ray, CT, MRI, and ultrasound, to guide minimally invasive procedures and treatments.*
>
> *Examples include angioplasty, embolization, biopsy, and tumor ablation.*

Indications

- Vascular interventions: IR procedures include angioplasty, stent placement, embolization, thrombolysis, and angiography to treat conditions such as peripheral artery disease, deep vein thrombosis, aneurysms, and arteriovenous malformations.

- Oncologic interventions: IR techniques such as tumor ablation, chemoembolization, radioembolization, and percutaneous biopsies are used in the diagnosis and treatment of cancer, including liver, lung, kidney, and bone tumors.

- Pain management: IR offers procedures such as nerve blocks, vertebroplasty, kyphoplasty, and radiofrequency ablation for pain relief in conditions such as spinal fractures, osteoarthritis, and cancer-related pain.
- Gastrointestinal interventions: IR procedures such as percutaneous gastrostomy, biliary drainage, abscess drainage, and transjugular intrahepatic portosystemic shunt (TIPS) are performed for conditions affecting the digestive system.
- Urologic interventions: IR techniques such as nephrostomy, ureteral stent placement, and percutaneous nephrolithotomy are used in the management of urinary tract obstruction, kidney stones, and other urologic conditions.
- Neurointerventions: IR procedures such as cerebral angiography, embolization of cerebral aneurysms, and thrombectomy for stroke treatment are performed for neurovascular disorders.
- Musculoskeletal interventions: IR offers procedures such as joint injections, bone biopsies, and treatment of musculoskeletal tumors or fractures using image-guided techniques.
- Other ultrasound-guided procedures: Aspiration and drainage of fluid collections or body cavities, placement of central venous catheters or PICCs, and fetal interventions such as biopsies or amniocentesis.

Advantages
- Minimally invasive: IR procedures are less invasive than traditional surgery, resulting in smaller incisions, reduced trauma to surrounding tissues, and faster recovery times.
- Precise targeting: Image guidance allows for precise localization of the target site, minimizing damage to healthy tissues and reducing complications.
- Outpatient or same-day procedures: Many IR procedures can be performed on an outpatient basis, allowing patients to return home the same day.
- Alternative to surgery: IR offers alternatives to traditional surgery for patients who are not candidates for surgery or prefer less invasive treatment options.
- Reduced risk of infection: Minimally invasive techniques reduce the risk of post-procedural infections and complications compared to open surgery.

22.8. Nuclear Medicine

> ➤ *Nuclear medicine is a medical specialty that uses small amounts of radioactive materials, known as radiopharmaceuticals or radiotracers, to diagnose and treat various diseases.*
>
> ➤ *These materials are either injected into the body, swallowed, or inhaled, depending on the type of examination or treatment.*

Diagnostic

Nuclear medicine is used for imaging to visualize the structure and function of organs. The radiotracers emit gamma rays that can be detected by special types of cameras (such as gamma cameras or PET scanners), creating detailed images.

- **Bone Scintigraphy (Bone Scan):** Used to detect abnormalities in bone metabolism, such as fractures, infections, tumors, or metastases.
- **Thyroid Scan:** Evaluates thyroid function and morphology, aiding in the diagnosis of conditions like hyperthyroidism, hypothyroidism, thyroid nodules, and thyroid cancer.
- **Myocardial Perfusion Imaging (MPI):** Assesses blood flow to the heart muscle, helping diagnose coronary artery disease, evaluate myocardial viability, and determine the extent of myocardial infarction.
- **Single-Photon Emission Computed Tomography (SPECT):** A 3D imaging technique that provides detailed functional information about organs and tissues, often used in conjunction with radiotracers for cardiac, neurological, and oncological evaluations.
- **Positron Emission Tomography (PET):** Uses radiotracers labeled with positron-emitting isotopes to visualize metabolic processes in tissues, aiding in cancer detection, staging, and monitoring, as well as neurological and cardiac assessments.
- **Gastric Emptying Study:** Measures the rate at which food leaves the stomach, helping diagnose gastroparesis and other gastric motility disorders.
- **Renal Scintigraphy:** Assesses renal function, blood flow, and urinary tract obstruction, commonly used in the evaluation of kidney function, renal artery stenosis, and urinary reflux.
- **Lung Perfusion and Ventilation Scans:** Evaluate pulmonary blood flow and ventilation, assisting in the diagnosis of pulmonary embolism, lung nodules, and other pulmonary conditions.

Therapeutic

Nuclear medicine also has therapeutic applications, particularly in treating certain types of cancer and thyroid disorders. In these treatments, radiopharmaceuticals are chosen for their ability to target specific cells and deliver a dose of radiation that destroys or damages diseased cells while sparing surrounding healthy tissue.

- Radioactive iodine therapy (I-131): Used to treat thyroid cancer and hyperthyroidism by destroying thyroid tissue.
- Radiopharmaceutical therapy for cancer: Such as the use of radium-223 for treating prostate cancer that has spread to the bones.

Safety and Risks

- Nuclear medicine procedures are generally safe and have been used for decades.
- The amount of radiation in most diagnostic tests is comparable to that of conventional radiology procedures. However, as with any medical procedure involving radiation, there is a small risk that the exposure could contribute to future cancer risk.
- The benefits of these procedures, though, often far outweigh the potential risks, especially when it comes to diagnosing serious conditions early and providing targeted treatments.

References

- Ballinger, P. W., & Frank, E. D. (2008). Merrill's atlas of radiographic positioning and procedures. Elsevier Health Sciences.
- Webb, W. R., Brant, W. E., & Major, N. M. (2016). Fundamentals of body CT. Elsevier Health Sciences.
- Edelman, R. R., Hesselink, J. R., Zlatkin, M. B., & Crues, J. V. (2010). Clinical magnetic resonance imaging. Elsevier Health Sciences.
- Rumack, C. M., Levine, D., & Rumack, C. M. (2011). Diagnostic ultrasound. Elsevier Health Sciences.
- Townsend, D. W., Carney, J. P., & Yap, J. T. (2013). PET/CT today and tomorrow. Journal of Nuclear Medicine Technology, 41(2), 96-106.
- Mettler Jr, F. A., & Guiberteau, M. J. (2018). Essentials of nuclear medicine imaging. Elsevier Health Sciences.
- Kaufman, J. A., & Lee, M. J. (2016). Vascular and interventional radiology: the requisites. Elsevier Health Sciences.
- Sandler, M. P., & Coleman, R. E. (2010). PET and PET/CT: a clinical guide. Thieme.

Chapter 23: Preventive Measurements in Primary Care

23.1. Colon Cancer Screening

> ➢ Colon cancer screening aims to detect precancerous polyps or early-stage cancer in the colon or rectum.
>
> ➢ Common methods include colonoscopy, fecal occult blood tests (FOBT), and stool DNA tests, with guidelines recommending regular screening starting at age 45 or earlier for those at increased risk.
>
> ➢ Early detection through screening can significantly reduce mortality rates by enabling timely intervention and treatment.

1. Indications
- Colonoscopy screening is recommended for patients at average risk for colorectal cancer starting at age 45 in most guidelines, including those from the American Cancer Society (ACS), the U.S. Preventive Services Task Force (USPSTF), and the American College of Gastroenterology (ACG).
- Patients with certain risk factors, such as a family history of colorectal cancer or polyps, may require earlier or more frequent screening.

2. Procedure
- During a colonoscopy, a thin, flexible tube with a camera (colonoscope) is inserted into the rectum and advanced through the entire length of the colon.
- The camera allows the gastroenterologist to visualize the lining of the colon and rectum, identify abnormalities such as polyps or tumors, and perform biopsies or remove polyps for further evaluation.

3. Preparation
- Before a colonoscopy, patients must undergo bowel preparation to clear the colon of stool, allowing for better visualization during the procedure.
- This typically involves a liquid diet, laxatives, and/or enemas to empty the colon completely.

4. Screening Interval

- For average-risk patients with normal colonoscopy results, repeat screening is typically recommended every 10 years. However, the screening interval may be shorter for patients with certain risk factors or findings such as a history of adenomatous polyps or a family history of colorectal cancer.

5. Benefits

- Early detection of colorectal cancer: Colonoscopy screening can detect colorectal cancer at an early stage when treatment is most effective, leading to improved outcomes and survival rates.

- Detection and removal of precancerous polyps: Colonoscopy allows for the identification and removal of precancerous polyps, reducing the risk of colorectal cancer development.

- Prevention of colorectal cancer: By removing precancerous polyps during colonoscopy, the risk of developing colorectal cancer can be significantly reduced.

6. Risks

- Complications: While colonoscopy is generally considered safe, there is a small risk of complications such as bleeding, perforation of the colon, or adverse reactions to sedation.

- Bowel preparation: The bowel preparation process can be uncomfortable and may cause nausea, bloating, or dehydration.

- Sedation risks: Sedation medications used during colonoscopy can cause side effects such as drowsiness, dizziness, or respiratory depression.

7. Alternatives

- Other screening modalities: In addition to colonoscopy, there are alternative screening modalities for colorectal cancer, including fecal immunochemical testing (FIT), fecal occult blood testing (FOBT), stool DNA testing (e.g., Cologuard), flexible sigmoidoscopy, and virtual colonoscopy (CT colonography). However, colonoscopy is considered the gold standard for colorectal cancer screening due to its ability to detect and remove precancerous polyps.

23.2. Cervical Cancer Screening

> ➤ *Cervical cancer screening aims to detect precancerous changes or early-stage cancer in the cervix.*
> ➤ *Common methods include Pap smears (Pap tests) to examine cervical cells for abnormalities and HPV testing to detect high-risk HPV strains.*

1. Indications

Cervical cancer screening is recommended for women aged 21 to 65 years, regardless of sexual activity or vaccination status against human papillomavirus (HPV). Routine screening may begin at age 21, regardless of sexual history, and continue every 3-5 years, depending on the screening method used.

Screening Methods:

- <u>Pap smear (Pap test):</u> During a Pap smear, cells from the cervix are collected and examined under a microscope to detect any abnormal changes. Pap smears can identify precancerous lesions or early-stage cervical cancer.
- <u>HPV test:</u> HPV testing detects the presence of high-risk HPV strains that are associated with cervical cancer. HPV testing may be performed alone or in combination with a Pap smear (co-testing).

Screening Schedule:

- For women aged 21 to 29: Pap smear alone every 3 years
- For women aged 30 to 65:
  - Pap smear alone every 3 years, or
  - HPV test alone every 5 years, or
  - Co-testing (Pap smear and HPV test) every 5 years

2. Guidance for Special Populations

- Women under 21: cervical cancer screening is not recommended as cervical cancer is rare in this age group.
- Women over 65: they may discontinue cervical cancer screening if they have had adequate prior screening and are not at high risk.
- Women who have had a hysterectomy: cervical cancer screening may not be necessary for those who have had a hysterectomy and do not have a history of cervical cancer or precancerous lesions.

3. Follow-up for Abnormal Results

- Abnormal Pap smear results may indicate the presence of precancerous or cancerous cells, prompting further evaluation with

colposcopy (examination of the cervix using a magnifying instrument) and biopsy (removal of tissue for pathological examination).
- Abnormal HPV test results may lead to further evaluation with colposcopy if high-risk HPV strains are detected.

4. Vaccination against HPV

In addition to cervical cancer screening, vaccination against HPV is recommended for both males and females to prevent HPV infection and reduce the risk of cervical cancer and other HPV-related cancers. HPV vaccination is typically administered to adolescents between the ages of 11 and 12, but it can be given as early as age 9 and up to age 26 for females and age 21 for males who have not previously been vaccinated.

23.3. Breast Cancer Screening

> ➢ Breast cancer screening involves methods like mammography, clinical breast exams, and breast self-exams to detect abnormalities in breast tissue.
>
> ➢ Regular screening, typically starting at age 40 or earlier for those at higher risk, aids in early detection and improves treatment outcomes.
>
> ➢ Guidelines recommend individualized screening plans based on age, risk factors, and personal preferences.

1. Indications
- Mammography is primarily used for breast cancer screening in asymptomatic women to detect tumors and other abnormalities that may not be palpable during a physical examination.
- It is also utilized for diagnostic purposes in women with breast symptoms such as lumps, pain, nipple discharge, or changes in breast size or shape.

2. Procedure
- During a mammogram, the breast is compressed between two plates while low-dose X-rays are used to create detailed images of the breast tissue.
- Mammography may be performed using either digital mammography or analog (film-screen) mammography systems.

3. Screening Guidelines
- Screening mammography guidelines vary by organization, but many recommend starting regular mammograms at age 40 or 50 for average-risk women and continuing every 1-2 years thereafter.

- Women at higher risk of breast cancer, such as those with a family history of the disease or certain genetic mutations (e.g., BRCA1/BRCA2), may require earlier or more frequent screening.

4. Benefits
- Early detection of breast cancer: Mammography can detect breast cancer at an early stage, often before symptoms are present, allowing for prompt treatment and improved outcomes.
- Reduction in breast cancer mortality: Regular mammography screening has been associated with a decrease in breast cancer mortality rates by facilitating earlier detection and treatment.
- Detection of precancerous lesions: Mammography can identify precancerous changes in breast tissue, such as ductal carcinoma in situ (DCIS), allowing for preventive measures to be taken to reduce the risk of invasive breast cancer.

5. Risks
- False positives: Mammography may produce false-positive results, leading to unnecessary follow-up tests (e.g., additional imaging, biopsies) and anxiety for patients.
- False negatives: Mammography may miss some breast cancers, particularly in women with dense breast tissue or certain tumor characteristics.
- Radiation exposure: While mammography uses low doses of radiation, repeated exposure over time may increase the cumulative radiation dose, although the benefits of screening typically outweigh the risks.

6. Alternatives
- Digital breast tomosynthesis (DBT): Also known as 3D mammography, DBT is a newer imaging technique that provides more detailed, three-dimensional images of the breast tissue, potentially improving cancer detection rates and reducing false-positive results.
- Breast MRI: Magnetic resonance imaging (MRI) of the breast may be recommended for women at high risk of breast cancer or those with dense breast tissue, as it can provide additional information beyond mammography.

23.4. Lung Cancer Screening

> ➢ *Lung cancer screening primarily utilizes low-dose computed tomography (LDCT) scans to detect early signs of lung cancer in high-risk individuals, such as long-term smokers.*
>
> ➢ *Screening aims to identify tumors at an early, more treatable stage, potentially reducing mortality rates.*

1. Indications

Lung cancer screening is recommended for patients at high risk of developing lung cancer.

- Current or former smokers aged 50 to 80 years old.
- Current smokers or former smokers who have quit within the past 15 years.
- patients with a history of heavy smoking, defined as a smoking history of at least 30 pack-years (pack-years = number of packs smoked per day multiplied by the number of years smoked).

2. Screening Method

- The primary screening modality for lung cancer is low-dose computed tomography (LDCT) scanning of the chest.
- LDCT scans use lower radiation doses than standard CT scans and can detect smaller abnormalities in the lungs.

3. Screening Schedule

- Screening should be conducted annually for patients who meet the high-risk criteria mentioned above.
- It's important to note that lung cancer screening is not recommended for patients who have never smoked or who have quit smoking more than 15 years ago, as the benefits of screening may not outweigh the potential harms in these populations.

4. Benefits of Screening

- Early detection: Lung cancer screening can detect lung cancer at an early stage when it is more likely to be treatable and potentially curable.
- Reduced mortality: Studies have shown that lung cancer screening with LDCT can reduce lung cancer mortality in high-risk patients by detecting tumors at an earlier, more treatable stage.
- Quality of life: Early detection and treatment of lung cancer may improve quality of life and prolong survival in affected patients.

5. Risks of Screening
- False positives: Lung cancer screening may lead to false-positive results, which can cause anxiety and may result in unnecessary follow-up tests or procedures.
- Overdiagnosis: Some lung cancers detected through screening may be slow-growing and may not have caused symptoms or harm during a person's lifetime. Overdiagnosis can lead to unnecessary treatments with potential side effects.

23.5 Prostate Cancer Screening

> ➤ Prostate cancer screening involves the use of prostate-specific antigen (PSA) blood tests and digital rectal exams (DRE) to detect potential signs of prostate cancer.
> ➤ Screening may lead to early detection and improved outcomes, but may also result in false positives and overdiagnosis.

1. Indications
- Prostate cancer screening is typically recommended for men who are at average or increased risk of developing the disease.
- The decision to undergo screening should be based on a discussion between the patient and their healthcare provider, taking into account factors such as age, family history, and overall health status.

2. Screening Methods
The two primary screening tests for prostate cancer are the prostate-specific antigen (PSA) blood test, and digital rectal examination (DRE):

- <u>PSA Blood Test</u>: Measures the level of PSA, a protein produced by the prostate gland, in the blood. Elevated PSA levels may indicate the presence of prostate cancer, although other conditions such as benign prostatic hyperplasia (BPH) or inflammation of the prostate (prostatitis) can also cause elevated PSA levels.
- <u>Digital Rectal Examination (DRE)</u>: Involves the healthcare provider inserting a gloved, lubricated finger into the rectum to feel for abnormalities in the prostate gland, such as lumps or nodules.

3. Screening Recommendations
- The United States Preventive Services Task Force (USPSTF) recommends individualized decision-making about prostate cancer screening for men aged 55 to 69 years, based on a discussion between the patient and their healthcare provider.

- For men at average risk, screening may be considered starting at age 55.
- For men at higher risk, such as those with a family history of prostate cancer or African American men, screening discussions may begin at age 45 or earlier.

4. Benefits of Screening

- Early detection: Prostate cancer screening can detect the disease at an early stage, when it is more likely to be treatable and potentially curable.
- Improved outcomes: Early detection and treatment of prostate cancer may lead to better treatment outcomes and survival rates.

5. Risks of Screening

- False positives: PSA testing can result in false-positive results, leading to unnecessary follow-up tests (e.g., biopsies) and anxiety for the patient.
- Overdiagnosis and overtreatment: Prostate cancer screening may detect slow-growing tumors that may not have caused symptoms or harm during a patient's lifetime. Treatment of these tumors may lead to unnecessary side effects and complications.

23.6. Osteoporosis Screening

> *Osteoporosis screening typically involves bone mineral density (BMD) testing, such as dual-energy X-ray absorptiometry (DXA), to assess bone strength and density.*
>
> *It helps identify patients at risk of fractures, particularly postmenopausal women and older adults, enabling early intervention with lifestyle modifications and medication to prevent fractures and manage osteoporosis.*

1. Indications

Osteoporosis screening is typically recommended for:

- Women aged 65 years and older
- Men aged 70 years and older
- Younger patients with risk factors for osteoporosis, such as a history of fractures, prolonged corticosteroid use, low body weight, smoking, excessive alcohol consumption, or certain medical conditions affecting bone health

2. Screening Methods

The primary screening tool for osteoporosis is dual-energy X-ray absorptiometry (DXA or DEXA) scanning:

- DXA Scan: This non-invasive imaging test measures bone mineral density (BMD) at various sites, typically the hip, spine, or forearm. The results are reported as a T-score, comparing the patient's BMD to that of a healthy young adult of the same sex.
- A T-score of -1.0 or higher is considered normal, between -1.0 and -2.5 indicates osteopenia (low bone mass), and -2.5 or lower indicates osteoporosis.
- Z-Score: This compares an individual's BMD to the average BMD of people of the same age, sex, and ethnicity. It helps assess bone density relative to peers.

3. Screening Recommendations

- The United States Preventive Services Task Force (USPSTF) recommends bone density testing with DXA for women aged 65 years and older and for younger women at increased risk of fracture based on their fracture risk assessment.
- Screening recommendations for men vary among different organizations, but most recommend DXA testing for men aged 70 years and older and for younger men at increased risk of fracture.

4. Benefits of Screening

- Early detection: DXA screening can detect osteoporosis and low bone density before fractures occur, allowing for early intervention to prevent fractures.
- Risk stratification: Screening helps identify patients at increased risk of fractures, allowing the APh to implement preventive measures and interventions to reduce fracture risk.

5. Risks of Screening

- Radiation exposure: DXA scanning involves low levels of radiation exposure, but the benefits of screening generally outweigh the risks.
- False positives and overdiagnosis: DXA testing may result in false-positive findings, leading to unnecessary worry and additional testing. Additionally, some patients may be diagnosed with osteopenia (low bone mass) without necessarily being at high risk of fracture.

6. Follow-Up and Management

- Patients diagnosed with osteoporosis or low bone density may require further evaluation to identify underlying causes and to assess fracture risk.
- Treatment and management options may include lifestyle modifications (e.g., calcium and vitamin D supplementation, weight-bearing exercise), pharmacological therapy (e.g., bisphosphonates, hormone replacement therapy), fall prevention strategies, and fracture risk reduction measures.

23.7. Skin Cancer Screening

> ➤ *Skin cancer screening involves visual examination of the skin by dermatologist or PCP to detect abnormal moles or lesions indicative of skin cancer.*
>
> ➤ *Regular screenings, often conducted during routine medical check-ups, help identify skin cancers early when they are most treatable, potentially improving outcomes and reducing mortality rates.*
>
> ➤ *Self-examinations for suspicious skin lesions at home, focusing on changes in moles, spots, or skin lesions, complement with professional screenings for a comprehensive skin cancer detection and prevention.*

1. Indications

Skin cancer screening is recommended for patients with risk factors for skin cancer, including:

- History of excessive sun exposure or sunburns
- Family history of skin cancer
- Personal history of skin cancer or precancerous lesions
- Fair skin, light hair, and blue or green eyes
- History of indoor tanning or use of tanning beds
- Presence of numerous moles or atypical moles (dysplastic nevi)
- Weakened immune system (e.g., due to organ transplantation, HIV infection, or immunosuppressive medications)
- Occupational exposure to sunlight (e.g., outdoor workers)

2. Screening Methods

- Skin cancer screening typically involves a visual examination of the skin by a healthcare provider such as APP, PCP, or a dermatologist.

- The provider examines the entire body, including areas not typically exposed to the sun, looking for any suspicious lesions, moles, or changes in existing moles.

3. Self-Examination

In addition to clinical skin exams, patients are encouraged to perform regular self-examinations of their skin at home.

- This involves inspecting the skin from head to toe, using mirrors or assistance from a partner for hard-to-see areas, and noting any changes in moles, freckles, or other skin lesions.

4. Screening Recommendations

- The American Academy of Dermatology (AAD) recommends regular skin cancer screenings for all adults, particularly those with risk factors for skin cancer.
- The frequency of screening may vary based on patient risk factors, but most experts recommend annual skin exams for high-risk patients and periodic exams for those at average risk.

5. Benefits of Screening

- Early detection: Skin cancer screening can detect skin cancers at an early stage when they are most treatable and have the highest likelihood of cure.
- Improved outcomes: Early detection allows for prompt treatment, reducing the risk of cancer progression, disfigurement, and metastasis.
- Prevention of advanced disease: Screening may identify precancerous lesions or early-stage skin cancers that can be treated before they develop into more advanced or invasive cancers.

6. Risks of Screening

- False positives: Skin cancer screening may lead to the identification of benign lesions or moles that are mistakenly thought to be cancerous, leading to unnecessary worry or biopsies.
- False negatives: Screening may miss some skin cancers or precancerous lesions, particularly if they are small, inconspicuous, or located in areas not easily visible during examination.

23.8. Depression Screening

> ➤ *Depression screening involves the use of standardized questionnaires or assessments to identify symptoms of depression, such as persistent sadness, loss of interest, or changes in sleep and appetite.*
>
> ➤ *It aims to detect depression early, allowing for timely intervention with counseling, therapy, medication, or other supportive measures to improve mental health outcomes.*
>
> ➤ *Depression screening may occur in various healthcare settings, including primary care offices, mental health clinics, or through online platforms, promoting accessibility and early intervention for individuals at risk.*

1. **Indication**
   - Routine Assessment: Routine screening may be recommended as part of preventive healthcare to identify individuals at risk for depression or those experiencing subclinical symptoms.
   - Clinical Suspicion: Screening may be indicated when patients present with symptoms suggestive of depression, such as persistent sadness, loss of interest or pleasure, changes in sleep or appetite, fatigue, or difficulty concentrating.
   - Chronic Medical Conditions: Individuals with chronic medical conditions, such as diabetes, cardiovascular disease, or chronic pain, are at increased risk for depression and may benefit from routine screening.
   - Medication Side Effects: Certain medications, such as corticosteroids, beta-blockers, and hormonal contraceptives, can cause or exacerbate depressive symptoms, warranting screening in individuals using these medications.

2. **Methods of depression screening in primary care**
   - Questionnaires: Validated self-report questionnaires, such as the Patient Health Questionnaire-2 or 9 (PHQ-2 or PHQ9), Beck Depression Inventory (BDI), or Hospital Anxiety and Depression Scale (HADS), are commonly used to assess depressive symptoms.
   - Structured Interviews: Clinician-administered structured interviews, such as the Primary Care Evaluation of Mental Disorders (PRIME-MD) or the Mini International Neuropsychiatric Interview (MINI), may be used for more comprehensive assessments.

- Electronic Screening Tools: Electronic health record (EHR)-integrated screening tools or online assessments may facilitate efficient screening and documentation of results.

3. Risks and benefits of depression screening include

Benefits:

- Early Identification: Screening can facilitate early identification of depression, allowing for prompt intervention and improved outcomes.
- Treatment Initiation: Positive screening results can prompt further evaluation and treatment, leading to appropriate management of depressive symptoms.
- Reduced Stigma: Routine screening may help reduce stigma associated with mental health conditions by normalizing discussions about depression in primary care settings.

Risks:

- False Positives: Screening tools may yield false-positive results, leading to unnecessary distress, stigma, and medicalization of normal variations in mood.
- False Negatives: False-negative results may occur, particularly in individuals who underreport symptoms or have atypical presentations of depression, leading to missed opportunities for intervention.
- Overdiagnosis and Overtreatment: Screening may lead to overdiagnosis and overtreatment of mild or transient depressive symptoms, potentially resulting in unnecessary use of antidepressant medications or psychotherapy.

References

- Wolf, A. M., Fontham, E. T., Church, T. R., Flowers, C. R., Guerra, C. E., LaMonte, S. J., ... & Doria-Rose, V. P. (2018). Colorectal cancer screening for average-risk adults: 2018 guideline update from the American Cancer Society. CA: a cancer journal for clinicians, 68(4), 250-281.
- Saslow, D., Solomon, D., Lawson, H. W., Killackey, M., Kulasingam, S. L., Cain, J., ... & Myers, E. R. (2012). American Cancer Society, American Society for Colposcopy and Cervical Pathology, and American Society for Clinical Pathology screening guidelines for the prevention and early detection of cervical cancer. Journal of lower genital tract disease, 16(3), 175-204.
- Smith, R. A., Andrews, K. S., Brooks, D., Fedewa, S. A., Manassaram-Baptiste, D., Saslow, D., ... & Wender, R. C. (2018). Cancer screening in the United States, 2018: A review of current American Cancer Society

guidelines and current issues in cancer screening. CA: a cancer journal for clinicians, 68(4), 297-316.

- Wender, R., Fontham, E. T. H., Barrera Jr, E., Colditz, G. A., Church, T. R., Ettinger, D. S., ... & Smith, R. A. (2013). American Cancer Society lung cancer screening guidelines. CA: a cancer journal for clinicians, 63(2), 106-117.
- Carter, H. B., Albertsen, P. C., Barry, M. J., Etzioni, R., Freedland, S. J., Greene, K. L., ... & Vickers, A. J. (2013). Early detection of prostate cancer: AUA guideline. The Journal of urology, 190(2), 419-426.
- Cosman, F., de Beur, S. J., LeBoff, M. S., Lewiecki, E. M., Tanner, B., Randall, S., ... & Naganathan, S. (2014). Clinician's guide to prevention and treatment of osteoporosis. Osteoporosis International, 25(10), 2359-2381.
- US Preventive Services Task Force, Bibbins-Domingo, K., Grossman, D. C., Curry, S. J., Barry, M. J., Davidson, K. W., ... & Tseng, C. W. (2016). Screening for skin cancer: US Preventive Services Task Force recommendation statement. Jama, 316(4), 429-435.

Chapter 24: Medical Ethics for the Advanced Pharmacist Practitioners

24.1. Ethical Principles

> ➤ *Ethical principles in healthcare decision-making include beneficence (doing good), nonmaleficence (avoiding harm), autonomy (respecting patient choices), and justice (fair distribution of resources).*
>
> ➤ *They guide clinicians in navigating complex medical dilemmas, ensuring patient well-being, dignity, and rights are upheld while balancing competing interests and priorities.*

Respect for Autonomy

- Respect patients' right to make informed decisions about their own healthcare, including the right to refuse treatment, express preferences, and participate in shared decision-making processes.
- Provide patients with accurate and understandable information about their medical condition, treatment options, risks, benefits, and alternatives to empower them to make autonomous decisions aligned with their values and preferences.

Beneficence

- Act in the best interests of patients and strive to promote their well-being and overall health outcomes through the delivery of high-quality, evidence-based care.
- Prioritize interventions and treatments that are likely to benefit patients, minimize harm, and maximize positive outcomes while considering patient needs, goals, and preferences.

Non-Maleficence

- Avoid causing harm or inflicting unnecessary suffering to patients by carefully assessing the risks and benefits of medical interventions, treatments, and procedures.
- Adhere to ethical standards and clinical guidelines to minimize the potential for adverse events, complications, and iatrogenic harm in the provision of healthcare services.

Justice

- Ensure fair and equitable distribution of healthcare resources, services, and opportunities to all patients, regardless of their socio-

economic status, race, ethnicity, gender, age, or other personal characteristics.
- Advocate for healthcare policies, practices, and systems that promote social justice, address health disparities, and eliminate barriers to access and quality care for vulnerable and marginalized populations.

Veracity
- Be truthful, honest, and transparent in all interactions with patients, colleagues, and other stakeholders, providing accurate and complete information about medical diagnoses, prognoses, treatment options, and expected outcomes.
- Respect patients' right to know and be fully informed about their healthcare status, including disclosing adverse events, errors, and unanticipated outcomes with compassion and empathy.

Confidentiality
- Safeguard patients' privacy and confidentiality by adhering to HIPAA regulations and ethical standards governing the collection, storage, and disclosure of protected health information.
- Obtain informed consent from patients before sharing their medical information with other healthcare providers or third parties and ensure secure transmission and storage of confidential data.

Professional Integrity
- Uphold professional integrity, honesty, and accountability in all aspects of clinical practice, research, education, and leadership roles.
- Avoid conflicts of interest, bias, or self-serving behaviors that could compromise the trust, integrity, or professionalism of the APh or the healthcare system.

Cultural Competence
- Demonstrate cultural humility, sensitivity, and awareness in interactions with patients from diverse cultural, linguistic, and religious backgrounds.
- Respect and honor patients' cultural beliefs, values, traditions, and preferences when making healthcare decisions and delivering culturally competent care.

Continuous Learning and Improvement
- Commit to lifelong learning, professional development, and ethical reflection to enhance clinical competence, critical thinking skills, and ethical decision-making abilities.

- Engage in ethical deliberation, consultation with colleagues, and ethical committees or review boards when encountering complex ethical dilemmas or moral uncertainties in healthcare practice.

24.2. Professional Integrity and Conflicts of Interest

> ➢ *Professional integrity in medicine entails upholding honesty, transparency, and ethical conduct while prioritizing patient welfare above personal gain.*
> ➢ *Conflicts of interest arise when financial, personal, or professional considerations potentially influence medical decisions, requiring disclosure and mitigation to safeguard patient trust and well-being.*
> ➢ *The APh should adhere to ethical guidelines, maintain transparency, foster professionalism and preserve the integrity of medical practice.*

Professional Integrity:
- Honesty and Transparency: Uphold honesty and transparency in all interactions with patients, colleagues, and stakeholders. Provide accurate information, communicate clearly, and disclose relevant information to patients to foster trust and informed decision-making.
- Accountability: Take responsibility for your actions, decisions, and the outcomes of patient care. Admit mistakes, learn from them, and strive to continuously improve the quality of care delivered to patients.
- Ethical Practice: Adhere to ethical principles such as beneficence, non-maleficence, respect for autonomy, and justice in all aspects of practice. Prioritize patient well-being, respect patient rights, and ensure that treatment decisions are based on clinical evidence and ethical considerations.

Conflicts of Interest
- Identification: Recognize situations where conflicts of interest may arise, including financial relationships with pharmaceutical companies, involvement in research or consulting activities, or personal biases that could influence decision-making.
- Disclosure: Disclose any potential conflicts of interest to patients, colleagues, or employers in a transparent manner. Provide clear and comprehensive information about financial relationships, research affiliations, or other relevant interests that may impact patient care.
- Management: Proactively manage conflicts of interest to prevent their influence on patient care. This may involve recusing oneself

from decision-making processes, seeking independent advice or consultation, or implementing safeguards to mitigate potential biases.

- Patient-Centered Decision-Making: Prioritize patient interests above personal or financial interests when making clinical decisions. Consider patients' values, preferences, and treatment goals, and ensure that recommendations are based on evidence-based practice and ethical principles.

- Organizational Policies: Familiarize yourself with organizational policies, professional codes of conduct, and legal regulations related to conflicts of interest. Adhere to institutional standards and guidelines for disclosing conflicts of interest and managing ethical dilemmas.

By upholding professional integrity and effectively managing conflicts of interest, the advanced pharmacist practitioners can maintain trust, integrity, and ethical practice standards in their professional roles.

24.3. Ethical Dilemmas in Pharmacy Practice

> ➤ *Ethical dilemmas in pharmacy practice may involve issues like medication errors, confidentiality breaches, or conflicts of interest.*
>
> ➤ *Resolution strategies include consulting ethical guidelines, seeking input from colleagues or supervisors, and prioritizing patient welfare while considering legal and professional obligations.*
>
> ➤ *Open communication, reflection, and adherence to ethical principles guide the APh in navigating complex dilemmas, ensuring ethical practice and patient-centered care.*

Medication Errors

- Dilemma: Discovering a medication error that has the potential to harm a patient.
- Resolution: Immediately inform the appropriate healthcare team members, report the error following organizational protocols, and take corrective actions to prevent harm to the patient. Apologize to the patient and family, provide necessary medical interventions, and offer support and follow-up care as needed.

Patient Confidentiality

- Dilemma: Balancing patient confidentiality with the need to share information with other healthcare providers for the patient's benefit.

- Resolution: Adhere to legal and ethical guidelines regarding patient confidentiality while collaborating with other healthcare professionals as necessary. Obtain informed consent from the patient before sharing confidential information and consider the patient's preferences and best interests when making disclosure decisions.

Access to Medications

- Dilemma: Addressing barriers to medication access, such as cost or insurance coverage limitations.
- Resolution: Advocate for the patient by exploring alternative medication options, assisting with prior authorization processes, and providing information about patient assistance programs or discount cards. Collaborate with other healthcare providers and insurance companies to find solutions that ensure the patient has access to necessary medications.

End-of-Life Care

- Dilemma: Supporting patients and families in end-of-life decision-making.
- Resolution: Respect patient autonomy by facilitating discussions about end-of-life care preferences, advance directives, and goals of care. Provide compassionate support, symptom management, and resources for palliative care or hospice services. Consult with ethics committees or palliative care specialists for guidance on navigating complex end-of-life decisions.

Pharmaceutical Marketing Practices

- Dilemma: Balancing the influence of pharmaceutical marketing with ethical prescribing practices.
- Resolution: Avoid conflicts of interest by critically evaluating pharmaceutical promotional materials and prioritizing evidence-based prescribing decisions. Disclose any potential conflicts of interest to patients and colleagues and adhere to professional codes of conduct and legal regulations governing interactions with pharmaceutical companies.

Cultural Competence

- Dilemma: Addressing cultural differences in healthcare beliefs and practices.
- Resolution: Cultivate cultural competence through ongoing education, training, and self-reflection. Respect patients' cultural beliefs, values, and preferences by providing culturally sensitive care and tailoring treatment plans to meet their patient needs. Collaborate

with interpreters or cultural liaisons when language or cultural barriers exist.

Off-Label Medication Use

- Dilemma: Considering the ethical implications of prescribing medications for off-label uses.
- Resolution: Engage in shared decision-making with patients, providing them with information about off-label use, including potential benefits, risks, and alternatives. Document the rationale for off-label prescribing and monitor patients closely for safety and efficacy. Follow institutional guidelines and consult with colleagues or clinical pharmacists for guidance as needed.

Scope of Practice

- Dilemma: Navigating professional boundaries and scope of practice limitations.
- Resolution: Respect professional boundaries and collaborate with other healthcare providers within the scope of pharmacy practice. Seek additional training or certifications to expand scope of practice opportunities and enhance clinical skills. Advocate for legislative changes or policy reforms that support expanded roles for pharmacists in healthcare delivery.

References

- Beauchamp, T. L., & Childress, J. F. (2019). Principles of biomedical ethics. Oxford University Press.
- Lo, B., & Field, M. J. (Eds.). (2009). Conflict of interest in medical research, education, and practice. National Academies Press.
- Brody, H. (1989). The Healer's Power. Yale University Press.

www.ingramcontent.com/pod-product-compliance
Lightning Source LLC
LaVergne TN
LVHW072117060526
838201LV00011B/258